Atlas of Experimental
Toxicological Pathology

To Cora P. Cherry
for sharing with us her wealth of
experience in the field of
toxicological pathology

Current Histopathology

Consultant Editor
Professor G. Austin Gresham, TD, ScD, MD, FRC Path.
Professor of Morbid Anatomy and Histology, University of Cambridge

Volume Thirteen

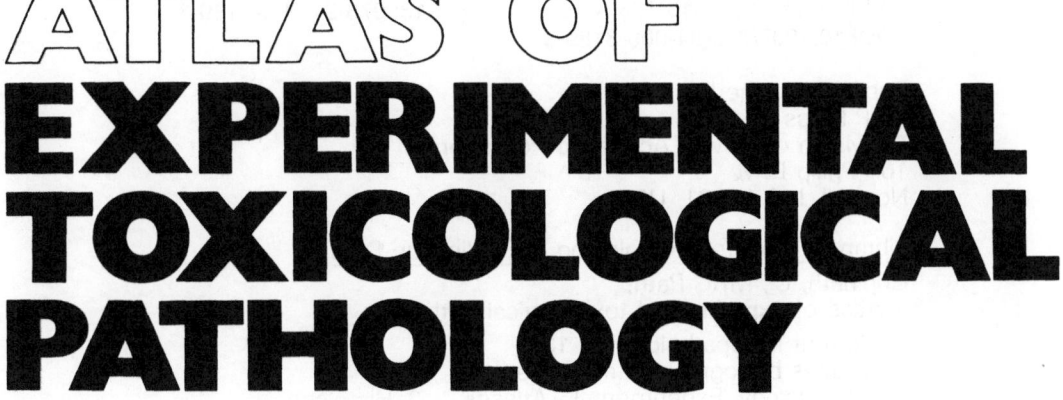

ATLAS OF EXPERIMENTAL TOXICOLOGICAL PATHOLOGY

BY

C. GOPINATH
Director of Pathology
Huntingdon Research Centre
Huntingdon, UK

D. E. PRENTICE
Head of Pathology Group
Deputy Head of Toxicology Department
Pharmaceutical Division
Sandoz Ltd
Basle, Switzerland

D. J. LEWIS
Deputy Head of Pathology
Huntingdon Research Centre
Huntingdon, UK

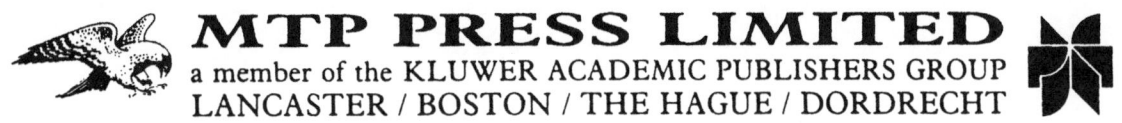

MTP PRESS LIMITED
a member of the KLUWER ACADEMIC PUBLISHERS GROUP
LANCASTER / BOSTON / THE HAGUE / DORDRECHT

Published in the UK and Europe by
MTP Press Limited
Falcon House
Queen Square
Lancaster, England

British Library Cataloguing in Publication Data
Gopinath, C.
    Atlas of experimental toxicological pathology. —
(Current histopathology; v.13)
    1. Toxicology — Technique
I. Title   II. Prentice, D. E.   III. Lewis, D. J.
IV. Series
    615.9'0028   RA1211

    ISBN-13: 978-94-010-7930-3   e-ISBN-13: 978-94-009-3189-3
    DOI:10.1007/978-94-009-3189-3

Published in the USA by
MTP Press
A division of Kluwer Academic Publishers
101 Philip Drive
Norwell, MA 02061, USA

Library of Congress Cataloging in Publication Data
Gopinath, C., MRC Path.
    Atlas of experimental toxicological pathology.

    (Current histopathology; v. 13)
    Includes bibliographies and index.
    1. Toxicology, Experimental—Atlases.   2. Histology,
    Pathological—Atlases.   3. Laboratory animals—
    Histology—Atlases.   4. Diseases—Animal
    models—Atlases.
I. Prentice, D. E.   II. Lewis, D. J.   III. Title.
IV. Series.   [DNLM: 1. Pathology—atlases.
2. Toxicology—atlases.
WI CU788JBA v.13 /QZ 17 G659a]
RA1199.G67   1987   615.9'07   87-21448

Phototypesetting by Titus Wilson, Kendal.
Colour origination by Laserscan, Stretford, Manchester.

Contents

Current Histopathology Series

Consultant Editor's Note

Toxicological pathology is a subject which attracts the interests of a wide variety of workers. Human and veterinary pathologists often need access to the information provided by this book. It will be of especial value to those working in the fields of drug testing, experimental pathology and clinical pharmacology.

This is a comprehensive volume dealing with changes that are induced by a wide variety of agents in many species of animals. An extensive bibliography has contributed greatly to the usefulness of this book.

Texts on toxicological pathology are not numerous. This is a welcome addition to the series and follows the tradition of being a bench manual for workers in the field.

G. Austin Gresham

Acknowledgements

We are greatly indebted to many people who have assisted us over several years in the preparation of this atlas. Our helpers are too numerous to mention individually, but we are particularly grateful to Huntingdon Research Centre and Sandoz pathologists for ideas and histological slides, and to the technical staff of both companies for excellent assistance.

We also wish to thank our wives for their tolerance during the long preparation of the book and we particularly wish to thank Mrs Ann Lewis for typing the various forms of the manuscript.

Introduction

Our aim in producing a colour atlas of toxicological pathology was to present a catalogue of histopathological lesions which we had encountered over the years in various laboratory animal species exposed to a vast range of pharmaceuticals, agrochemicals and industrial chemicals. While we believe a colour atlas is the ideal way to share our experiences with others, it quickly became clear to us that for the atlas to be meaningful the associated text must be comprehensive and contain ample literature references.

The atlas is intended for both the trainee and the experienced toxicological pathologist working with laboratory animals in the pharmaceutical, agrochemical or chemical environment. In addition, it is aimed at experimental pathologists, toxicologists and pharmacologists who may wish to obtain further insights into toxicological pathology. It may also be of value to veterinary pathologists in academic institutes who may encounter toxic lesions from time to time in domestic animals or who may be required to deal occasionally with laboratory animals.

The history of modern toxicology and therefore of toxicological pathology is relatively short and, as a consequence, the number of books and texts dealing solely with the subject are few. Those books which are available to the practitioner tend to concentrate on spontaneous and induced neoplasia in laboratory rodents. This atlas deals exclusively with induced, non-neoplastic, morphological lesions in the tissues and organs of laboratory animals. Although most of the photomicrographs used in this book were taken from routine haematoxylin and eosin stained paraffin sections, a small number of special stains, enzyme histochemical preparations, resin sections and electron micrographs are also included.

We wish to emphasize that the lesions presented in this atlas were encountered during the histopathological evaluation of routine toxicity studies. These studies were undertaken to assess whether a substance could present a health hazard to man and his environment. In essence, toxicity tests are considered as safety assessment studies. The types of compound involved in testing and the immediate aims of the assessment vary considerably. Studies with novel pharmaceutical preparations, for example, are designed to predict possible side effects in human patients, while studies with industrial chemicals are performed to determine whether worker contamination constitutes a health hazard. Although the requirements for and the conduct of toxicity studies are today controlled by governmental regulatory bodies and health authorities, the aims were, and are, to ensure human safety from potentially noxious chemicals. Guidelines on the conduct and design of toxicity studies are issued by governmental authorities. These guidelines itemize the investigations to be carried out during the course of the study and they normally include: clinical observations and behaviour; food intake and body weight measurements; serum biochemistry; haematology; ECG and ophthalmology. At the end of a study, full macroscopic and microscopic examinations of the organ weight analyses together with tissues are essential. By far the greater part of the material used in this book is from toxicity studies conducted in recent years and performed in compliance with the Good Laboratory Practice standards of governmental regulatory bodies in Europe, Japan and North America.

Toxicity studies are commonly carried out in rats, mice, dogs or monkeys, but the range of species used is extensive and may include larger animals such as sheep and pigs or non-mammalian species like the domestic hen. The selection of species, dose levels, route of administration (oral, parenteral, inhalation) and duration of study are all determined by the proposed use of the compound and the perceived potential risk. Conventionally, studies have an untreated control group and three groups of animals exposed to low, intermediate and high levels of the test compound. The rationale for using three dose levels in toxicity studies is well established. The highest dose utilized should show some evidence of toxicity, ideally identifying target organs and thereby indicating the area of risk for man. The lowest dose, on the other hand, should be free of toxicity as this is often close to the level of expected exposure for man. The intermediate dose may either be free of toxicity or show toxic changes similar to the highest dose, but minor in degree. The majority of the photomicrographs in this atlas are examples of high dose effects on target organs. The establishment of a clear 'no toxic effect level' (NTEL) in a toxicity study is of paramount importance; it allows the calculation of a safety factor for use of the compound in the human situation. For a pharmaceutical preparation, for example, the NTEL from the toxicity study, expressed as mg of compound per kg body weight per day, should ideally be at least several times the proposed therapeutic dose in man.

The full nature of toxic change is beyond the scope of this book. We do not attempt to give details of basic pathological responses to injury, but when the pathogenesis of a particular lesion is known it is mentioned and referenced in the text. Here we are dealing primarily with morphological changes which follow administration of test substances. Toxicity manifesting as morphological changes is produced by numerous pharmaceuticals and industrial chemicals. In fact, in our experience, there are few completely inert industrial chemicals or indeed pharmaceuticals. Most compounds will induce a toxic reaction under experimental conditions in which a susceptible species is exposed at a sufficiently high dose level via a specific route of administration. There are, however, some toxic manifestations which have no histopathological counterpart. The interpretation of a morphological response may be difficult for the toxicologist as there is often only a fine distinction between a toxic response, an exaggerated pharmacological response and a physiological response. In a few well publicized examples evidence of induced toxicity in man has been established in the absence of similar findings in laboratory animal species. However, it should perhaps be stressed that toxicity studies are on the whole predictive for man and that the majority of induced morphological changes encountered in these studies do have counterparts in man.

This book has been compiled with material from numerous sources and because of the confidential nature of the work we are unable to divulge the chemical names of many compounds. For many of the lesions illustrated the individual chemical or pharmaceutical agent responsible is, therefore, not named but whenever possible we have given the general class of the compound, e.g. novel corticosteroid, contraceptive steroid, neuroleptic. In a few other instances we have only been able to use extremely vague terms such as agrochemical or industrial chemical. As our aim was to include the widest possible spectrum of induced lesions, it is hoped that this constraint does not detract from the value of the atlas.

The Cardiovascular System

1

Lesions of the cardiovascular system in routine toxicity studies are, in general, uncommon. However, the search for more and more cardioactive drugs has brought to light its share of cardiotoxic manifestations. Myocardial lesions in experimental animals have recently been reviewed[1]. There are a number of chemicals, metallic compounds and pharmacologically active drugs which are known to exert their toxic influence on the heart. Although cardiotoxicity involves a wide area of malfunction of the heart, of necessity the present work deals only with those involving pathomorphological abnormalities. In routine investigation the importance of a thorough and detailed macroscopic examination of the heart at necropsy cannot be overstressed. In several instances the myocardial lesions induced by a cardiotoxic agent are focal leaving large areas of the myocardium unaffected. A good anatomical knowledge is also essential, especially when lesions of coronary vasculature are suspected. In such cases, the use of perfusion techniques for fixation is recommended as the intramural vessels undergo collapse and marked distortion in unperfused, immersion-fixed samples.

The myocardium, by virtue of its high energy and oxygen demand, is particularly vulnerable to anoxic injuries. In addition, direct cardiotoxicity is exerted by some antineoplastic antibiotics where there is chemical interaction of a reactive intermediary metabolite with cellular macromolecules. A number of cardioactive drugs (certain catecholamines and vasodilating anti-hypertensive drugs) exert their cardiotoxic lesions as a result of exaggerated pharmacological responses. In these instances the cardiac lesions are believed to be due to multiple factors such as: excessive myocardial stimulation resulting in increased oxygen demand; exaggerated vasodilation and consequent drop in coronary blood pressure; reflex tachycardia and reduced perfusion time. All these factors contribute to local ischaemia and the lesions develop at the most vulnerable sites of the myocardium. In cardiotoxicity the correlation between functional abnormalities and myocardial lesions is not always good. In several instances functional alterations such as bradycardia, tachycardia and arrhythmias are not accompanied by pathological lesions. The cardiotoxic lesions recorded are, in general, multi-focal myocardial necrosis, intrasarcoplasmic appearance of contraction bands, excessive sarcoplasmic granularity, focal myolysis, vacuolation, calcification, varying degrees of inflammatory and fibroblastic responses and haemorrhage. The lesions may or may not be accompanied by coronary vascular changes. Although predilection sites for certain types of compounds are reported, generally speaking hypoxic injuries are localized, whilst cytotoxic lesions are more widespread[2]. It must be pointed out that in the context of cardiotoxic myocardial lesions, myocardial injury can also be secondary to renal failure, to lesions in the central nervous system and to stress. In recent times the search for potent immunomodulators has increased and, in our experience, the cardiovascular system is a major target organ in toxicity studies with many of these compounds.

Vascular lesions as a toxic end-point are rare. Toxic doses of mercurial compounds, pyrrolizidine alkaloids, some immunostimulant drugs and high fat diets are among those which are known to induce lesions in the vasculature. The important and characteristic responses of the cardiovascular system to toxic doses of a number of differing agents are listed in Table 1.1 and described in the following sections.

Table 1.1 Induced cardiovascular lesions

Heart
  Myocardial necrosis
  Myocardial necrosis with vascular lesions
  Myocardial vacuolation
  Myocardial fatty degeneration
  Myocardial lipofucsinosis
  Myocardial calcification
  Myocardial hypertrophy
  Pericarditis

Vasculature
  Degenerative arteriopathy
  Thrombosis
  Aneurysms
  Vasculitis
  Atherosclerosis

Multi-focal myocardial necrosis and haemorrhage, located mainly in the subendocardial area of the left ventricle and in the papillary muscles, are induced by catecholamines in several species including dogs, rats and rabbits. The most frequently studied compound in this respect is isoproterenol. Several others, including endogenous catecholamines are known to induce similar changes in the myocardium. Histologically, the lesion appears as foci of myocardial fibres with dense eosinophilic sarcoplasm and loss of cross striations (Figure 1.1). The sarcoplasm of some fibres shows excessive granularity, fragmentation and sometimes characteristic condensation of contractile materials into transverse bands (Figure 1.2). The lesions also show fibres with focal myolysis (Figure 1.3), pyknosis and loss of nuclei. Initially there is a mild inflammatory cell response soon followed by marked histiocytic and fibroblastic proliferation (Figure 1.4). During the late stages myocardial fibrosis develops (Figure 1.5). Phosphotungstic acid haematoxylin (PTAH) staining is a valuable additional technique for the detection of small foci of myocardial

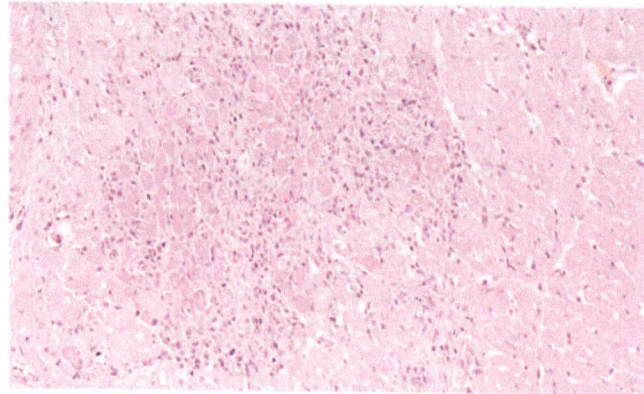

Figure 1.1 Myocardial necrosis in the left ventricle of a dog induced by administration of a cardioactive drug. The affected fibres appear more eosinophilic with loss of striations. The necrotic area is surrounded by a mild inflammatory response. H & E

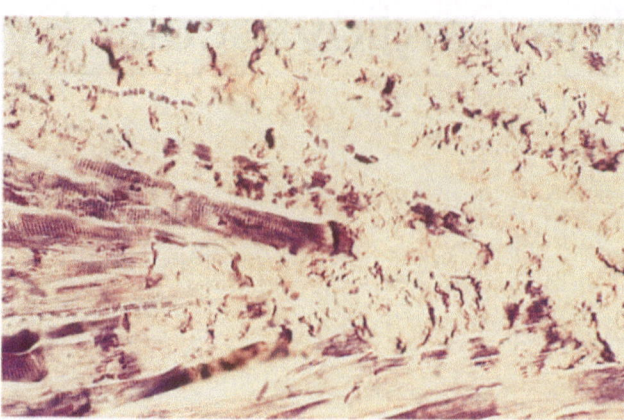

Figure 1.2 Myocardial necrosis in the left ventricle of a dog treated with isoprenaline. The affected fibres show loss of cross-striations and reveal the presence of contraction bands. Phospho-tungstic acid–haematoxylin

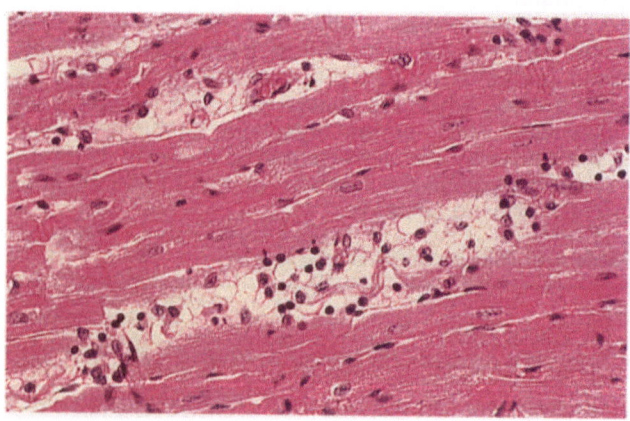

Figure 1.3 Focal vacuolation and myolysis in the ventricular myo-cardium of a dog. A minimal inflammatory reaction is present and the affected fibres reveal nuclear pyknosis. H & E

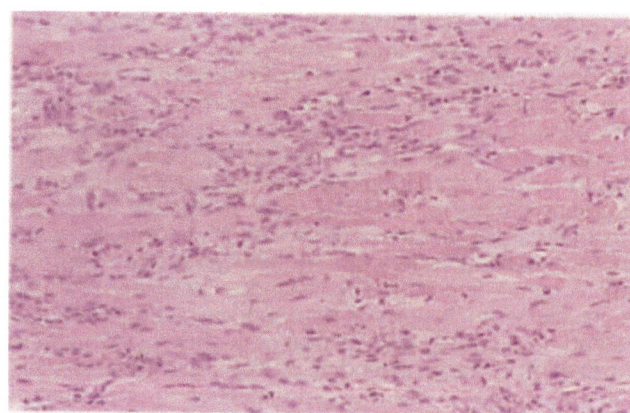

Figure 1.4 Focal myocardial necrosis found in the left ventricle of a dog following administration of a novel cardiovascular drug. A marked histiocytic and fibroblastic reaction is associated with eosinophilic necrotic myocardial fibres. H & E

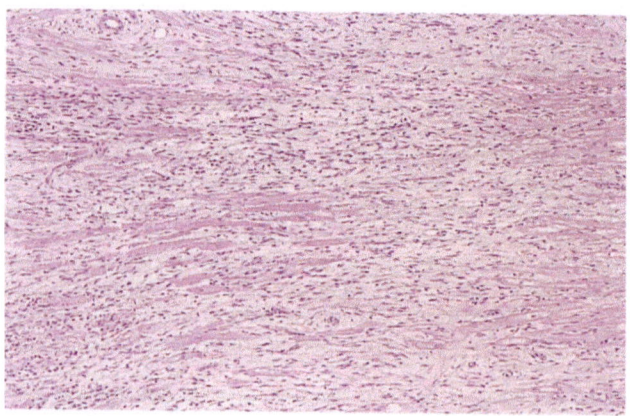

Figure 1.5 An area of myocardial fibrosis in the left ventricle of a dog treated with a cardio-active compound. Necrotic fibres have been replaced by fibrosis. H & E

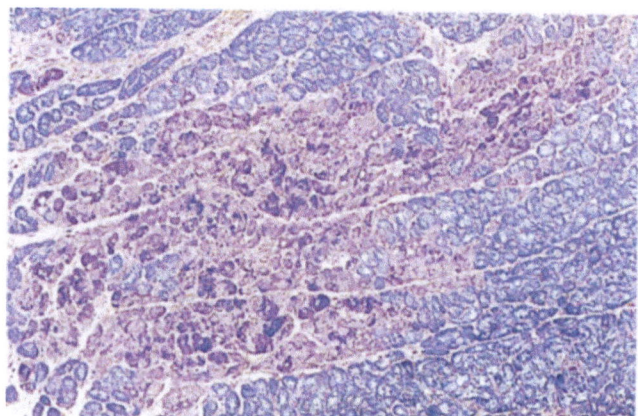

Figure 1.6 Areas of myocardial necrosis in the left ventricle of a dog treated with a cardio-active drug. Note the distinct loss of blue staining from necrotic fibres. The necrotic foci are clearly delineated. Phosphotungstic acid–haematoxylin

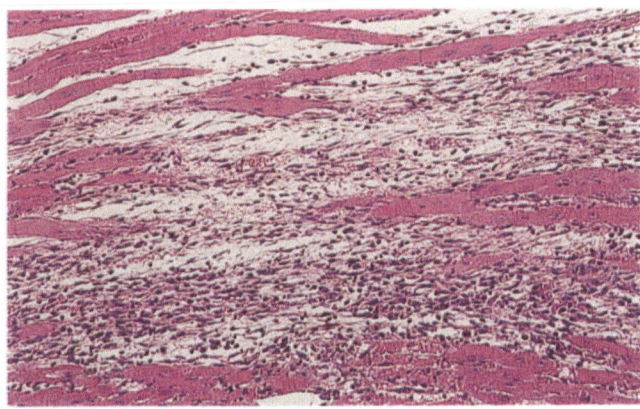

Figure 1.7 An area of myocardial fibrosis and oedema in the left ventricle of a dog treated with a cardiovascular drug. Foci of necrosis were present in other areas of the heart. H & E

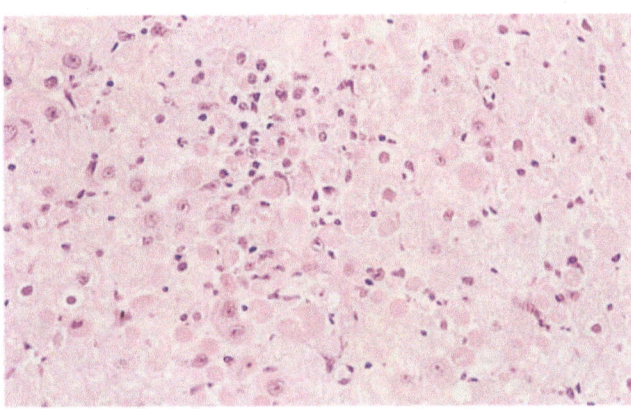

Figure 1.8 Focal necrosis in the ventricular myocardium of a monkey from a toxicity study with gossypol. Note swollen fibres with increased eosinophilia, sarcoplasmic vacuolation and a minimal inflammatory reaction. H & E

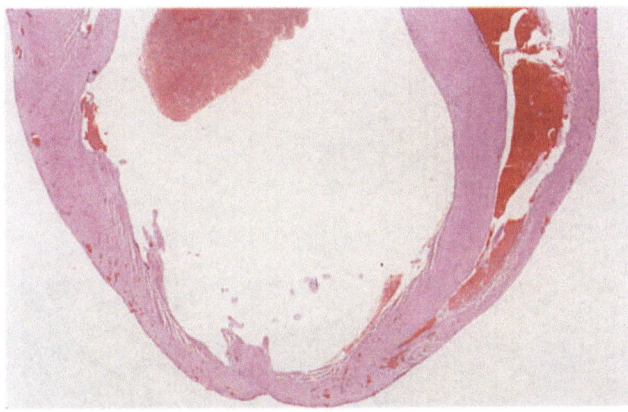

Figure 1.9 Dilated ventricles in a rat given prolonged doses of a cardiotoxic compound. Note the thin ventricular walls. Dilatation is probably a sequel to widespread focal myocardial degeneration. H & E

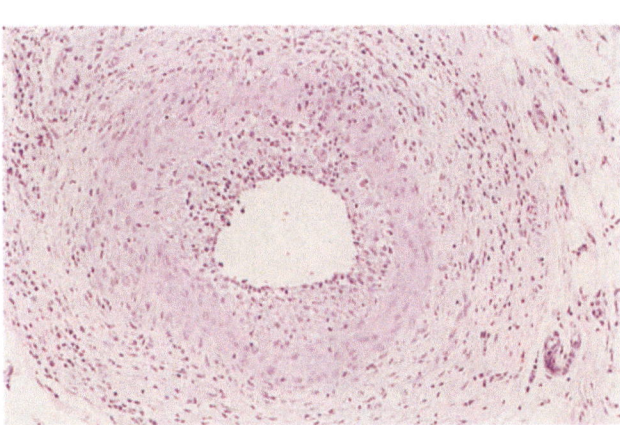

Figure 1.10 Arteritis in a coronary artery of a dog treated with a cardio-active drug. Medial necrosis, inflammation of the arterial wall and peri-arterial connective tissue are prominent. The lesion was associated with foci of myocardial necrosis. H & E

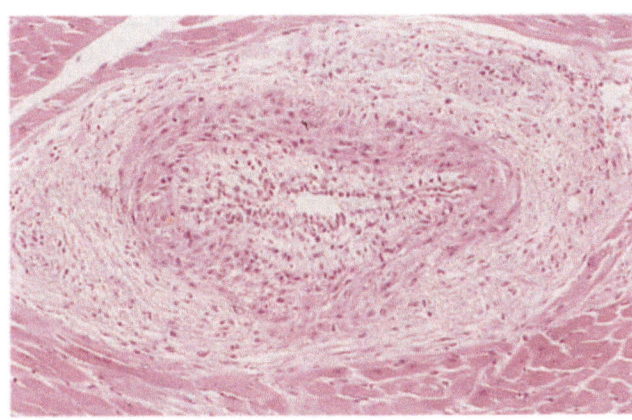

Figure 1.11 Medial degeneration and hypertrophy of an intramural artery in the left ventricle of a dog from a toxicity study with a novel cardiotonic drug. Note the smooth muscle cell proliferation in the tunica media, subintimal intercellular oedema and increase in periarterial connective tissue. H & E

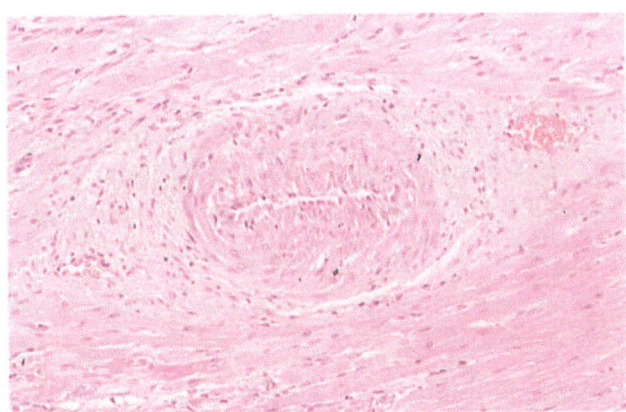

Figure 1.12 Medial hypertrophy of intramural arteries in the left ventricular myocardium of a dog from a toxicity study with a cardiotonic agent. The tunica media is thickened due to prominent and proliferating smooth muscle cells. The lesion was accompanied by focal myocardial necrosis. H & E

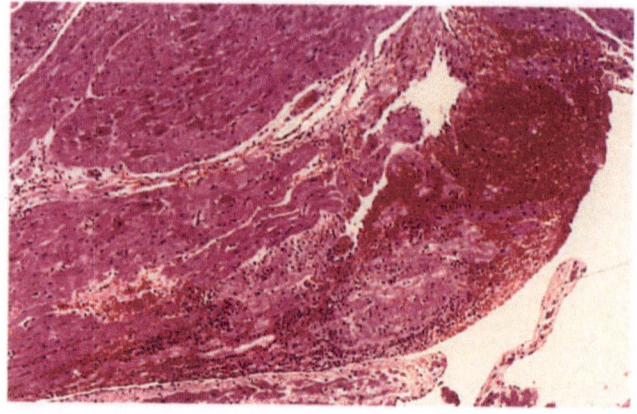

Figure 1.13 Marked fibrosis of the right atrium of a dog. The lesion was associated with inflammatory changes of the coronary arteries. This type of lesion may be induced by compounds such as theobromine.   H & E

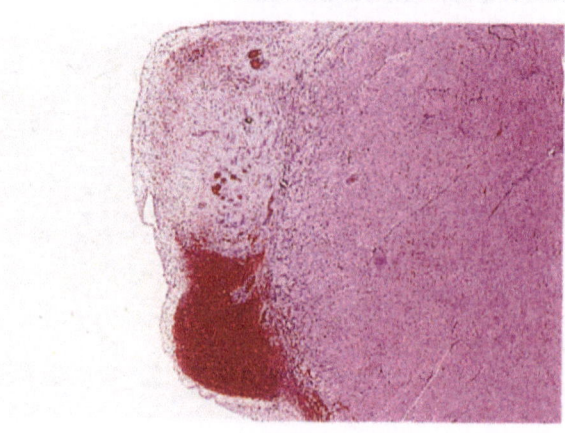

Figure 1.14 An area of endocardial haemorrhage in the left ventricle of a baboon treated with high doses of a cardio-active drug. Foci of myocardial necrosis were present elsewhere.   H & E

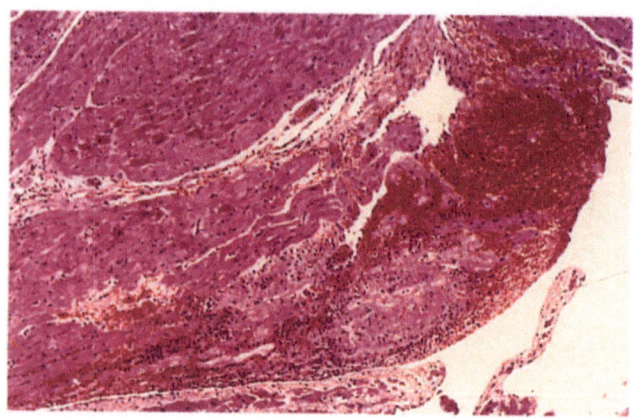

Figure 1.15 An area of myocardial (subendocardial) haemorrhage and inflammation in the left ventricle of a baboon from a toxicity study with a cardio-active drug.   H & E

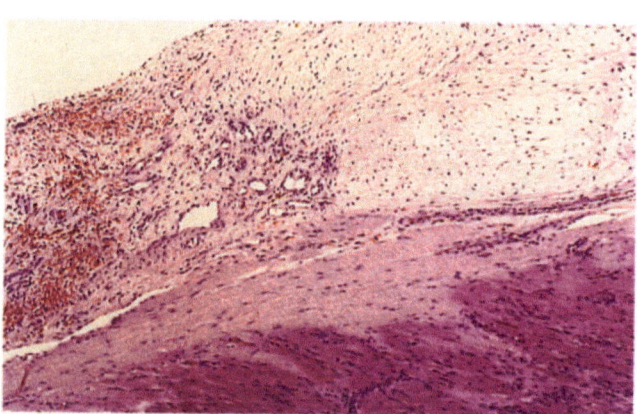

Figure 1.16 A focus of haemorrhage, inflammation and fibrosis in the endocardium of a dog treated with high doses of a cardiotonic drug probably as a sequel to endocardial haemorrhage. This is a relatively common finding with this type of drug.   H & E

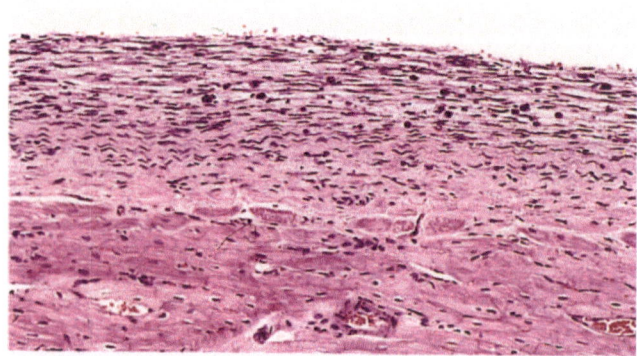

Figure 1.17 Endocardial fibrosis and inflammatory cell infiltration in a dog. This case is from the same study as Figure 1.16, and probably represents a later stage.   H & E

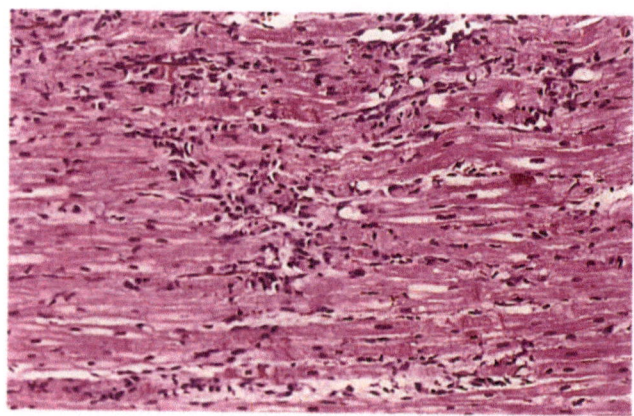

Figure 1.18 Focal myocarditis and myocardial scarring in the left ventricle of a rat from a chronic toxicity study with a β-adrenergic agonist. This change is typical for the class of drug, but may be detected only as an exacerbation of the spontaneous background myocardial changes which occur in older rats.   H & E

fibre degeneration or necrosis (Figure 1.6). Serum aspartate aminotransferase and creatine phosphokinase estimations and electrocardiogram can contribute to the assessment of early cardiac lesions in dogs, but are not particularly useful in the later stages of isoproterenol toxicity[3,4]. The myocardial necrosis is caused by ischaemia and appears infarct-like, although the ischaemia is not due to changes in the coronary vasculature. This type of lesion is produced by a number of adrenergic β-receptor stimulants and vasodilating antihypertensives and their lesions are due to exaggerated functional effects rather than to direct toxicity[5]. The adrenergic stimulation augments transmembrane calcium influx, which in turn increases the rate and force of contraction and increases utilization of energy and oxygen. Hypoxic changes develop in the least well perfused areas of the myocardium, such as the subendocardial locations of the left ventricle and the papillary muscles.

Various other unrelated agents also produce multifocal myocardial necrosis. Histamine in rabbits produces myocardial necrosis with the presence of contraction bands, haemorrhage and oedema. The lesions mainly occur in the right ventricle and papillary muscles and are not mediated by catecholamines[1]. Metallic compounds such as lead and cobalt are also capable of inducing myocardial injury. Cobalt cardiotoxicity has been demonstrated in several experimental animal species and the role of coexisting protein deficiency in the development of the cardiomyopathy has been established. Cobalt toxicity in piglets produces diffuse myocardial necrosis and calcification, mainly affecting the atria. The affected areas reveal necrosis, with contraction bands and myocytes with basophilic granular cytoplasm due to mitochondrial calcification. Macrophagic infiltration, interstitial oedema and fibroblastic proliferation (Figure 1.7) are accompanying features. Ultrastructurally, characteristic dilation of sarcoplasmic reticulum, focal myofibrillar lysis, mitochondrial damage and ruptured plasma membranes are recorded[1]. Gossypol is another agent which is known to produce focal myocardial necrosis (Figure 1.8) in experimental animals[6]. In pigs, gossypol toxicity results in ventricular dilation, congestive heart failure and pulmonary oedema. In pathological cardiac dilation, the affected ventricular walls are thin and the chambers are distended (Figure 1.9). Cardiac dilation leads to circulatory failure due to inefficient contraction. A type of haemorrhagic necrosis of the myocardium is reported in dogs and monkeys given high doses of cyclophosphamide[1]. Myocardial vacuolation and necrosis with contraction bands associated with macrophage response, are induced in several species of animals given high doses of ionophores like monensin. Other agents known to induce focal myocardial necrosis in experimental animals include the rodenticide, fluoroacetate, and antimetabolites such as 5-fluorouracil[1].

A number of agents induce both vascular lesions (Figure 1.10) and myocardial necrosis. Cardioactive compounds including digitoxin, theobromine and certain antihypertensive drugs are among this group of agents. Digitoxin given to dogs induces subendocardial haemorrhage, and myocardial necrosis of the right ventricle which are associated with arteritis and thrombosis of intramural coronary arteries. The affected arteries show medial haemorrhage, fibrinoid necrosis, and leukocyte infiltration of the tunica media and adventitia[7]. Theobromine given to dogs results in characteristic haemorrhage and necrosis of right atrial appendages with leukocytic infiltration. Associated vascular lesions include thickening of the tunica media of arteries due to smooth muscle hyperplasia and swelling (Figures 1.11 and 1.12). The

adventitia reveals a thick band of connective tissue containing inflammatory cells[8]. In a prolonged dosage regime this results in marked replacement fibrosis, which is usually confined to the right atrium (Figure 1.13). Vasodilating antihypertensive drugs like minoxidil also produce haemorrhagic right atrial lesions in dogs[1]. Necrosis of left ventricular papillary muscles, endocardial and epicardial haemorrhages are also seen. The atrial lesions are associated with endothelial swelling, fibrinoid necrosis of arterioles, perivascular inflammation, myocyte damage and epicardial inflammation. These lesions eventually progress to fibrosis[1]. Physical endothelial injury due to marked haemodynamic changes, plasma leakage into the vascular layers and functional demands exerted on the smooth muscle cells must all play a role in the production of these lesions[2]. A number of cardiotonic drugs produce endocardial and myocardial haemorrhage (Figures 1.14 and 1.15). Foci, or areas of haemorrhages, are often accompanied by areas of inflammation and fibrosis (Figures 1.16 and 1.17). The lesion often reveals pigmented macrophages containing stainable iron. In allylamine toxicity, multifocal subendocardial necrosis and fibrosis are reported in the myocardium of rats[1]. The lesion is sometimes associated with vascular changes in larger arterioles showing smooth muscle cell hyperplasia especially in the scarred areas. It is suggested that myocardial necrosis is the primary lesion[9]. Prolonged administration of certain β-stimulants to rats induces an increased incidence of focal myocarditis and scarring (Figure 1.18).

Prominent sarcoplasmic vacuolation, disorganization and hyalinization, loss of myofibrils and myocytolysis are the distinctive features of a cardiotoxicity induced by some anthracycline antibiotics such as daunomycin and adriamycin. There is interstitial oedema, infiltration of macrophages and proliferation of fibroblasts. Myocyte vacuolation is due to distension of sarcoplasmic reticulum and T-tubules and loss of myofibrils. The myocardial lesions induced in rabbits have been described in detail[10], and are accompanied by cardiac dilation. Toxic responses to these types of compounds are seen only after prolonged exposures. The type of toxicity induced by these anthracycline antibiotics is an example of direct cardiotoxicity. Adriamycin-induced cardiac lesions are reported in several species of experimental animals and man.

Fatty degeneration, myofibrillar fragmentation and myocytolysis in rats are produced by prolonged administration of high doses of brominated vegetable oils used in the food industry[1]. Lipid droplet accumulation and myofibrillar lysis are seen in rats and mice given large doses of glucocorticoids[1].

Myocardial lipofuscinosis is seen in rats given Brown FK, a food colouring agent. Lipofuscin occurs intracellularly at the poles of the myocardial fibres. At larger doses Brown FK produces necrosis of myocardial fibres[1].

Multi-focal myocardial necrosis and calcification (Figure 1.19) and focal calcification of smooth muscle cells in the walls of intramyocardial arteries are observed in vitamin D toxicity of rats.

A diet-induced atrial thrombosis is reported in certain strains of mice[11]. Thrombosis is preceded by damage to the endocardium and myocardium.

Myocardial hypertrophy is occasionally seen in toxicity studies. Increased heart weight, associated with enlargement of myocardial fibres, is reported in dogs and rats given prolonged doses of oxfenicine[12] and in dogs treated with a certain novel calcium channel blocker. Ventricular hypertrophy is induced in experimental animals given thyroxine[13]. Necrosis of subepicardial fat has been observed in the hearts of primates treated with high doses of novel glucocorticoids (Figure 1.20).

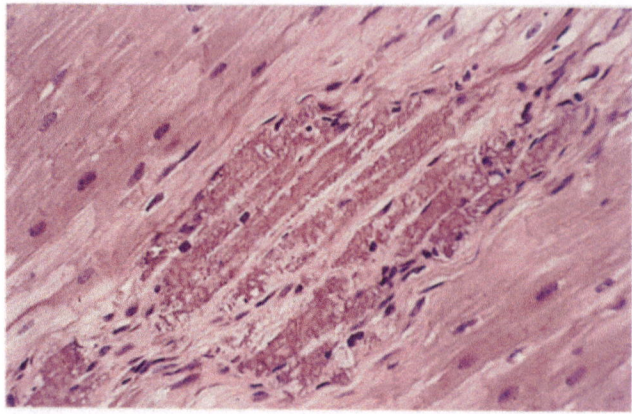

Figure 1.19 A focus of myocardial necrosis and calcification in the papillary muscle of a dog. Note the intrasarcoplasmic basophilic granular staining of the affected fibres. H & E

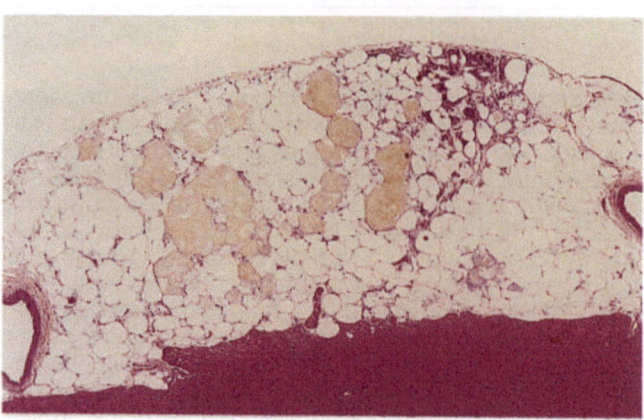

Figure 1.20 Prominent subepicardial adipose tissue with focal fat necrosis from a monkey treated with a novel gluco-corticosteroid. H & E

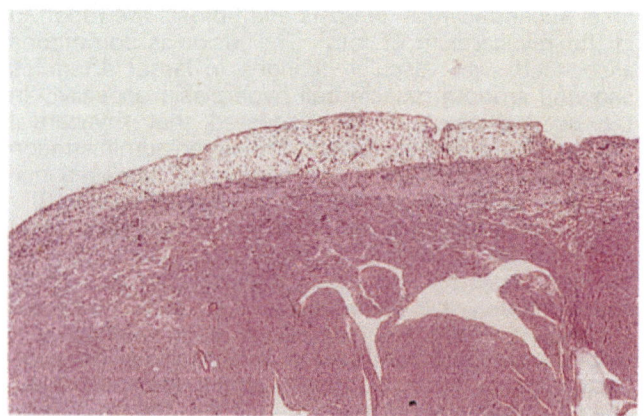

Figure 1.21 An area of epicarditis in a dog treated with high doses of a novel immunostimulant drug. Note the area of oedema and inflammation. H & E

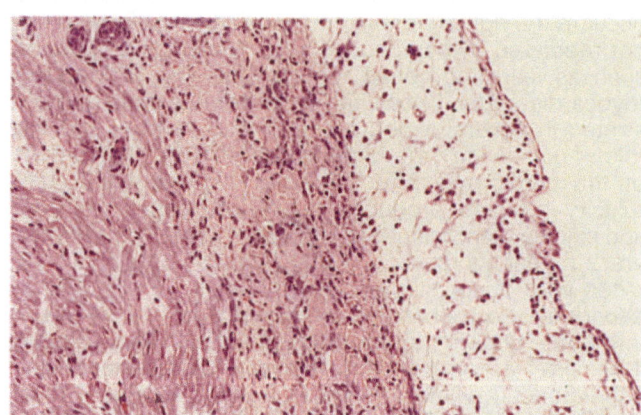

Figure 1.22 This is from the same slide as Figure 1.21 but at higher magnification. The inflammation extends to the superficial layers of the myocardium. H & E

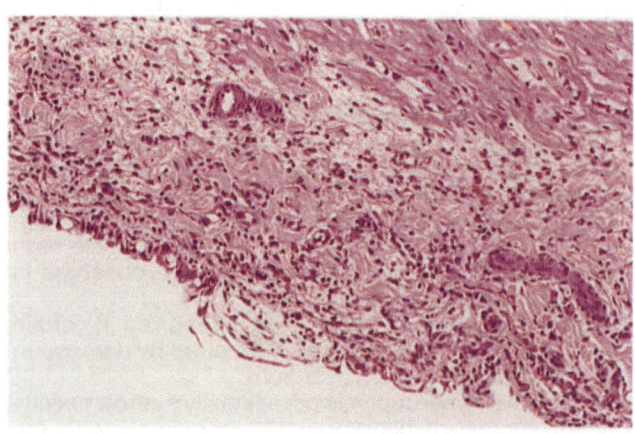

Figure 1.23 Epicarditis in a dog. Note the prominent mesothelial cells, inflammation and proliferating fibroblasts. The dog is from a toxicity study with an immunostimulant drug. H & E

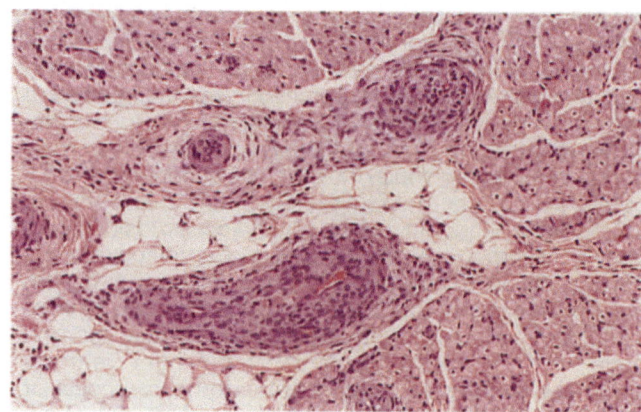

Figure 1.24 Vasculitis in the myocardium of a dog from a toxicity study with a novel immunostimulant drug. H & E

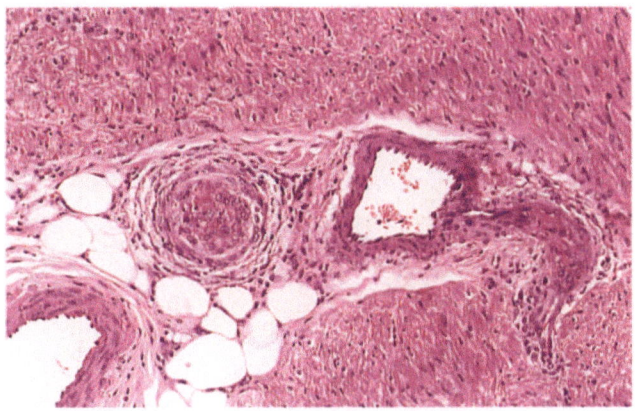

Figure 1.25 Vasculitis and thrombosis affecting arterioles of the ventricular myocardium of a dog treated with a novel immunostimulant drug. Note the luminal occlusion. Such lesions bear similarity to thromboangitis obliterans in man. In the present case the lesion was associated with haemorrhagic necrosis in the myocardium. H & E

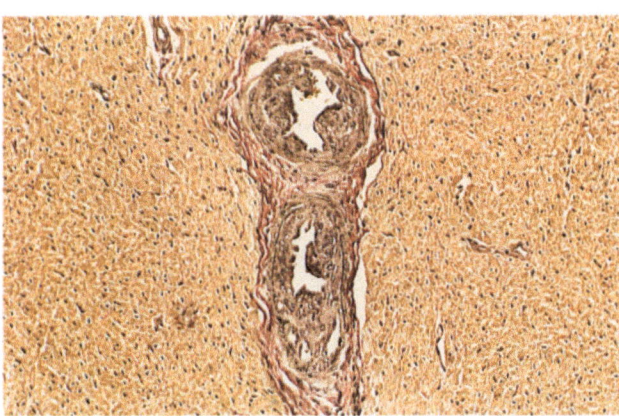

Figure 1.26 Intramural arterioles showing intimal proliferation in the myocardium of a dog from a toxicity study with an immunostimulant drug. Elastic van Gieson

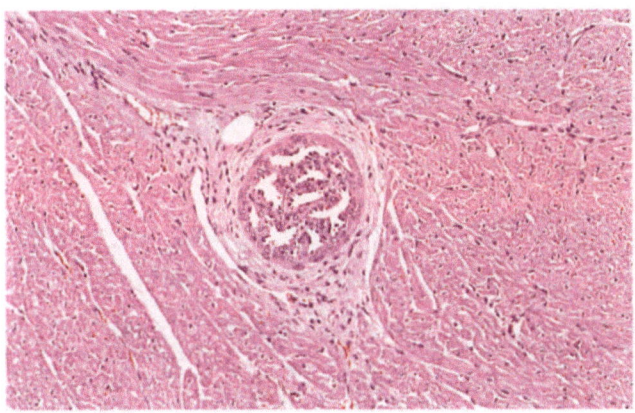

Figure 1.27 Endothelial proliferation and recanalization in a myocardial intramural artery from a dog treated with a novel immunostimulant drug. H & E

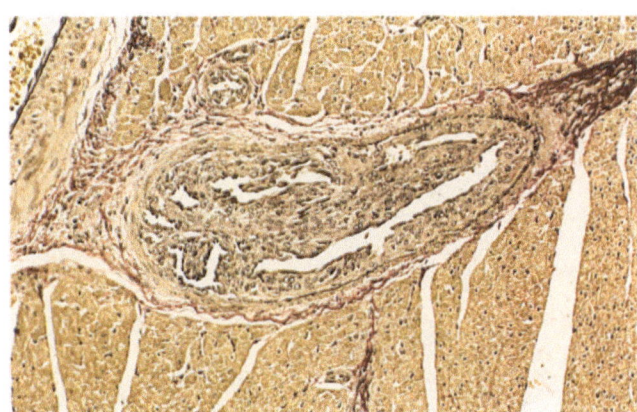

Figure 1.28 From the same study as Figure 1.26. The recanalization of the occluded lumen is clearly depicted by the elastic staining. Elastic van Gieson

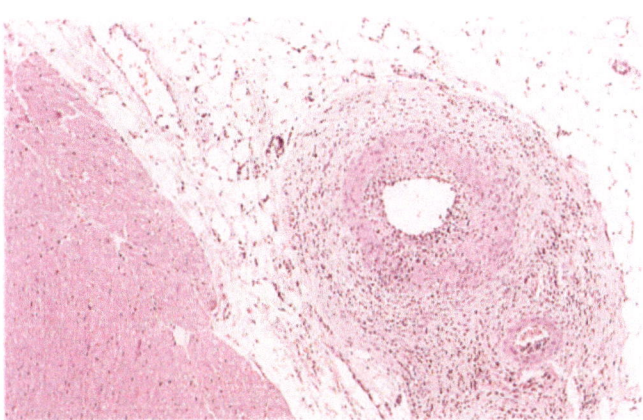

Figure 1.29 Arteritis involving a coronary artery of a dog treated with a potential immunomodulator drug. The inflammation affects all the layers and peri-arterial connective tissue. H & E

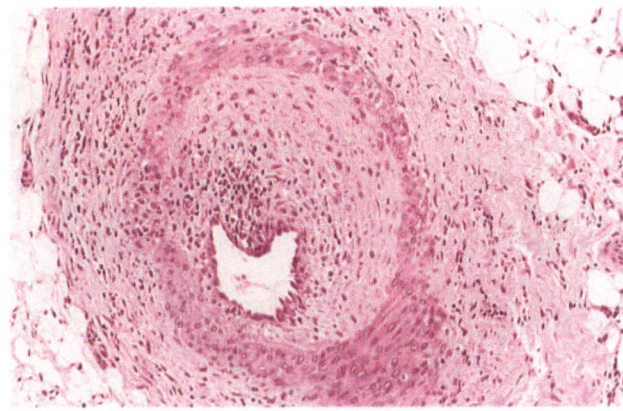

Figure 1.30 From the same study as Figure 1.29 but at a higher magnification. In this case there is narrowing of the lumen with evidence of intimal proliferation. H & E

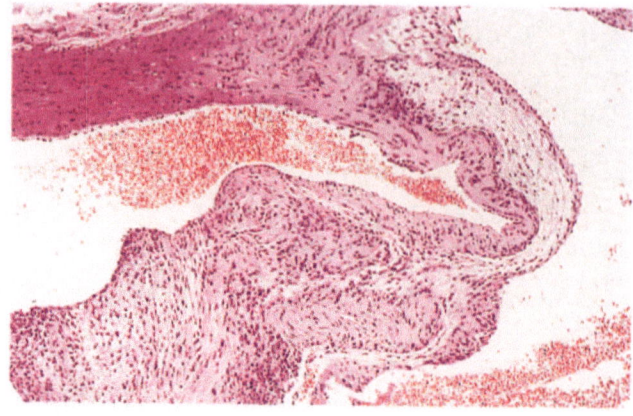

Figure 1.31 Valvular thickening in an atrio-ventricular valve of a rat from a toxicity study with an immunomodulatory drug. Increased cellularity and inflammatory cell infiltration of the valvular stroma.   H & E

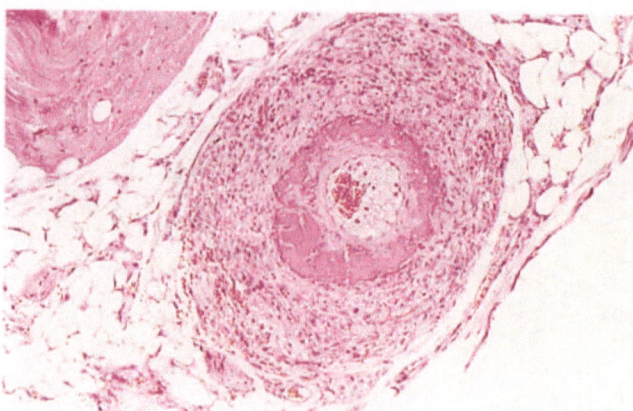

Figure 1.32 Necrotizing arteritis in a peritoneal artery of a dog treated with an immunomodulatory drug. Medial necrosis and inflammation affect all layers of the artery and the peri-arterial connective tissue.   H & E

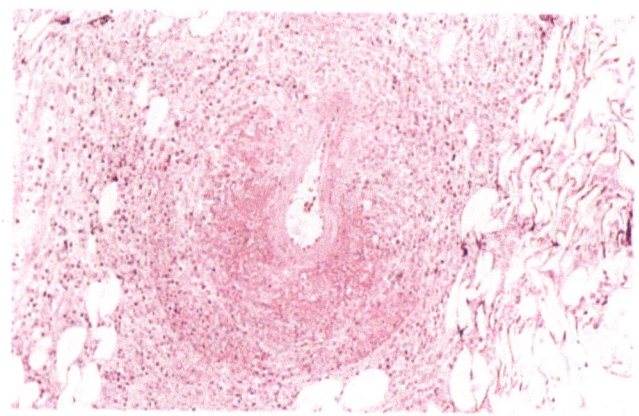

Figure 1.33 Necrotizing arteritis in a mesenteric artery of a dog treated with an immunomodulatory drug. Fibrinoid necrosis of the tunica media. Inflammatory reaction spreads into the peri-arterial connective tissue.   H & E

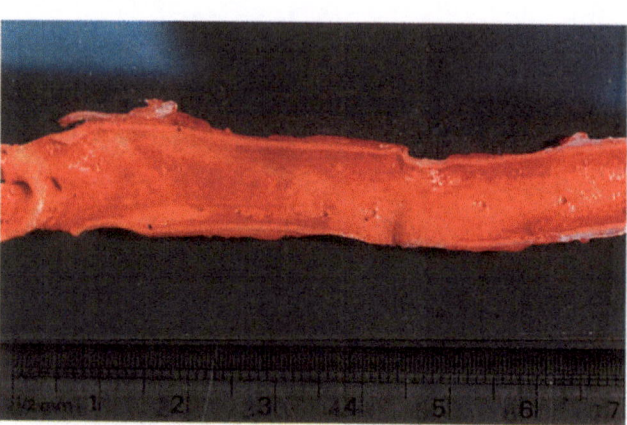

Figure 1.34 Dietary study. Fatty streaks seen macro-scopically on the aortic endothelium of a monkey fed a high fat, high cholesterol diet for a period of 52 weeks. The lesion represents an early stage in the development of diet-induced atherosclerosis. Oil red O

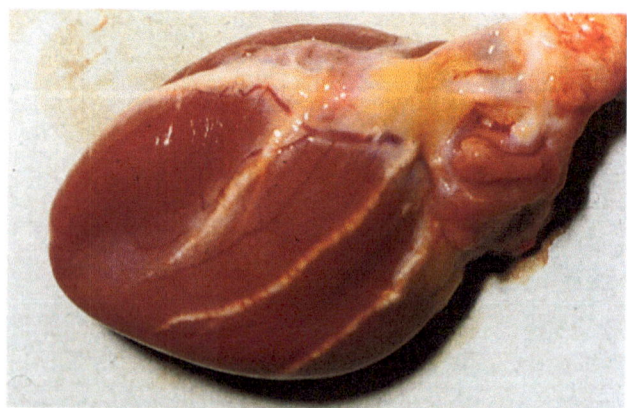

Figure 1.35 Dietary study. Atherosclerotic changes in a monkey heart. Note the opaque-white tortuous and nodular appearance of the coronary arteries. This represents an advanced stage of diet induced atherosclerosis

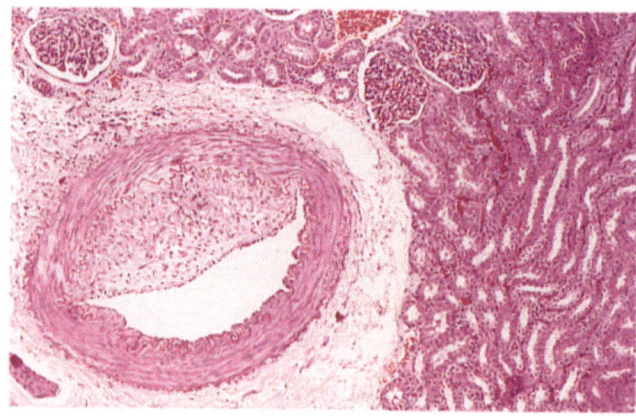

Figure 1.36 Dietary study. Intimal plaque in a renal artery of a monkey. The plaque projects into the lumen.   H & E

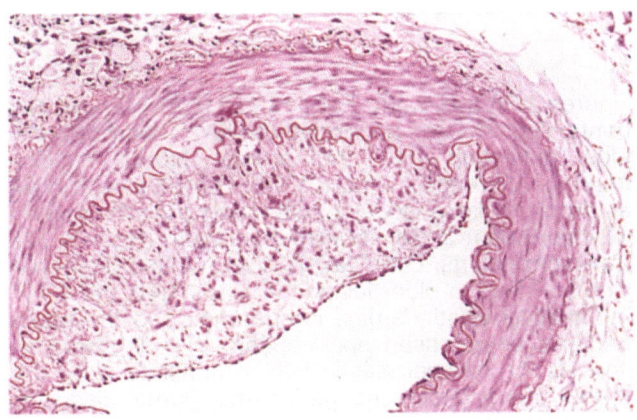

Figure 1.37 Dietary study. Atherosclerotic plaque in a peripheral artery of a monkey. The elastic lamina is intact and the plaque reveals proliferating smooth muscle cells, vacuolated macrophages and a homogeneous eosinophilic matrix. H & E

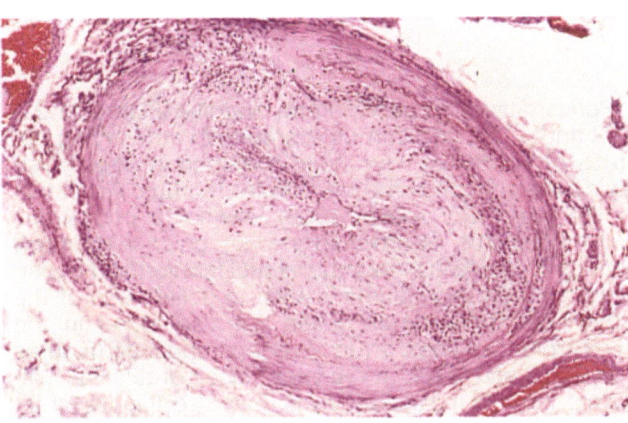

Figure 1.38 Dietary study. Advanced atherosclerotic lesion in a peripheral artery of a monkey showing complete stenosis. The plaque reveals fibrosis and lipophages and the lesion extends into the media. H & E

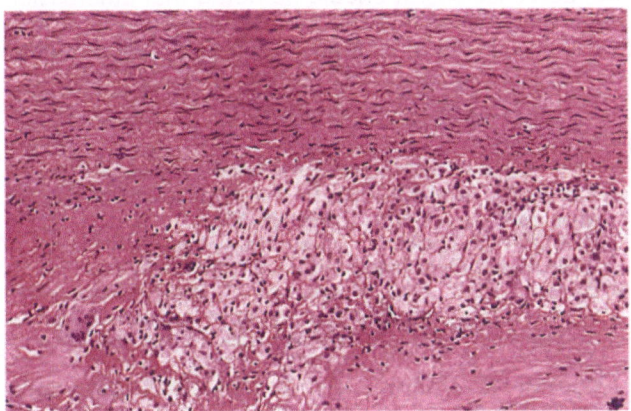

Figure 1.39 Dietary study. Advanced atherosclerotic changes affecting the aorta of a monkey. Note the group of lipophages, fibrosis and hyalinized matrix. The lesion extends into the medial layers. H & E

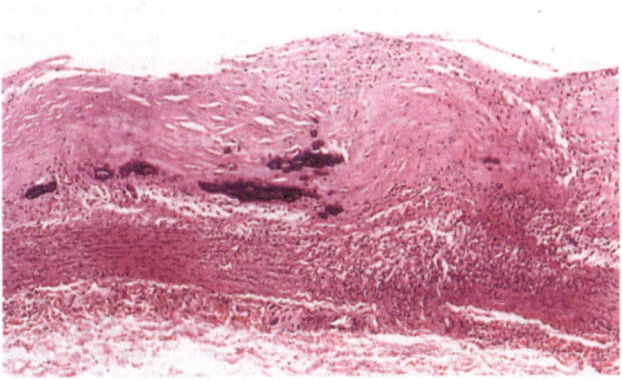

Figure 1.40 Dietary study. Advanced atherosclerotic lesion in the aorta of a monkey showing fibrosis, hyalinization and focal calcification. H & E

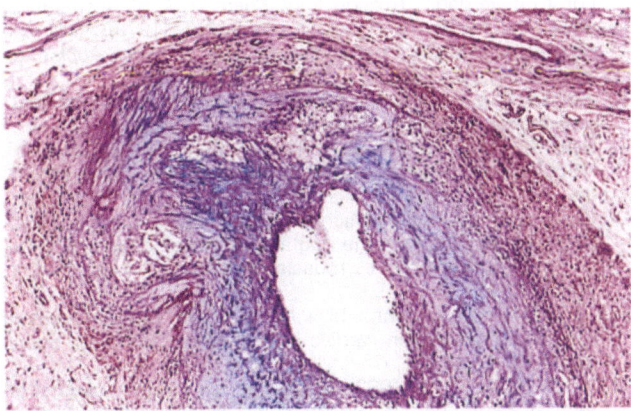

Figure 1.41 Dietary study. Advanced atherosclerotic lesion in a coronary artery of a monkey. The lesion extends to involve all layers of the artery. Hyaline matrix reveals glycoproteins, cholesterol clefts and fibrous tissue. PAS–Alcian Blue

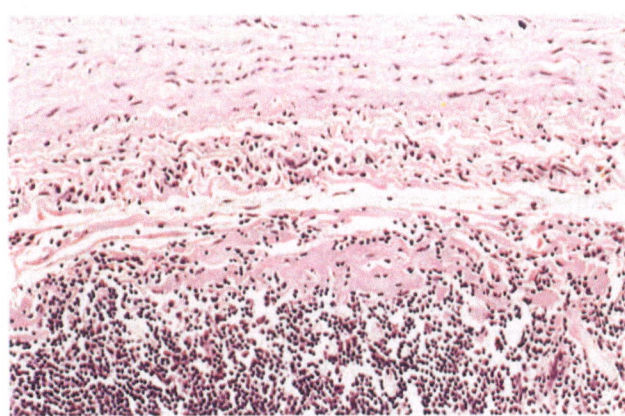

Figure 1.42 Dietary study. Peri-aortic lymphoid accumulation associated with advanced atherosclerotic lesion of the aorta in a monkey. H & E

Pericarditis and underlying myocarditis (Figures 1.21, 1.22 and 1.23), sometimes associated with varying degrees of vasculitis, have been observed in dogs given toxic doses of some immunostimulant drugs. Activation of the pericardial mesothelium leading to pericarditis and myocarditis, is reported in dogs given a muramyl peptide[14]. Vasculitis, endothelial proliferation and hyperplasia of the tunica intima leading to obliteration of the lumen of intramural arterioles are also found in the myocardium of dogs given similar compounds (Figures 1.24, 1.25 and 1.26). In the later stages of this vascular lesion, luminal recanalization is observed (Figures 1.27 and 1.28). In the early stages vascular lesions are also associated with myocardial necrosis. Periarteritis and arteritis affecting the extramural coronary arteries are encountered in dogs treated with some novel immunomodulating drugs (Figures 1.29 and 1.30). Treatment of rats with novel immunostimulants in our laboratories has also resulted in proliferative lesions in the stroma of auriculoventricular valves (Figure 1.31).

Several induced vascular lesions have already been described along with cardiac lesions, and vascular changes by themselves as end-points in toxicity studies are uncommon. A degenerative arteriopathy affecting arteries in the meninges, oesophagus and stomach is reported in young pigs given mercurial compounds[15]. Proliferation of the tunica adventitia, thickening of the intima and media, re-duplication of the elastic lamina, narrowing of the lumina, and subintimal fibrinoid deposits are among the salient features of this arterial lesion. Capillary thrombosis, arteriolar medial and endothelial hypertrophy and panarteritis are induced in the pulmonary vasculature of stump-tailed monkeys treated with monocrotaline, a pyrrolizidine alkaloid[16]. Similar vascular lesions are reported in rats given monocrotaline[17].

Thrombosis, although an uncommon toxic response, has been observed at the site of intravenous infusions using irritant drugs which produce phlebitis and thrombosis in experimental animals.

Aneurysms are induced in rats by β-amino-propionitrile and are also reported in lathyrism[18].

Toxicity studies with certain immunostimulant compounds in dogs result in acute necrotizing vasculitis with fibrinoid necrosis and marked inflammatory cell infiltration of the tunica adventitia (Figures 1.32 and 1.33). Immune-mediated vasculitis affects smaller vessels and is associated with deposition of immune complexes in the vessel wall and with activation of the complement system. It must be pointed out that dogs, and to a lesser extent rats, show this type of lesion spontaneously, albeit at a low incidence.

Arterial intimal proliferation and medial degeneration of the peripheral arteries are reported in ergotamine intoxication[18].

Atherosclerotic lesions can be induced in several species of experimental animals. Diet-induced hyperlipidaemia causes direct injury to vascular endothelium without any additional factors[19]. Patchy areas of vascular de-endothelialization are induced in baboons by infusion with homocystine. Carbon disulphide is known to enhance coronary atherosclerosis in experimental animals[20]. Carbon monoxide accelerates atherogenesis in rabbits fed a diet rich in cholesterol[21]. In diet-induced atherosclerosis of primates the lesions are seen in the abdominal aorta, coronary arteries (Figures 1.34 and 1.35) and many of the other larger arteries. The affected coronary arteries appear opaque, white, nodular and tortuous. Histologically, the lesion is characterized by a focal intimal thickening, which is due to accumulation of lipoid materials along with other tissue constituents (Figures 1.36 and 1.37). Fat and connective tissue elements accumulate, subendothelially as localized plaques projecting into the arterial lumen causing progressive stenosis (Figure 1.38). The plaques contain fat droplets, lipophages, proliferating smooth muscle cells, fibroblasts and a ground tissue matrix (Figure 1.39). Cholesterol clefts, calcification, collagen and proteoglycans are seen in older lesions (Figures 1.40 and 1.41). The internal elastic lamina is stretched and the tunica media is compressed and appears thin. In some instances the internal elastic lamina appears to be disrupted, allowing the changes in the intimal plaque to spread into the deeper layers. Ulceration of the endothelium and thrombosis, although frequent complications in man, are uncommon in experimental atherosclerosis. Stenosis of affected arterioles is frequently seen in induced primate lesions. Extension of the intimal lesion into the tunica media and even the tunica adventitia is not uncommon in the older lesions. In some of these instances foci of lymphoid cells in the adventitia are occasionally seen (Figure 1.42) associated with aortic lesions. It should be noted that atherosclerosis involves a multi-stage process and it is not feasible to see all aspects of changes in the same experimental lesion.

References

1. Van Vleet, J. F. and Ferrans, V. J. (1986). Myocardial diseases of animals. *Am. J. Pathol.*, **124**, 95–178
2. Glaister, J. R. (1986). Cardiovascular system. In *Principles of Toxicological Pathology*, p. 116. (London: Taylor and Francis)
3. Balazs, T., Earl, F. L., Beerbower, G. W. and Weinberger, M. A. (1973). The cardiotoxic effect of pressurised aerosol isoproterenol in the dog. *Toxicol. Appl. Pharmacol.*, **26**, 407–417
4. Gopinath, C., Thuring, J. and Zayed, I. (1978). Isoprenaline-induced myocardial necrosis in dogs. *Br. J. Exp. Pathol.*, **59**, 148–157
5. Balazs, T. and Ferrans, V. J. (1978). Cardiac lesions induced by chemicals. *Environ. Health Perspect.*, **26**, 181–191
6. Smith, H. A. (1957). Pathology of gossipol poisoning. *Am. J. Pathol.*, **33**, 353–365
7. Teske, R. H., Bishop, S. A., Righter, H. F. and Detweiler, D. K. (1976). Subacute digitoxin toxicosis in beagle dogs. *Toxicol. Appl. Pharmacol.*, **35**, 283–301
8. Gans, J. H., Korson, R., Cater, M. R. and Ackerly, C. C. (1980). Effects of short-term and long-term theobromine administration to male dogs. *Toxicol. Appl. Pharmacol.*, **53**, 481–496
9. Boor, P. J., Moslen, M. T. and Reynolds, E. S. (1979). Allylamine toxicity: sequence of pathological events. *Toxicol. Appl. Pharmacol.*, **50**, 581–592
10. Jaenke, R. S. (1974). An anthracyclin antibiotic-induced cardiomyopathy in rabbits. *Lab. Invest.*, **30**, 292–304
11. Ball, C. R., Clower, B. R., Willams, W. L. and Jackson, M. (1965). Dietary-induced atrial thrombosis in mice. *Arch. Pathol.*, **80**, 391–396
12. Greaves, P., Martin, J., Michel, M. C. and Mompon, P. (1984). Cardiac hypertrophy in the dog and rat induced by oxfenicine, an agent which modifies muscle metabolism. *Arch. Toxicol.*, Suppl. 7, 488–493
13. Skelton, C. L. and Sonnenblick, E. H. (1974). Heterogeneity of contractile function in cardiac hypertrophy. *Circ. Res.*, Suppl. 34–35, **2**, 83–96
14. Wachsmuth, E. D. (1983). Evaluating immunopathological effects of new drugs. In Gibson, G. G., Hubbard, R. and Parke, D. V. (eds.) *Immunotoxicology*. p. 237. (London: Academic Press)
15. Tryphonas, L. and Nielson, N. O. (1973). Pathology of chronic alkyl mercurial poisoning in swine. *Am. J. Vet. Res.*, **34**, 379–392
16. Chesney, C. F. and Allen, J. R. (1973). Cardiopulmonary disease. *Am. J. Pathol.*, **70**, 489–492
17. Lalich, J. J., Johnson, W. D., Raczniak, T. J. and Shumaker, R. C.

(1977). Fibrin thrombosis in monocrotaline, pyrrole-induced Cor Pulmonale in rats. *Arch. Path. Lab. Med.*, **101**, 69–73

18. Balazs, T., Hanig, J. P. and Herman, E. (1986). Toxic responses of cardiovascular system. In Klassen, C. D., Amdur, M. O. and Doull, J. (eds) *Casarett and Doull's Toxicology.* 3rd Edition, p. 387. (New York: Macmillan Publishing Co.)

19. Harker, L. A., Ross, R., Slichter, S. J. and Scott, C. R. (1976). Homocystine-induced arteriosclerosis. The role of endothelial cell injury and platelet response in its genesis. *J. Clin. Invest.*, **58**, 731–741

20. Wronska-Nofer, T., Szendzikowki, S. and Laurman, W. (1978). The effect of carbon disulfide and atherogenic diet on the development of atherosclerotic changes in rabbits. *Atherosclerosis*, **31**, 33–39

21. Astrup, P., Kjeldsen, K. and Wanstrup, J. (1967). Enhancing effect of carbon monoxide in development of atherosclerosis in cholesterol fed rabbits. *J. Atherosclerosis Res.*, **7**, 343–354

The Respiratory System

2

Considerable attention has been focused in recent years on the pulmonary effects of airborne pollutants such as SO_2, NO_2 and cigarette smoke, and occupationally inhaled chemicals and dusts such as solvents, asbestos, cements, glass fibre and silica[1]. With current rapid industrial and technological developments which involve the production and use of new products and processes the potential risk of toxic effects by inhalation is constantly increasing[2]. Similarly, the increasingly widespread use of household products in aerosol form, such as hairsprays, deodorants, perfumes, furniture polishes, oven cleaners, insecticides, leather sprays and upholstery cleaners, also offers a large and perhaps alarming potential for pulmonary damage. In addition, an increasing number of pharmaceutical preparations such as antibiotics, mucolytics, anti-asthmatics, anaesthetics, anti-allergics and decongestants have been developed for administration by inhalation[1]. This vast use of clinical aerosols is emphasized by the estimated 14 million prescriptions for inhalant bronchial therapies, dispensed in the USA alone in 1983[3].

Due to this rapidly expanding atmospheric, occupational and clinical exposure in man, the field of inhalation toxicology has become of major importance.

In addition to pulmonary changes induced by inhalation, a large number of drugs and chemicals have been found to produce lung damage following systemic administration[4]. The best known of these compounds are paraquat and the cytotoxic drugs such as bleomycin, busulfan and cyclophosphamide. Drug-induced pulmonary disease in man has recently been reviewed in detail[5,6].

In our experience few if any compounds result in unique or specific pathological changes in pulmonary tissues. Indeed, it should be emphasized that there are only a limited number of ways in which pulmonary tissue can react to toxic insults and many different compounds appear to induce pulmonary changes with similar morphological features. In many cases the toxicologically induced pathologies observed at any one time are to some extent dependent upon the time scale of the experiment involved (and the dose levels employed).

The following review describes and classifies the lesions encountered in the pulmonary tissues of experimental animals exposed to atmospheric, occupational, household and therapeutic agents during safety evaluation tests involving both systemic and inhalation exposure.

Nasal Chambers

The distribution of lesions within the nasal chambers varies with the compound under test, the test species and the mode of administration. Some chemicals only affect olfactory epithelium, others only respiratory epithelium, and yet others both types[7].

The nasal chambers are the first structures of the respiratory tract to be subjected to inhaled insults and are therefore a common site for induced change. In order to detect and identify these changes consistently, a systematic histopathological examination, such as that described by Young[7], is essential. This allows the accurate assessment of changes in epithelial types at specific sites.

Commonly encountered induced lesions of the nasal chambers are listed in Table 2.1.

Table 2.1 Induced lesions of the nasal chambers

Epithelial inclusions
Olfactory epithelial atrophy/degeneration
Goblet cell proliferation
Epithelial hyperplasia
Epithelial squamous metaplasia
Epithelial ulceration

An unusual epithelial response to irritant compounds in rodents is the production of eosinophilic globular inclusions in the sustentacular cells of the olfactory epithelium (Figure 2.1), and to a lesser extent in the respiratory epithelium and cells of the subepithelial glands and ducts. These inclusions are PAS negative and occupy both sub-nuclear and supra-nuclear positions. They are described in rodents following dimethylamine exposure[8] and in our laboratory with several irritant compounds including both industrial chemicals and pharmaceuticals. The significance of these inclusions is uncertain but they may represent a defence response[8]. In one study in our laboratories they were shown to persist in the epithelium even after a 12-week recovery period. Electron microscopy showed the inclusions were confined to the sustentacular or supporting cell and corresponded to membrane-bound elipsoid bodies (Figure 2.2). These bodies sometimes had a slightly irregular contour with a homogeneous, moderately electron-dense matrix. There was no evidence of degenerative changes within the affected cells.

Atrophic, degenerative or even necrotic changes in the olfactory epithelium are found following inhalation of numerous chemicals including[9] SO_2, 3-methylfuran[10], acetaldehyde[11], and 1,2-dibromo-3-chloropropane and 1,2-dibromoethane[12]. Depending on the compound and the dose levels employed, the histological appearance of the olfactory mucosa may range from minor disorganization of the cellular layers (Figure 2.3), through various degrees of atrophic change (Figures 2.4–2.6) to complete necrosis or ulceration (Figure 2.7). In addition the picture

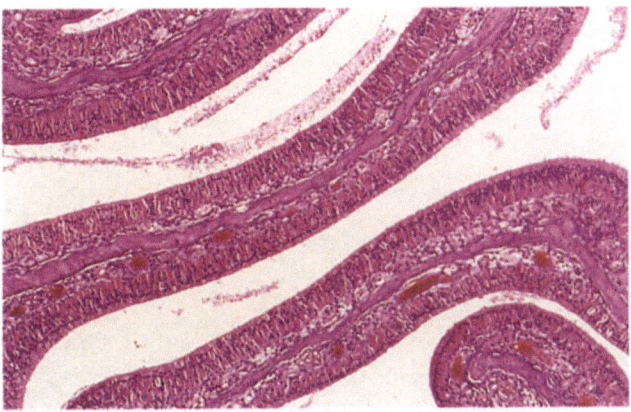

Figure 2.1 Olfactory epithelial cells of the nasal turbinates of a rat containing numerous homogeneous, eosinophilic cytoplasmic inclusions. These inclusions are a non-specific response to inhaled irritant materials and may persist after cessation of administration of the test compound. H & E

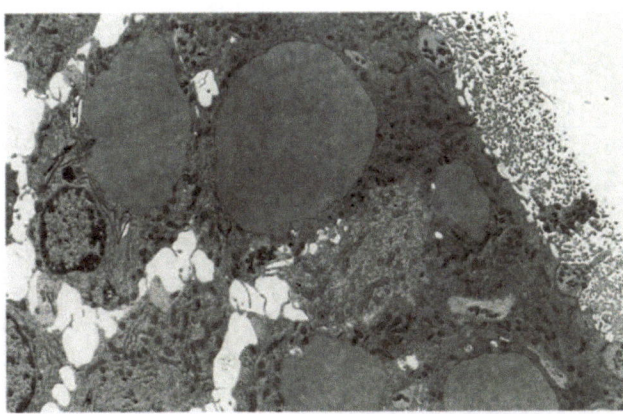

Figure 2.2 Homogeneous inclusions in the sustentacular (supporting cells) of the olfactory epithelium in a rat. These inclusions correspond with those shown in Figure 2.1. The olfactory cells with ciliated apical olfactory vesicles appear unaffected. Electron micrograph

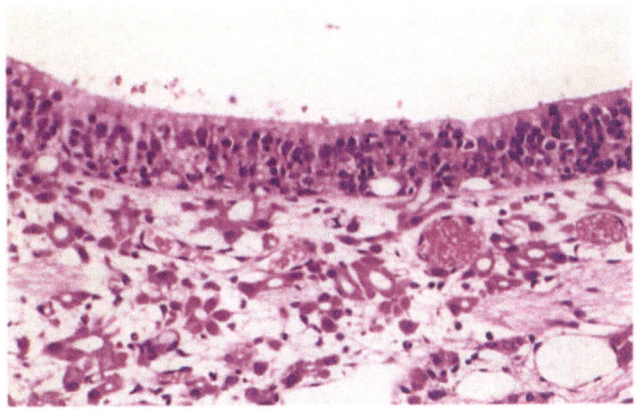

Figure 2.3 Mild disorganization of the olfactory epithelium in a rat following inhalation of an irritant compound. Subepithelial nerve fibres and glands are unaffected. H & E

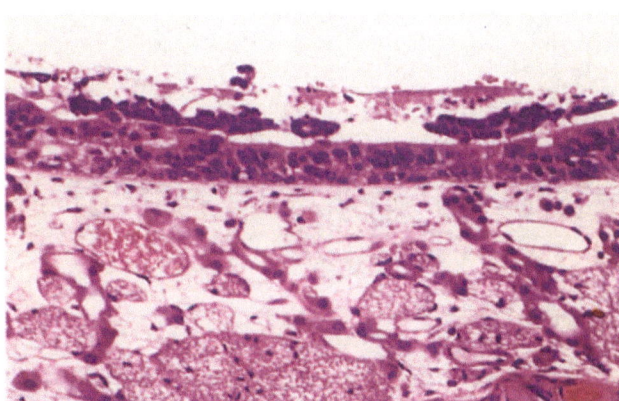

Figure 2.4 Moderate atrophy with exfoliation of damaged cells from the olfactory epithelium of a rat following inhalation of an irritant compound. Subepithelial glands and nerve fibres appear normal. H & E

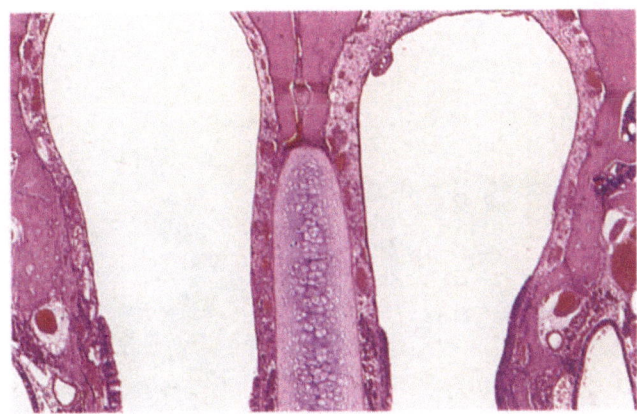

Figure 2.5 Transverse section through nasal chambers of a rat exposed, by inhalation, to an irritant compound. Severe atrophy of the olfactory epithelium. Note the distinct junctions with the ciliated respiratory epithelium which is unaffected. H & E

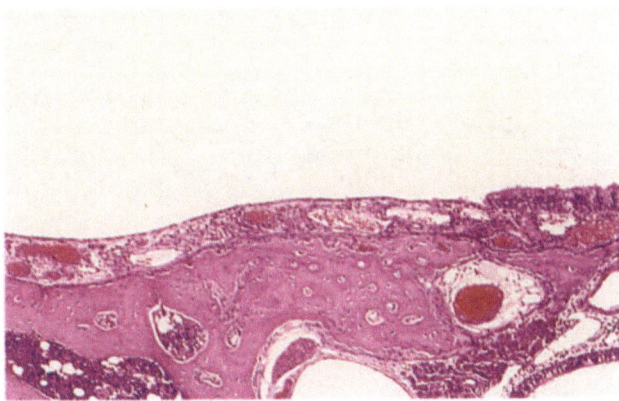

Figure 2.6 Higher magnification of Figure 2.5. The olfactory epithelium is reduced to a single cell layer. The adjacent respiratory epithelium appears normal. H & E

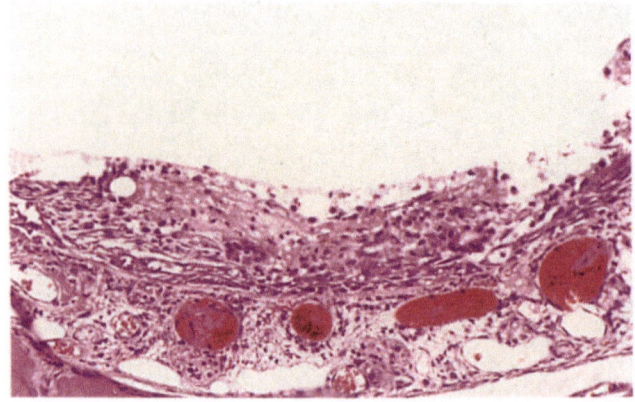

Figure 2.7 Severe damage to the olfactory epithelium with ulceration, inflammation and exudation in a rat exposed to an inhaled industrial chemical.   H & E

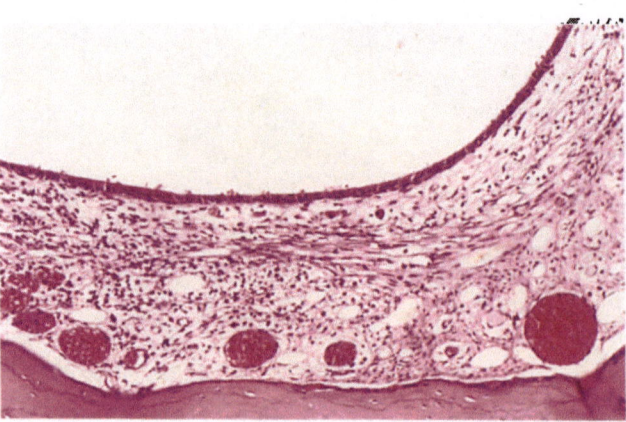

Figure 2.8 Olfactory region from a rat exposed by inhalation to an industrial chemical. The epithelium is mainly composed of low cuboidal cells. The subepithelium is grossly thickened with oedema, congestion and fibroblasts. Subepithelial nerve fibres and glands are absent.   H & E

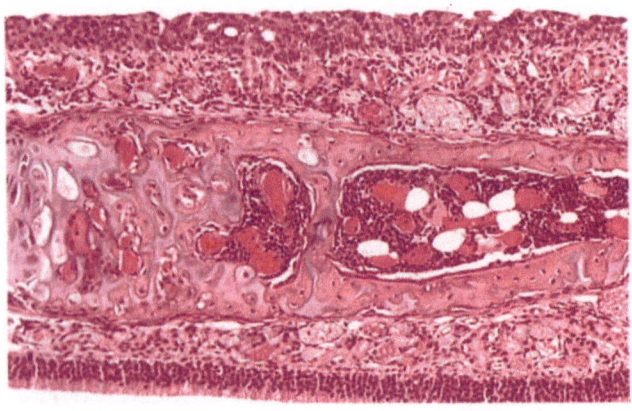

Figure 2.9 Transverse section through the central septum of the nasal chambers of a rat exposed by inhalation to an irritant pharmaceutical preparation. On one side of the septum, the olfactory epithelium is unaffected. On the contralateral side the epithelium shows hyperplasia with slight basophilia and loss of the normal orderly cellular arrangement.   H & E

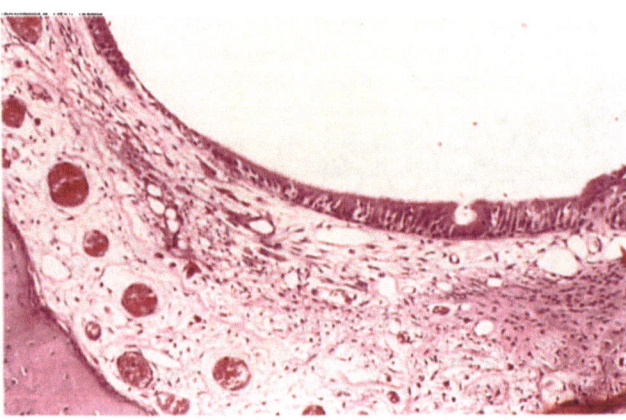

Figure 2.10 Olfactory epithelium from a rat exposed by inhalation to an irritant compound and subsequently allowed a recovery period. The epithelium is composed of columnar ciliated cells. There is no evidence of regeneration of subepithelial nerve fibres or glands. This metaplastic transformation to a ciliated epithelium represents attempted repair, but a normal olfactory epithelium did not develop in any animal from this study.   H & E

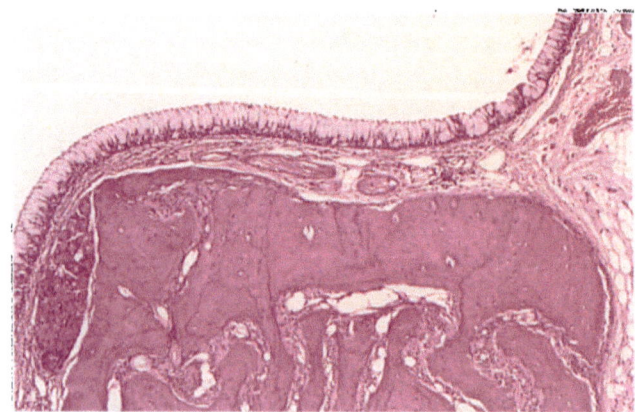

Figure 2.11 The respiratory epithelium in the nasal chambers of a rat exposed to a mildly irritant material by inhalation shows markedly increased numbers of goblet cells.   H & E

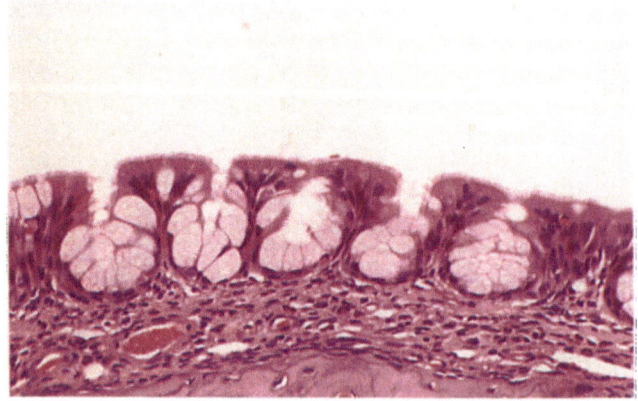

Figure 2.12 Goblet cell proliferation with a pseudoglandular pattern in the nasal chambers of a rat. This represents a more pronounced response to an irritant than Figure 2.11. The goblet cells are located in groups at the base of the epithelium within the basement membrane and are in contact with the nasal lumen via a short pseudoduct. The epithelium in this region of the nasal chambers is normally ciliated columnar in type.   H & E

is inevitably complicated by stages of attempted repair, which may vary from a single layer of thin cuboidal elongate cells (Figure 2.8), through degrees of hyperplasia (Figure 2.9) to squamous, sometimes highly keratinized metaplasia. The sensory nerve cells of the olfactory epithelium possess the ability to regenerate[8] following withdrawal of an insult. However, in our experience, regeneration often results in the production of ciliated respiratory epithelium (Figure 2.10). This respiratory metaplasia probably represents attempted repair. Replacement of damaged olfactory epithelium by respiratory epithelium is reported in mice exposed to formaldehyde[13]. The degenerative changes in olfactory epithelium are usually accompanied by rhinitis, with, in severe cases, pronounced inflammatory exudation into the nasal chambers. Also, in severe reactions, the subepithelium becomes thickened and oedematous with fibrosis and loss of Bowman's glands and nerve bundles (Figures 2.8 and 2.10). The few remaining glands often appear hypertrophic. In addition to damage to the olfactory epithelium induced by inhalation studies, a few compounds also cause degenerative changes when administered systemically. An example is 3-methylindole which causes damage to the olfactory epithelium in mice[14]. Manipulation of the mixed function oxidase system by the cytochrome P-450 inhibitor β-diethylaminoethyldiphenylpropyl acetate decreases the epithelial damage.

A common, non-specific reaction in the nasal chambers is the proliferation of goblet cells in the respiratory epithelium. The epithelium becomes hypertrophic with typical goblet cells distended with secretory droplets (Figure 2.11). In cases of marked, prolonged exposure, goblet cells may form intra-epithelial crypts in which they are located around a short 'pseudoduct' or 'crypt-like' invagination of the epithelium (Figure 2.12). These structures remain within the epithelial basement membrane and may be termed 'pseudoglands'. They are readily produced by relatively high doses of cigarette smoke, but are also seen with industrial chemicals, atmospheric pollutants and occasionally pharmaceuticals.

The respiratory epithelium of the nasal chambers also commonly illustrates degenerative, inflammatory, proliferative and reparative changes (Figures 2.13–2.18). Dependent on the compound and dose levels, epithelial degeneration, erosion, ulceration, hyperplasia and metaplasia may all be produced.

The ability of some compounds, such as nasal decongestants, solvents, essences and air pollutants, to cause damage to the nasal epithelium has been given a possible explanation[15]. Of 32 substances tested, 18 were metabolized to produce formaldehyde by microsomal activity in the cells of the nasal cavity. When the inhalation of formaldehyde itself was studied, rhinitis, squamous metaplasia and eventually squamous cell carcinomas were produced in the nasal chambers of rats and mice[13].

The vomeronasal organ (VNO) or organ of Jacobson is normally composed of specialized olfactory and columnar epithelia. Rarely, inhaled compounds induced degenerative (Figure 2.19) and subsequently proliferative changes in the VNO. The susceptible olfactory epithelium degenerates and is replaced by a squamous metaplastic type.

Larynx

A summary of induced laryngeal lesions is given in Table 2.2.

Table 2.2 Induced lesions of the larynx

Epithelial hyperplasia
Epithelial squamous metaplasia
Epithelial ulceration
Epithelial/subepithelial necrosis
Submucosal gland degeneration

In our experience, the larynx is a major site of induced changes in rodents exposed by inhalation to industrial chemicals, pharmaceuticals, cigarette smoke and even some propellants. However, laryngeal changes are rarely seen with dusts.

The distribution of aerosol-induced lesions in the rodent larynx shows distinct predilection sites. These sites include the ventrolateral regions, anterior and lateral to the ventral pouch or pit, which are covered with respiratory/cuboidal epithelium, and the inner aspects of the arytenoid projections which are lined by squamous epithelium[16]. Induced laryngeal lesions commonly involve degeneration of original epithelial cells with hyperplasia and squamous metaplasia of the ciliated or cuboidal epithelium (Figures 2.20 and 2.21) and hyperplasia of squamous epithelium (Figure 2.22). As in the nasal chambers, a thorough knowledge of the normal laryngeal anatomy and histology, and consistent detailed histological sampling, are essential to allow interpretation of subtle changes in epithelial type distribution. A squamous metaplastic epithelium induced at one site may be completely indistinguishable, histologically, from a normal squamous epithelium at another site.

In more severe reactions, the larynx illustrates epithelial erosion or ulceration with pronounced inflammatory exudation (Figures 2.23 and 2.24). Alternatively, the mucosa may undergo necrosis (Figure 2.25) without an appreciable inflammatory component, and in some cases necrosis of a preformed hyperplastic or metaplastic epithelium is observed. Repair of ulcerative or necrotic epithelia initially involves the development of a single layer of flattened, elongated cells (Figure 2.26).

The reason for the susceptibility of the rodent larynx to aerosol formulations is uncertain, but probably involves several interacting factors[17]. Examples of substances found to cause laryngeal lesions include: 1,2-dibromo-3-chloropropane and 1,2-dibromoethane[12]; acetaldehyde[11]; and, in our experience, pharmaceuticals such as isoprenaline and xylometazaline and many industrial chemicals. The comparative ease and frequency with which laryngeal epithelial squamous metaplasia may be induced in rodents with chemicals, and especially pharmaceuticals, presents a difficult interpretative problem of extrapolation to man. Metaplastic changes are sometimes regarded as 'preneoplastic' lesions and thus their production by intended therapeutic agents may be disturbing. However, squamous metaplasia is probably only a defence mechanism by which a susceptible epithelium is replaced by a more resistant type. In our experience the compounds in question usually do not produce similar lesions in primates. Thus, it would appear that the rodent larynx is particularly sensitive to aerosol damage[17].

Lesions are rarely encountered in the submucosal glands (SMG) of the larynx or pharynx. However, they may undergo changes which appear to be secondary to damage to the overlying surface epithelium. Following epithelial erosion or ulceration we have observed the subsequent squamous metaplastic epithelium apparently, in some instances, 'seal over' the SMG duct openings (Figure 2.27). This duct obstruction initially

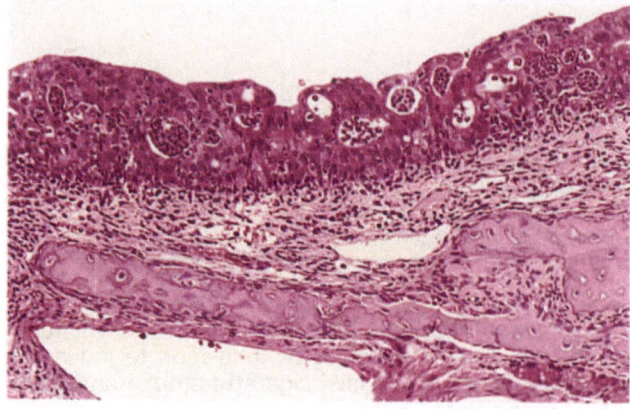

Figure 2.13 Pronounced hyperplasia of the respiratory epithelium from the nasal chambers of a rat following inhalation of an irritant compound. The epithelium is greatly increased in height, with neutrophil infiltration. H & E

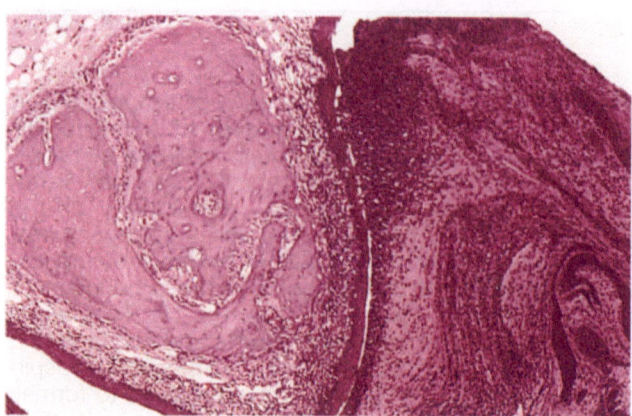

Figure 2.14 Following inhalation of an irritant material the nasal chambers of this rat contain a purulent exudate. The underlying epithelium has undergone squamous metaplasia. H & E

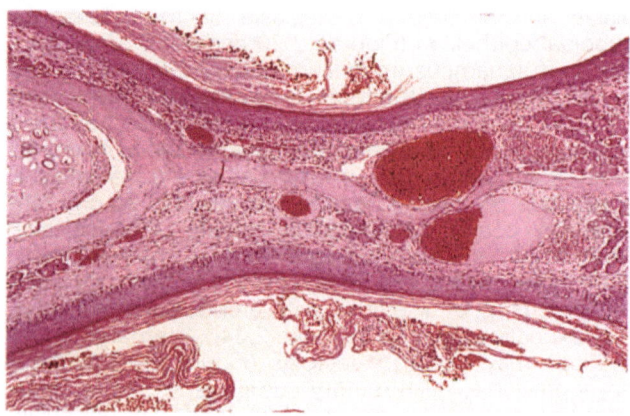

Figure 2.15 Central septum of the rat nasal chambers showing bilateral epithelial squamous metaplasia with superficial keratinization, following exposure to tobacco smoke. H & E

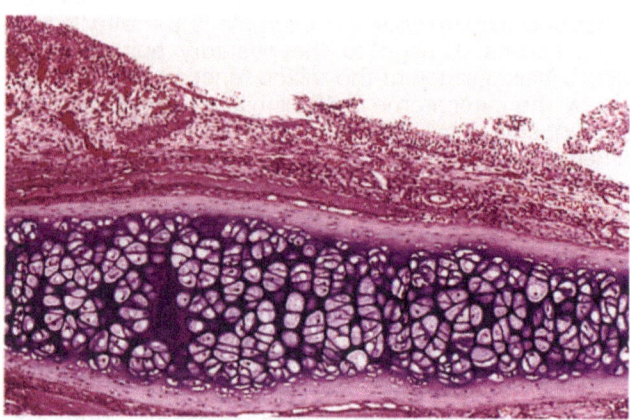

Figure 2.16 Severe ulceration of the respiratory epithelium along the central septum of the rat nasal chambers. The ulceration is associated with congestion and acute inflammatory cell infiltration. H & E

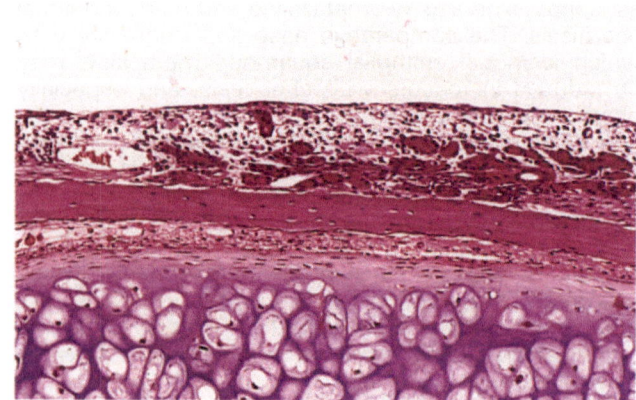

Figure 2.17 Early epithelial regeneration and repair along the central septum of rat nasal chambers. The epithelium is composed of a single layer of elongated, flattened cells which have restored epithelial continuity. H & E

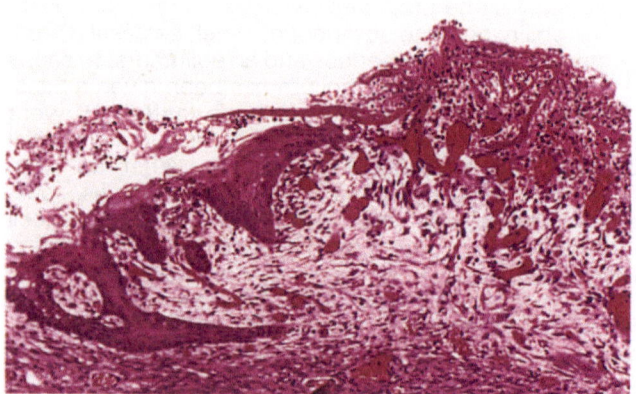

Figure 2.18 Area of epithelial ulceration in the nasal chambers of a rat. There is marked congestion with inflammatory cells and early attempts at epithelial repair by squamous cells. H & E

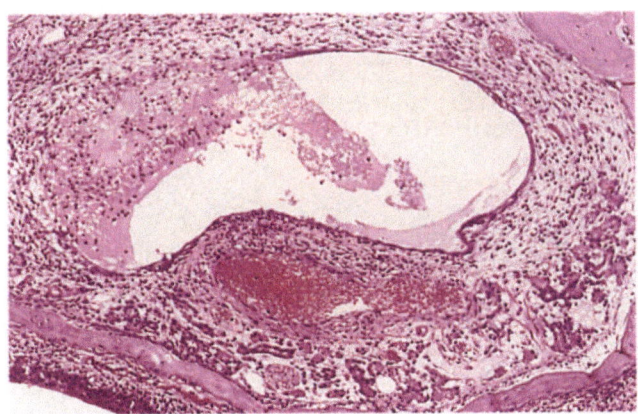

Figure 2.19 Vomeronasal organ (organ of Jacobson) from the nasal chambers of a rat exposed by inhalation to a novel pharmaceutical. This organ is normally composed of olfactory and respiratory types of epithelia. The photomicrograph shows ulcerative, necrotic and atrophic changes.   H & E

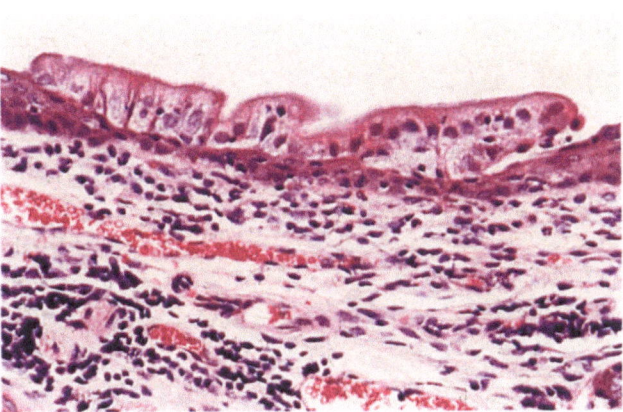

Figure 2.20 Early squamous metaplasia in rat larynx following exposure to tobacco smoke. The original columnar epithelial cells are in the process of being 'lifted' from the basement membrane by newly formed squamous metaplastic cells.   H & E

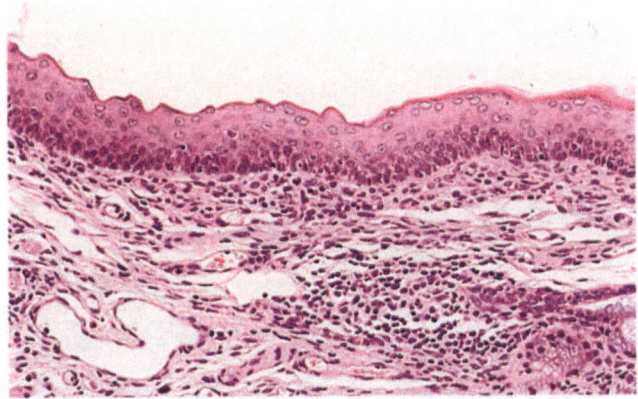

Figure 2.21 Epithelial squamous metaplasia in the ventrolateral aspect of a rat larynx following exposure to tobacco smoke. This site is normally occupied by a cuboidal type of epithelium but, following injury, readily undergoes squamous transformation. The change is usually reversible on cessation of treatment.   H & E

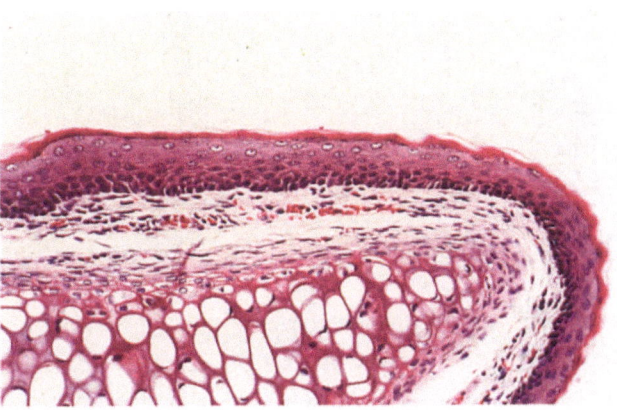

Figure 2.22 Epithelial hyperplasia with keratinization of the inner aspects of the arytenoid projections of the rat larynx. This change is relatively common in inhalation studies. The epithelium at this site is normally squamous, one to three cell layers thick, and non-keratinized.   H & E

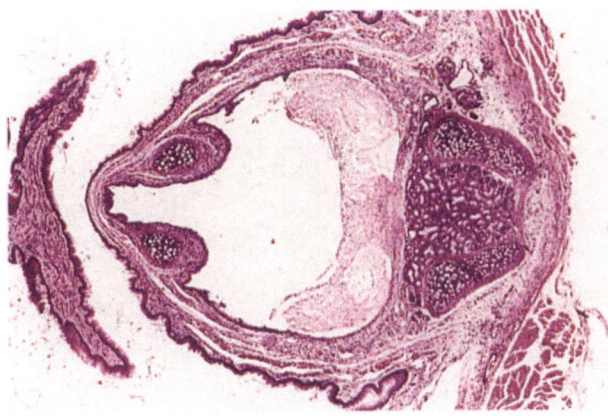

Figure 2.23 Low power photomicrograph of a transverse section through a rat larynx. The ventral and ventrolateral aspects show severe ulceration with pronounced exudation. These are predilection sites for induced change in inhalation studies. Note absence of change in the lateral and dorsal aspects.   H & E

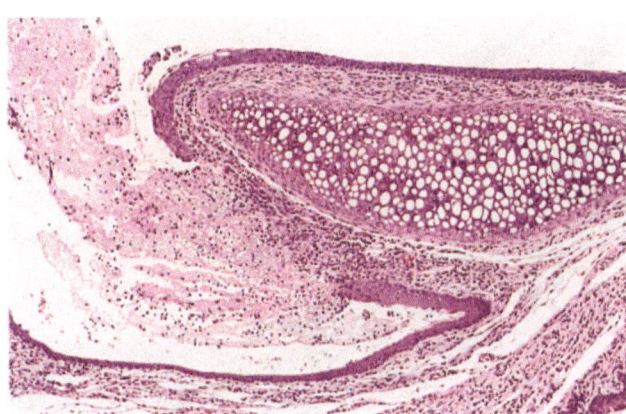

Figure 2.24 Epithelial ulceration along the lateral aspects of the arytenoid projection of the rat larynx with inflammatory exudation into the lumen. This is a relatively unusual site for induced change in the rat.   H & E

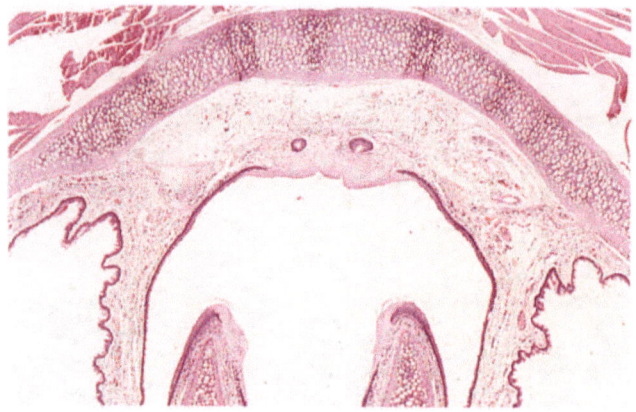

Figure 2.25 Transverse section through a rat larynx. Acute epithelial necrosis in the ventral region and focally along the inner aspects of the arytenoid projections, following administration of a pharmaceutical compound. These are the most common sites for induced change in inhalation studies in the rat.   H & E

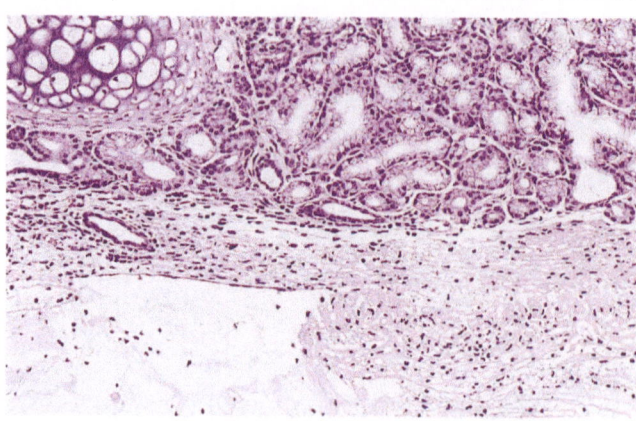

Figure 2.26 Early attempted epithelial repair in the ventrolateral region of the larynx of a rat, 24 hours after cessation of treatment. Focally, flattened epithelial cells form a single layer adjacent to ulceration and exudation.   H & E

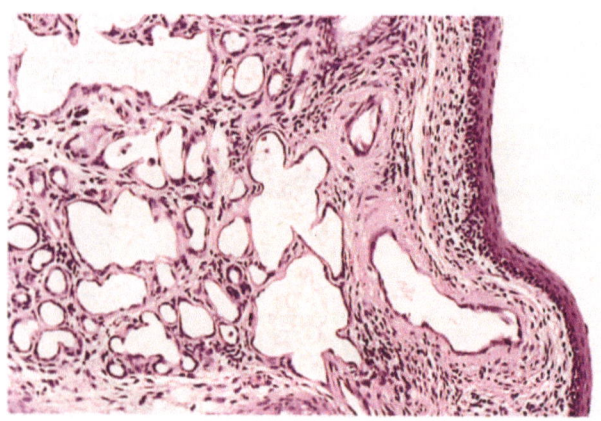

Figure 2.27 Cystic atrophy of submucosal glands from the ventral aspect of a rat larynx following inhalation of an industrial chemical. In this study, epithelial ulceration was initially followed by squamous metaplasia. In this case the newly formed squamous epithelium appears to have 'sealed over' the opening of the submucosal gland duct with consequent dilatation and atrophy.   H & E

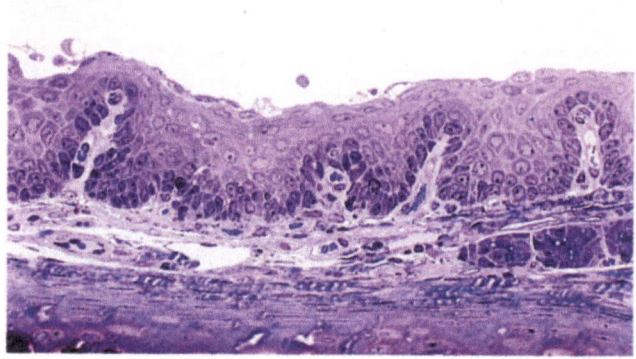

Figure 2.28 Squamous metaplasia of tracheal epithelium following smoke exposure. The metaplastic epithelium has developed into folds which project down between capillaries. 1 μm resin section. Toluidine Blue

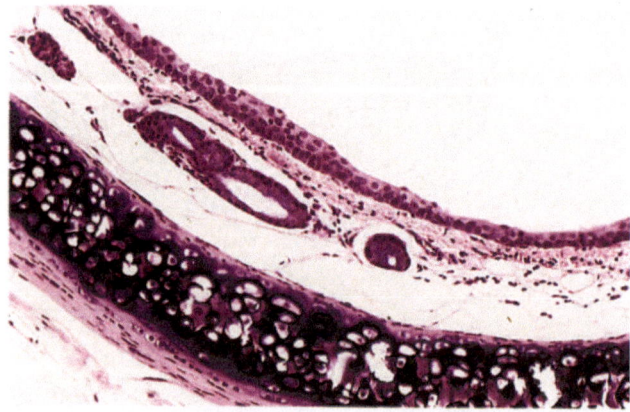

Figure 2.29 Development of a hyperplastic non-ciliated epithelium in the trachea of a rat following smoke exposure.   H & E

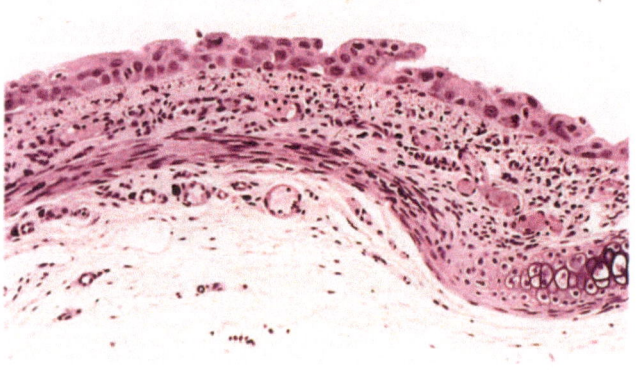

Figure 2.30 Hyperplasia of a non-ciliated tracheal epithelium showing mild nuclear pleomorphism in a rat exposed to an industrial chemical by inhalation.   H & E

leads to cystic distension by mucus and then to atrophy of the glands.

Trachea

Induced tracheal lesions are listed in Table 2.3.

Induced changes are less frequently found in the

Table 2.3   Induced lesions of the trachea

Epithelial hyperplasia
Epithelial squamous metaplasia
Epithelial ulceration
Submucosal gland hypertrophy

tracheal epithelium than in either the nasal chambers or the larynx, but hyperplastic and squamous metaplastic changes do occur. An unusual feature sometimes observed with squamous metaplasia of the tracheal epithelium is the apparent incorporation of capillaries into the epithelium. However, observations from 1 μm plastic sections (Figure 2.28) and at the ultrastructural level in our laboratory, have established that the capillaries, although surrounded by epithelial cells, remain outside the epithelial basement membrane. The appearance is in fact due to tortuous epithelial folding.

Squamous metaplasia, suppurative inflammation and submucosal fibrosis are detected in mice exposed to formaldehyde[13]. In some cases fibrous bands project into the tracheal lumen, show neovascularization and are covered by altered respiratory epithelium. Cellular atypia may also be detected.

Exposure of guinea pigs to toluene diisocyanate causes the development of cyst-like structures within ciliated cells[18]. The electron microscope shows these cysts contain cilia. Another unusual change was recorded in our laboratory in dogs exposed to a novel mucolytic. In these animals, light microscopy showed that extensive areas of the respiratory airways were denuded of cilia. Ultrastructurally, the ciliated cells were found to contain shortened cilia which appeared to have been 'clipped off'. The limiting ciliary membrane was intact over the foreshortened tip.

Following erosive or ulcerative changes, the tracheal epithelium may be composed solely of a single layer of regenerative cuboidal or elongated spindle-shaped epithelial cells. A hyperplastic non-ciliated epithelium then develops (Figures 2.29 and 2.30) and nuclear atypia and pleomorphism may be detected.

Changes in submucosal glands are difficult to assess in rats as normally such glands are sparse in the trachea and completely absent in bronchioles. This means that the rat is of limited value in the assessment of bronchitis-like conditions and other animal species are more suitable. However, the electron microscope detects features suggestive of hyperactivity and hypersecretion in submucosal glands of rats exposed to tobacco smoke for up to 2 years[19].

When sectioned longitudinally (as a 'Y' shape), the tracheal bifurcation is another site at which epithelial changes may be detected. The reaction usually involves a mild hyperplasia, but squamous metaplasia (Figure 2.31) may also occur. The lesions are often confined to the 'tip' of the carina, an obvious point of impaction of inhaled materials.

Bronchi and Bronchioles

A summary of induced bronchial/bronchiolar lesions is given in Table 2.4.

Table 2.4   Induced lesions of the bronchi and bronchioles

Bronchi and bronchioles
  Goblet cell proliferation
  Epithelial single cell degeneration
  Epithelial hyperplasia
  Epithelial squamous metaplasia
  Epithelial ulceration
  Bronchiolitis obliterans
  Neuroepithelial cell proliferation

Terminal bronchioles
  Epithelial atrophy
  Epithelial hyperplasia
  Epithelial necrosis

Mild irritation of the bronchioles, as with tobacco smoke and SO_2, results in changes in the mucin-secreting cells of the bronchiolar epithelium. In untreated Specific Pathogen Free barrier maintained rats, these mucin cells are predominantly of a serous type and stain red with combined Alcian Blue/PAS stain. Mucin-secreting cells are only rarely encountered in terminal bronchioles. Following exposure to irritant compounds such as SO_2 and cigarette smoke, goblet cells replace the serous cells and the tinctorial properties of the mucin change, becoming predominantly blue with Alcian Blue/ PAS. The cells also become enlarged, typically 'goblet' shaped and the epithelium appears hypertrophic. In addition, mucin-secreting cells extend into the terminal bronchioles where they replace Clara cells[20]. Changes in the number of goblet cells in bronchiolar epithelium are also reported following systemic injections of isoprenaline and pilocarpine to rats[21]. Isoprenaline causes the extension of goblet cells into terminal bronchioles, but salbutamol, which acts on β_2 receptors has no effect[22].

In comparison with the larynx, bronchiolar degenerative, hyperplastic (Figure 2.32) and metaplastic epithelial changes are found only in cases of more irritant compounds. In one instance an inhaled industrial chemical induced single-cell degeneration of the mouse bronchiolar epithelium (Figure 2.33).

In cases of inhalation of highly irritant compounds or by intratracheal instillation of substances such as crocidolite, bronchiolar epithelial ulceration and marked intraluminal fibrinous inflammatory exudation (Figure 2.34) may be seen[23]. The exudate becomes organized with infiltration of fibroblasts (Figure 2.35) and leads to variable degrees of bronchiolitis obliterans. Within the fibrous tissue, focal epithelial proliferations develop which form isolated ducts of undifferentiated cells (Figures 2.36 and 2.37). These may represent attempts at 're-canalization' (Figure 2.37). When complete or partial blockage occurs in bronchioles, mucus stasis and accumulation may occur distally. In severe cases this bronchiolar mucus may 'back flow' into peribronchiolar alveoli (Figure 2.38).

Alteration of the morphology of the Clara cells of the terminal bronchioles is a relatively common finding in inhalation toxicity studies. The characteristic apical 'bleb' is absent from these cells and they usually appear more basophilic (Figure 2.39). This appearance may represent either an atrophic or a regenerative change. The Clara cell is known to respond to injury by regression[24] and is also the progenitor cell of the terminal bronchioles. The terminal bronchioles are the main target of ozone and NO_2 which at high dose levels may cause complete necrosis[25]. Necrosis of Clara cells is also reported with carbon tetrachloride[26], and epithelial cytomegaly and metaplasia are observed in mice following 1,2-dibromo-

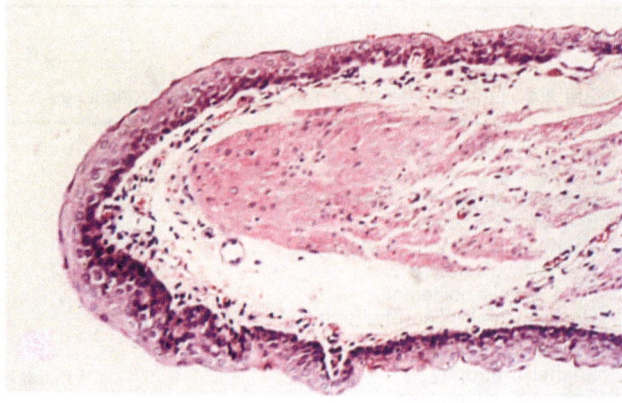

Figure 2.31 A longitudinal section taken through the tracheal bifurcation of a rat exposed to tobacco smoke, showing squamous metaplasia. The tip of the carina is a predilection site for induced changes in inhalation studies. In many cases the lesions are more focal and restricted to the tip of the carina, than in the example shown. H & E

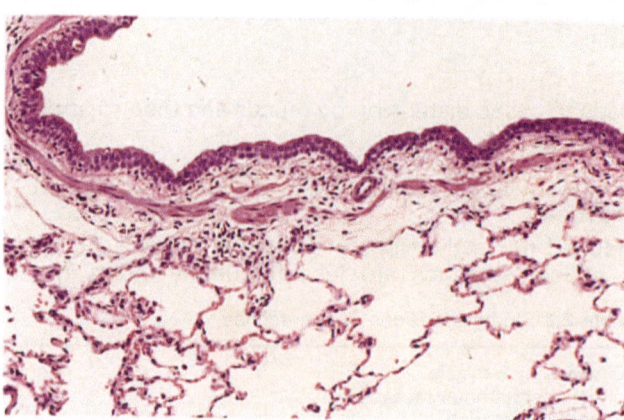

Figure 2.32 The epithelium of a major bronchiole in the rat is normally cuboidal/columnar with ciliated and serous cells. In this photomicrograph, epithelial hyperplasia with slight basophilia is shown. This developed following exposure to an inhaled industrial chemical. H & E

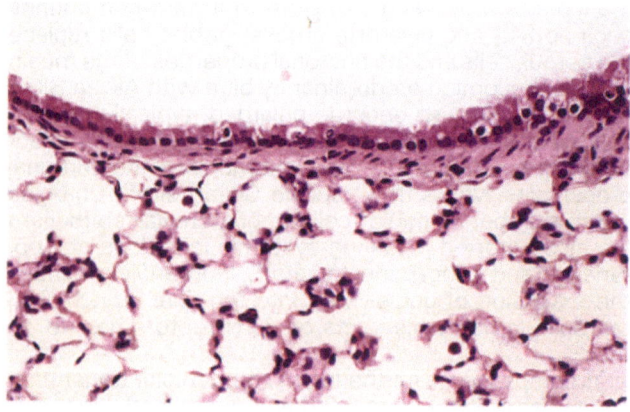

Figure 2.33 Single cell degeneration in a bronchiole of a mouse following smoke exposure. The degenerate cells appear shrunken with pyknotic nuclei. H & E

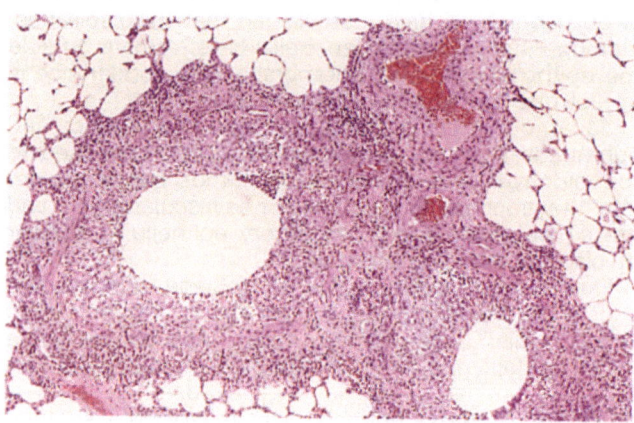

Figure 2.34 Transverse section through a bronchiole. This and the three following figures demonstrate the development of bronchiolitis obliterans in the rat following inhalation of an industrial chemical. Initially, as shown in this photomicrograph, ulceration of the bronchiolar epithelium occurs and an inflammatory exudate partially obscures the bronchiolar lumen. H & E

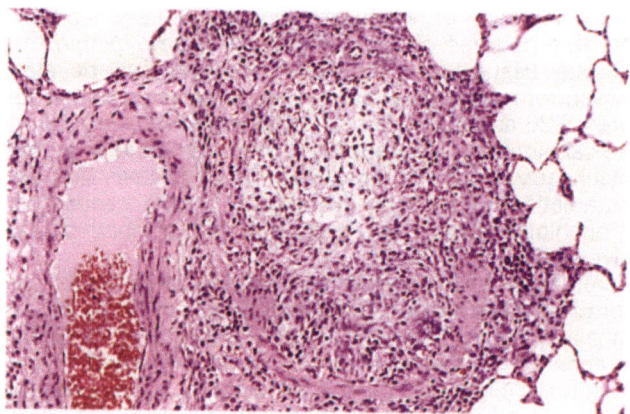

Figure 2.35 Transverse section through a bronchiole. The intraluminal inflammatory exudate begins to organize with fibroblast infiltration. The bronchiolar lumen is completely obliterated. H & E

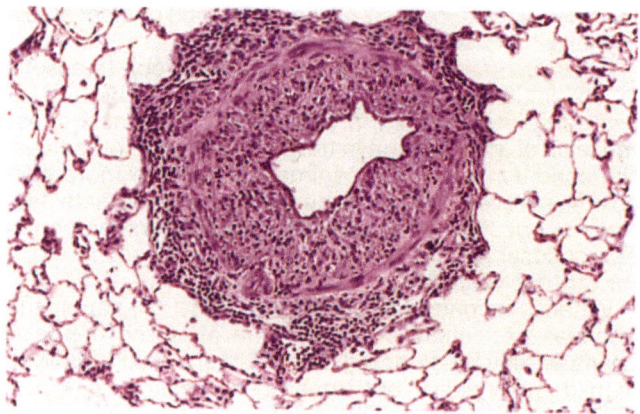

Figure 2.36 Transverse section through a bronchiole. A narrow lumen is lined by undifferentiated epithelial cells. The size of the original bronchiole may be assessed by reference to the position of the circular muscle layer. H & E

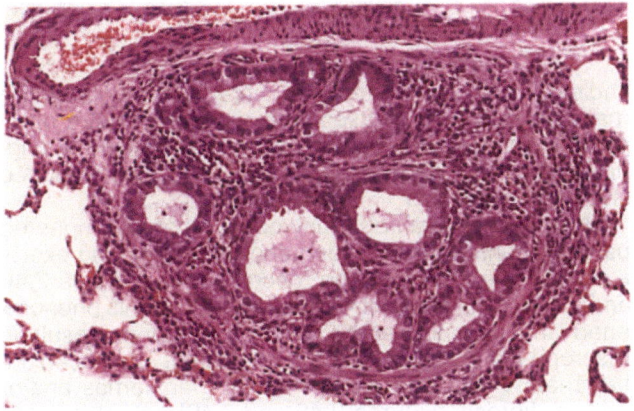

Figure 2.37 Transverse section through a bronchiole. In this example, the bronchiole contains several newly formed narrow lumina lined by cubiodal epithelial cells. Fibrous tissue remains between the epithelial channels. The size of the original bronchiole may again be assessed by the position of the band of circular muscle. H & E

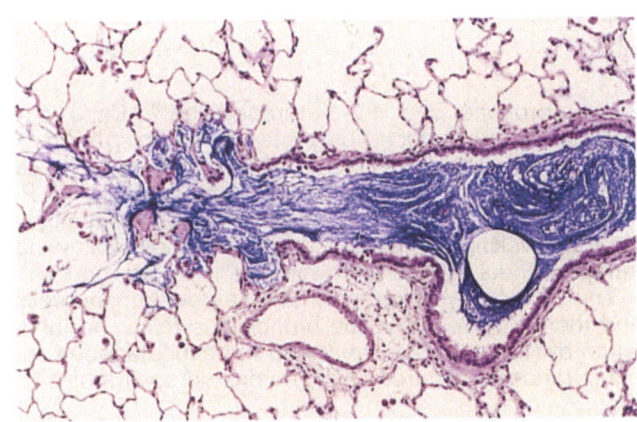

Figure 2.38 Terminal bronchiole of a rat, peripheral to induced bronchiolitis obliterans. Mucus has consequently accumulated in the lower regions of the bronchiolar tree with local extension into the alveoli where it has induced a mild inflammatory reaction. The staining of the mucus with Alcian Blue, in this SPF rat, demonstrates a change from the normal serous type (which stains preferentially with PAS), and indicates exposure to an irritant or infectious agent. Alcian Blue–PAS

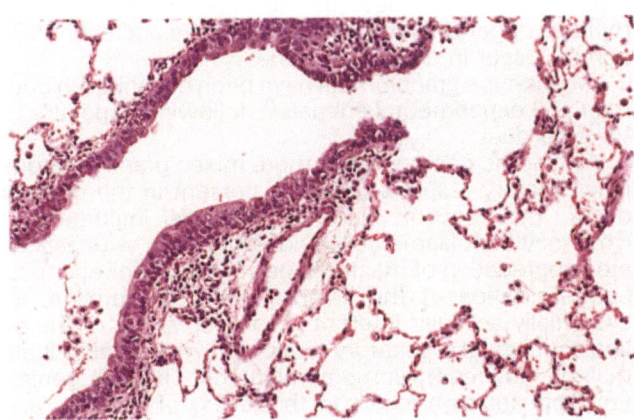

Figure 2.39 Terminal bronchiole from a rat treated with an industrial chemical by inhalation. The epithelium at this site is normally composed of cuboidal ciliated and Clara cells, which have characteristic apical projections. In this example the epithelium is slightly increased in height and basophilic, with complete loss of typical Clara cells. H & E

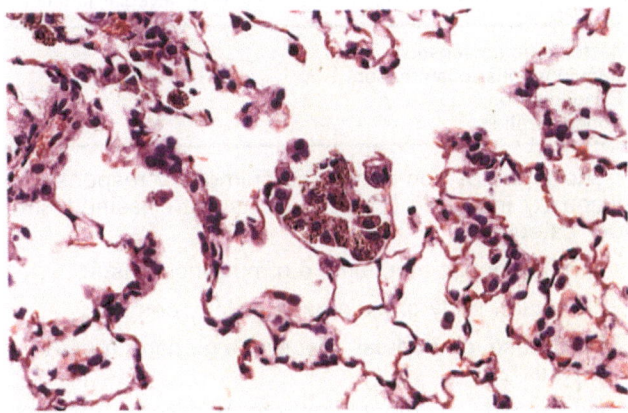

Figure 2.40 Alveolar macrophages in rat lung containing ingested brown particles following inhalation of a dust. No evidence of degenerative changes either in the macrophages or alveolar walls. H & E

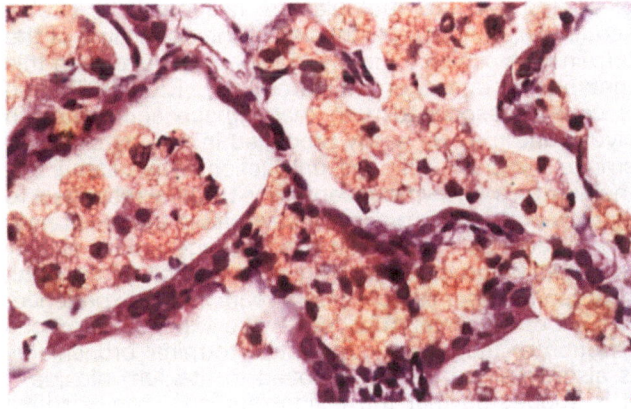

Figure 2.41 Aggregation of 'golden-brown' macrophages in lung of rat exposed to tobacco smoke. In one area the macrophages fill an alveolar space. Adjacent alveolar walls are thickened and focally lined by cuboidal cells (Type II pneumonocytes). H & E

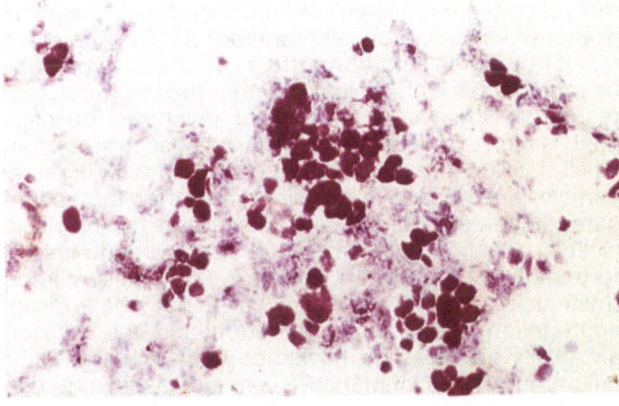

Figure 2.42 Prominent lysosomal enzyme activity in macrophages from the lung of a rat exposed to tobacco smoke. Acid phosphatase

3-chloropropane and 1,2-dibromoethane[12]. Clara cell necrosis is also induced by systemic administration of some furans. The mechanism for this toxicity is believed to be due to bioactivation by Clara cell cytochrome P-450[4]. A similar mechanism is thought to be responsible for the swelling and exfoliation of Clara cells following intraperitoneal injection of naphthalene in the mouse[27].

The pulmonary airways contain neuroendocrine cells and these proliferate in the bronchioles following inhalation of NO_2 and asbestos[28] and the subcutaneous administration of N-nitroso-bis-(2-hydroxypropyl) amine[29].

Bronchiolar–alveolar junction

This region is also a common site of reaction to inhaled insults. Anatomically it includes the junctions of the terminal bronchioles, respiratory bronchioles, alveolar ducts and adjacent alveoli. The lesions which may be encountered therefore reflect both airway and alveolar characteristics. A summary of induced lesions is given in Table 2.5.

Table 2.5 Induced lesions of the bronchiolar–alveolar junction

Macrophage aggregation
Granulomatous inflammation
Collagenization
Bronchiolization

The types of non-neoplastic pulmonary response induced by inorganic (mineral) dusts are classified[2] into four categories:

(i) macrophage reactions, e.g. nuisance dusts;

(ii) foreign body granuloma, e.g. talc, cement;

(iii) diffuse or nodular fibrosis, e.g. hard metals or quartz;

(iv) sarcoid-type granuloma, e.g. beryllium, Bakelite.

Although these reactions may be found throughout the lung parenchyma, they are most frequently found at the bronchio-alveolar junction and for the purpose of this review will be described here.

Increased numbers of alveolar macrophages are probably the most common reaction to inhaled materials. In terms of pulmonary response there are no 'inert' dusts[2]; inhaled particles are inevitably detectable within alveolar macrophages (Figure 2.40). We have observed this minimal response with so-called 'nuisance dusts'[2], such as plaster of Paris, photocopier toners and PVC. They rarely result in adverse long-term effects, and should probably be regarded as a physiological rather than a pathological response. However, if the level of an inhaled 'nuisance dust' is high or if substances such as tobacco smoke are inhaled, macrophages become engorged with ingested particles and lysosomal inclusions, and often form aggregates (Figures 2.41 and 2.42), usually at the bronchio-alveolar junction. With more reactive compounds the formation of granulomata (Figure 2.43), with or without multinucleate giant cells may occur. In both macrophage aggregation and granulomata formation the adjacent alveolar walls become thickened with mild interstitial inflammatory cell infiltration; slight increases in demonstrable reticulin and collagen fibres; and focal epithelialization (Type II pneumonocyte proliferation).

Aggregates of alveolar macrophages sometimes show cholesterol clefts and may form cholesterol granulomas. These are reported in rats following exposure to titanium dioxide[30]. They are also reported in rats exposed to shale dust, but are not found in monkeys when exposed to the same concentration. We have observed cholesterol clefts in rats associated with aggregated macrophages from studies with several different compounds and conditions, including tobacco smoke (Figures 2.44 and 2.45), phospholipidosis and quartz-induced alveolar proteinosis.

More severe reactions may occur when the ingested particles cannot be degraded and the compound exerts a direct toxic effect on the macrophages (Figures 2.46 and 2.47). Silica is a well known example of this phenomenon and this and some other compounds result in macrophage degeneration[2], consequent enhanced inflammatory reaction and ultimately granulomas and/or nodular fibrosis (Figures 2.48 and 2.49).

In prolonged inhalation studies involving exposures to relatively high concentrations of dusts such as quartz, dust-containing macrophages are often found in the peribronchiolar lymphoid aggregates (BALT) and also in the regional (hilar or bronchial) lymph nodes. A similar reaction is found with tobacco smoke exposure in which golden-brown pigmentation of alveolar macrophages occurs. Pigmented macrophages are often abundant in the bronchial lymph nodes. In the case of quartz, macrophage degeneration, granulation tissue and eventually fibrosis occur in the lymph nodes.

Sarcoid-type granulomata have been described in both man and experimental animals[31], following exposure to Bakelite dust.

With some compounds a more mixed granulomatous inflammatory response may be present in the alveolar ducts. This reaction involves interstitial infiltration of lymphocytes, plasma cells and neutrophils with associated aggregation of macrophages in the alveoli and focal epithelialization of the alveolar walls. In addition, an essentially acellular interstitial collagenization of the alveolar duct and respiratory bronchiole walls (Figure 2.50) may be induced by some compounds. This collagenization appears as a localized thickening of the wall and persists after cessation of exposure. In contrast to this acellular collagenization, active fibrosis occurs in this region either in association with foreign body reactions or following inhalation of highly toxic compounds or irritant particles. This will be discussed later, with reference to lung parenchymal changes.

At the bronchio-alveolar junction the walls of the respiratory bronchioles, alveolar ducts and adjacent alveoli may become lined by cuboidal ciliated cells (Figures 2.51 and 2.52). This change is termed bronchiolization[32] or ciliated cuboidal metaplasia[33]. It appears to involve sequential, peripheral extension of the epithelium of the terminal bronchioles. Rarely, goblet cells develop in this metaplastic epithelium (Figure 2.53). Bronchiolization is usually associated with macrophage aggregates in alveoli and may be easily produced in rats by cigarette smoke (Figure 2.54). The production of a ciliated epithelium at a known susceptible site as a response to injury is perhaps surprising. Elsewhere in the respiratory tract ciliated cells are sensitive to damage and are quickly replaced, whereas in these areas of metaplastic bronchiolization they persist for up to 2 years, in our experience, in spite of continued tobacco smoke exposure. Bronchiolization of the alveoli adjacent to terminal bronchioles is also detected in rats exposed to titanium dioxide[30]. It is suggested that the lesion represents an adaptive response to dust exposure by which the mucociliary escalator extends into the alveoli in an attempt to facilitate increased particulate removal.

Lung parenchyma

The lung parenchyma manifests one of the most diverse ranges of induced histopathological lesions of all organ

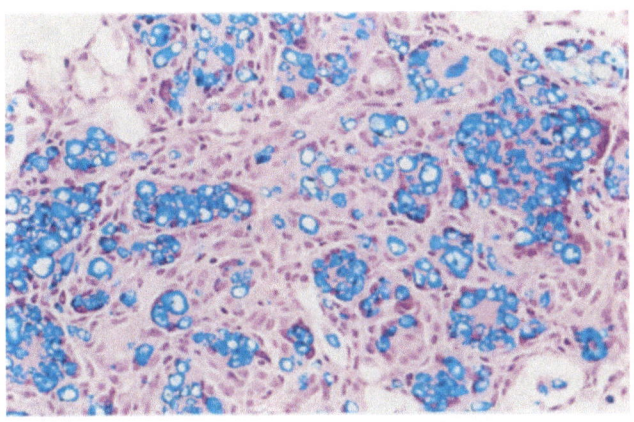

Figure 2.43 Lung of a rat exposed to coloured particulate dust by inhalation. The blue dust particles have been ingested by macrophages with subsequent development of a granuloma. The blue coloration has been preserved during routine histological processing.   H & E

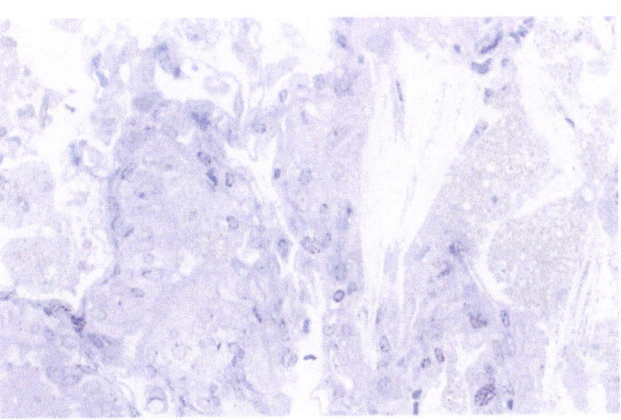

Figure 2.44 Cholesterol clefts associated with pigmented alveolar macrophages from the lung of a rat exposed to tobacco smoke. An area of alveolar bronchiolization is also present. 1 µm resin section. Toluidine Blue

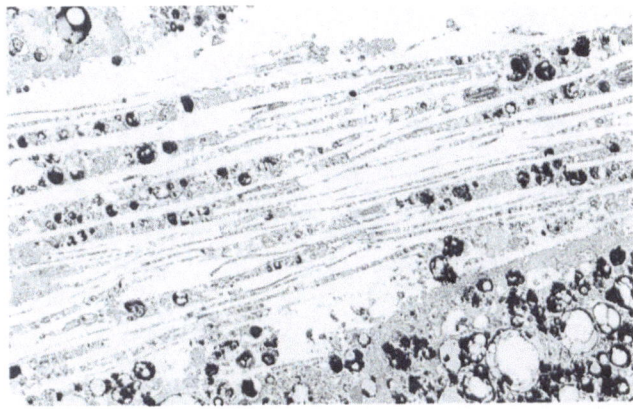

Figure 2.45 Cholesterol clefts, in a rat lung from the same study as Figure 2.44, appear as thin elongate areas distorting the cell debris and multilamellar bodies in the alveolar lumen. Adjacent alveolar macrophages contain heterogeneous inclusions typical of tobacco smoke exposure. Electron micrograph

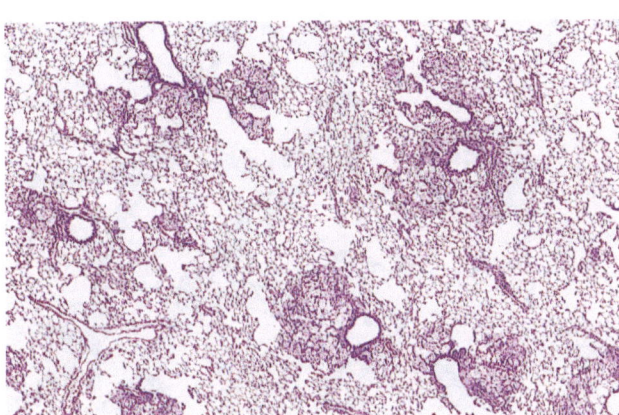

Figure 2.46 Rat lung showing typical distribution of lesions encountered in inhalation studies. Large aggregates of macrophages located around terminal bronchioles. Some of the aggregated macrophages appear pale and are degenerate.   H & E

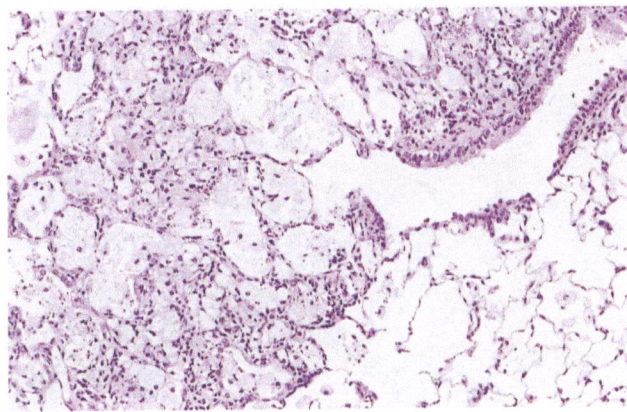

Figure 2.47 Similar macrophage aggregate to those shown in Figure 2.46. In this case, the inhaled substance has clearly induced macrophage degeneration and an associated inflammatory cell infiltration.   H & E

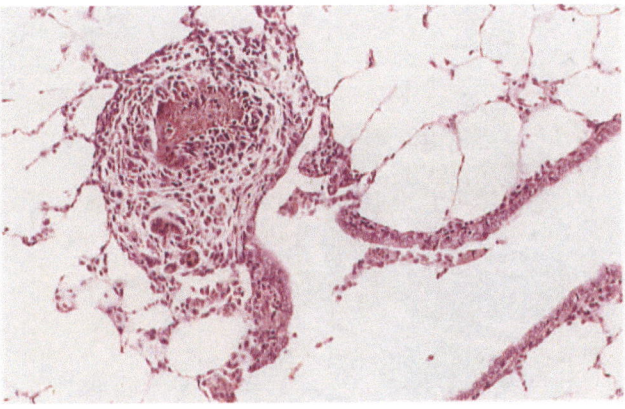

Figure 2.48 Granuloma in the alveolar duct of a rat following intratracheal administration of particulate material. A large deposit is present in the centre of the granuloma.   H & E

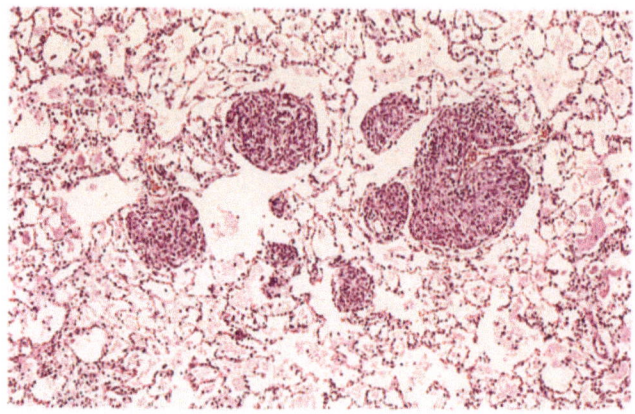

Figure 2.49 Granulomatous lesions in a rat lung following inhalation of quartz particles. H & E

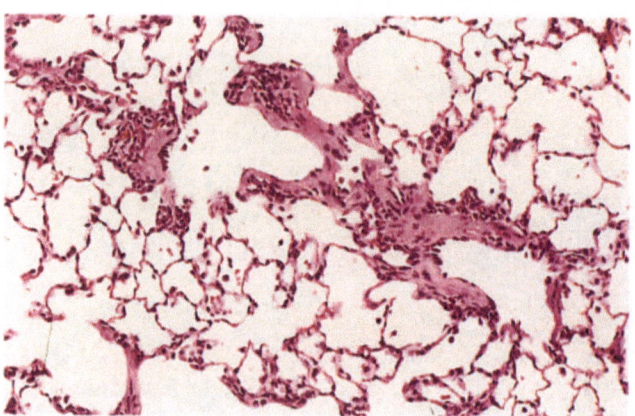

Figure 2.50 Focal interstitial collagen deposition in the walls of alveolar ducts of a rat following inhalation of an industrial chemical. The lesion is generally devoid of fibroblasts. H & E

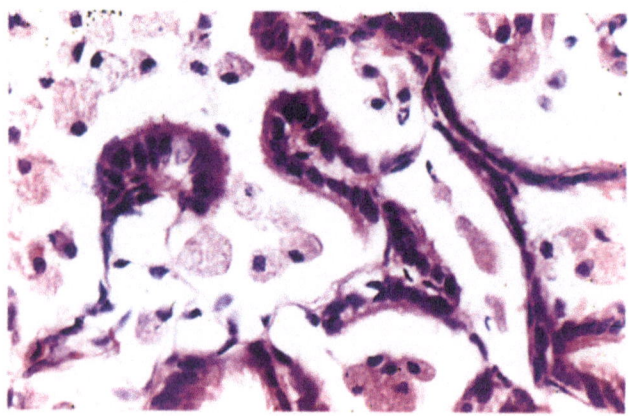

Figure 2.51 Focal bronchiolization of alveolar walls from a rat exposed to tobacco smoke. The alveolar walls are lined by ciliated cells. H & E

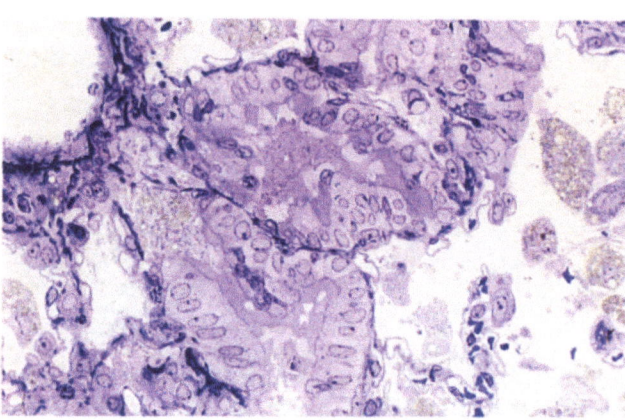

Figure 2.52 Bronchiolization (cuboidal ciliated metaplasia) of alveolar walls adjacent to a terminal bronchiole. This lesion involves the sequential extension of the bronchiolar epithelial cells into the alveolar ducts and alveoli where they replace the normal epithelial cells. This example is from a rat exposed to tobacco smoke, hence the characteristic pigmented macrophages. 1 μm resin section. Toluidine Blue

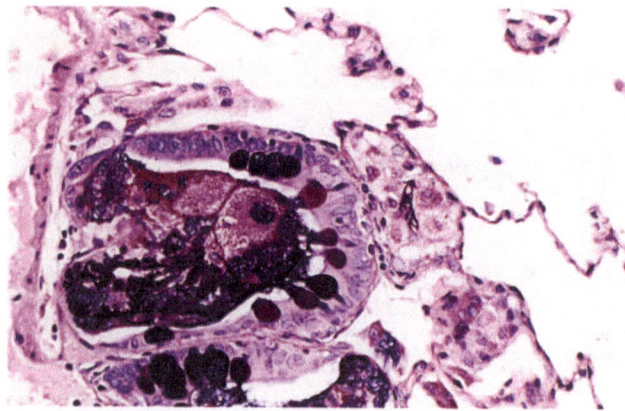

Figure 2.53 Bronchiolization of alveolar walls in the rat. This lesion, in contrast to previous and subsequent figures, involves goblet cells. The latter discharge mucus into the alveoli and provoke a macrophage reaction. Alcian Blue–PAS

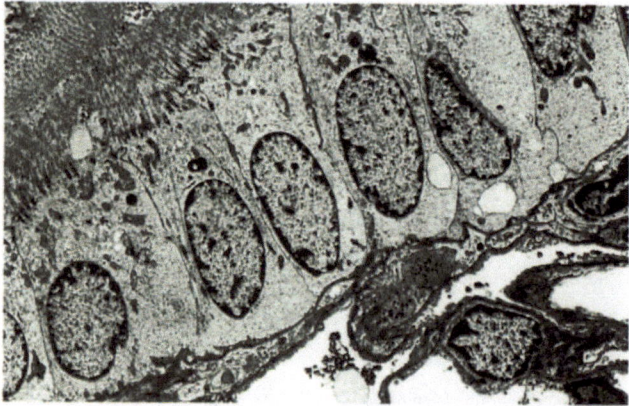

Figure 2.54 Alveolar bronchiolization showing ciliated epithelial cells lining one side of an alveolar wall, from a rat exposed to tobacco smoke. The cells are ultrastructurally indistinguishable from ciliated cells of the bronchiolar epithelium. Electron micrograph

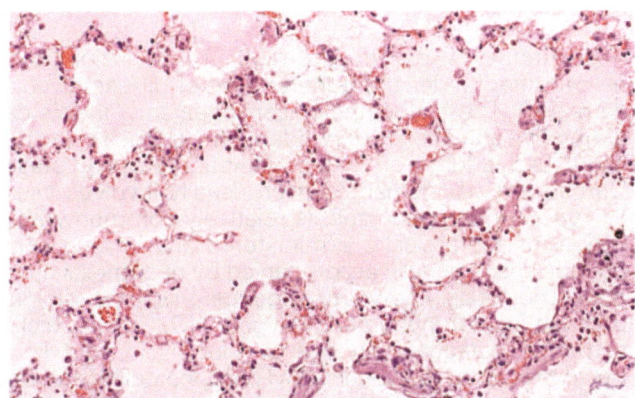

Figure 2.55 Pulmonary oedema in a rat from an acute inhalation study. The alveoli are filled with weakly eosinophilic material. The alveolar wall capillaries appear dilated. A slight inflammatory reaction is present but little evidence of degenerative change is detected.   H & E

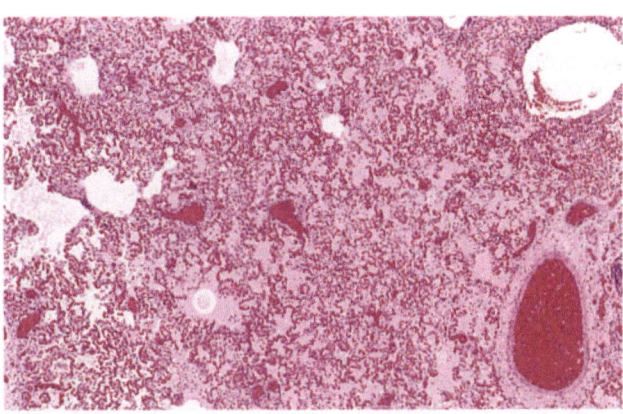

Figure 2.56 Pulmonary oedema in a rat from an acute inhalation study. In this case the lesion is associated with a pronounced inflammatory reaction and congestion.   H & E

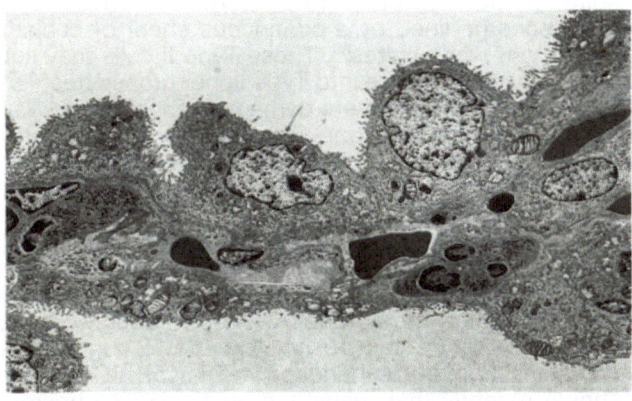

Figure 2.57 Epithelialization of the alveolar walls in a dog following systemic administration of an agrochemical product. The alveoli are lined by continuous cuboidal Type II pneumonocytes which contain characteristic multilamellar bodies. Electron micrograph

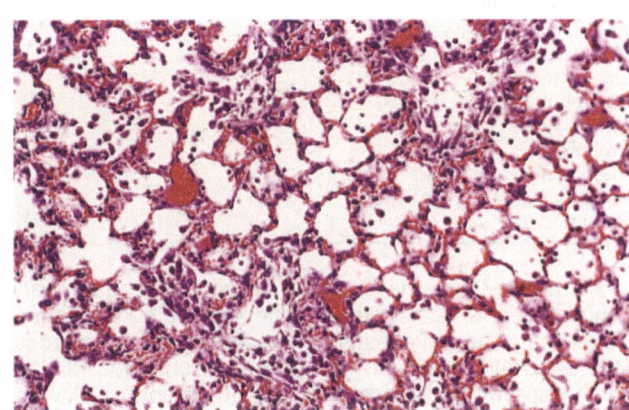

Figure 2.58 Rat lung from an acute inhalation study with an industrial chemical showing congestion, inflammation, alveolar wall degeneration and focal fibroblast proliferation.   H & E

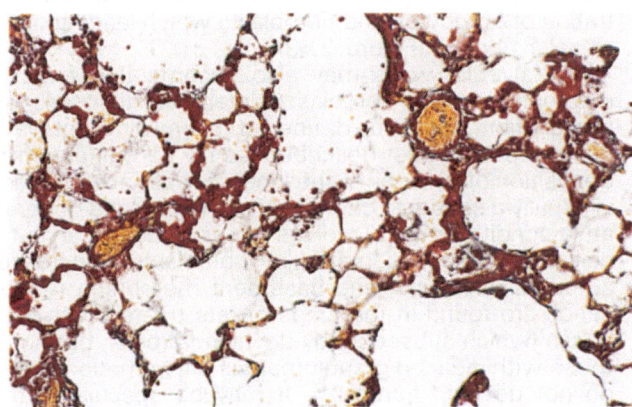

Figure 2.59 A similar study to Figure 2.58. Rat lung with fibrin deposition in alveolar walls, associated with inflammatory cell infiltration. Martius Scarlet Blue

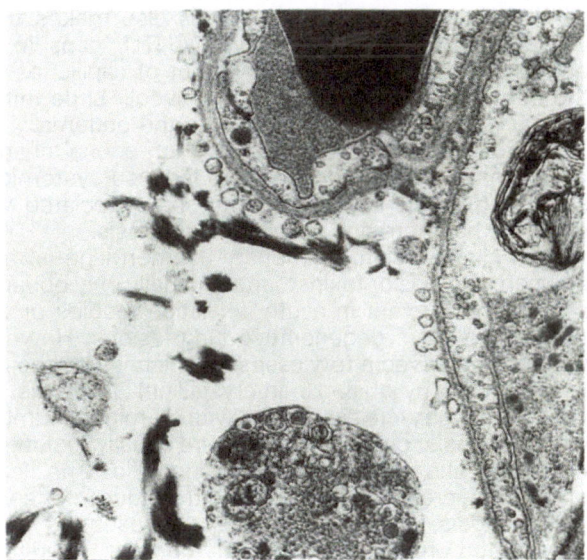

Figure 2.60 Lung from a dog treated with paraquat. The Type I pneumonocytes of the alveolar wall are lost exposing the basal lamina. The alveolar lumen contains cell debris and fibrin. The endothelial cells of the alveolar capillaries appear oedematous. Electron micrograph

systems (Table 2.6). In addition, the histological features are often complicated by the simultaneous presence of multiple lesions. Following acute damage by agents such as paraquat, for example, admixed degeneration, epithelialization (repair) and early fibrosis may all appear. Similarly, following administration of quartz, macrophage infiltration, macrophage necrosis, lipoproteinosis, granuloma formation and nodular fibrosis may all be identified concurrently. Thus, the overall histological picture may be potentially confusing unless a thorough understanding and identification of each component lesion is possible. Lesions are described individually, in the following text, but whenever possible reference is made to progression or regression and to involvement in more complex reactions.

Table 2.6 Induced lesions of the lung parenchyma

Pulmonary oedema
Pulmonary congestion
Alveolar haemorrhage
Diffuse alveolar damage
Interstitial fibrosis
Intra-alveolar fibrosis
Alveolar epithelialization
Alveolar adenomatous hyperplasia
Lipoproteinosis
Phospholipidosis
Emphysema
Embolism
Interstitial histiocytosis
Aspiration pneumonia
Pneumonitis

Pulmonary oedema (Figure 2.55) is produced by many drugs and chemicals, but is often associated with more severe degenerative lesions. However, it may also occur in the virtual absence of degenerative changes, e.g. by the intraperitoneal injection of α-napthylthiourea (ANTU), subcutaneous adrenaline, or with ethylchlorvynol[4,25,34]. The microscopic detection of slight pulmonary oedema is sometimes difficult in preparations from lungs fixed by intratracheal instillation. This instillation may displace and dilute or even completely obscure the oedema fluids[34]. Methods of avoiding this problem involve either fixation by vascular perfusion or by vapour fixation. The most important factor in the development of oedema is capillary damage. The endothelial cells represent the first target for toxic agents in the blood and their close proximity to the alveolar air spaces also makes them vulnerable from this route. With ANTU, gaps in the endothelium allow fluids to pass out of capillaries into the interstitium and then into the alveoli. Little inflammatory response is associated with the oedema[4].

Pulmonary congestion is a common agonal change, which may be seen secondary to induced systemic lesions, e.g. heart failure, and may be associated with oedema, haemorrhage and haemosiderosis.

As a single lesion, pulmonary haemorrhage is rarely induced by drugs or toxins[35] and is usually only observed as a terminal event in acute inhalation studies or with the more severe degenerative lung lesions. However, we have observed a few cases in which it was the only lesion caused by inhaled (non-crystalline) chemicals. The haemorrhages were associated with prominent numbers of intra-alveolar crystals. These were usually rectangular or needle-like and strongly eosinophilic. The lesion showed macrophage infiltration with evidence of crystal phagocytosis. No haemosiderin was present.

As noted previously, pulmonary oedema, congestion and haemorrhage may be associated with more severe

degenerative lesions (Figure 2.56). These lesions may be classified under the general term of diffuse alveolar damage[35]. The histopathological appearance in this degenerative condition is dependent on the time scale after injury, and is followed by a proliferation or repair stage. Diffuse alveolar damage, which usually involves injury to Type I pneumonocytes, is relatively common with a variety of systemically administered and inhaled compounds and is usually accompanied by endothelial changes. Chemicals known to produce this type of lung damage include hyperbaric oxygen. NO_2, ozone, nickel carbonyl, paraquat, phosgene, bleomycin, butylated hydroxytoluene, O,O,S-trimethyl-phosphorodithioate, and cyclophosphamide[4,25,36,37]. Diffuse alveolar damage is also induced in dogs and baboons by the intra-vascular administration of oleic acid[38]. Free fatty acids are known to be toxic to pulmonary cells and lead to rupture of the alveolar–capillary wall. In addition they inhibit surfactant activity which causes alveolar collapse. Oral administration of trialkylphosphorothioate to rats also causes a form of diffuse alveolar damage[39].

If the basement membrane remains intact following the initial damage to the alveolar walls then a period of epithelialization occurs (Figure 2.57) in which the alveolar walls become lined by a continuous sheet of cuboidal Type II pneumonocytes[36]. These Type II cells may subsequently differentiate into Type I pneumonocytes[4,25,36].

In cases of more severe damage to the alveolar walls the basement membrane is disrupted and exudation from the capillaries occurs producing an inflammatory reaction (Figure 2.58). Fibrin deposition may occur focally in the alveolar walls (Figure 2.59). The alveoli become filled with inflammatory cells, cell debris, macrophages and fibrin (Figure 2.60). This material may become oriented along the walls of the alveoli and alveolar ducts forming hyaline membranes[40]. These strongly eosinophilic membranes stain positively with PAS (Figure 2.61) and, variably in our experience, with MSB. It has been shown recently that respiratory epithelial cell necrosis is the initial lesion in the development of hyaline membranes[40]. This finding may explain the often weak MSB staining of hyaline membranes which were previously considered to be predominantly composed of fibrin. In time the hyaline membranes fragment, become displaced from the alveolar wall and may be phagocytosed by macrophages. These fragments appear as deeply eosinophilic material. The intra-alveolar fibrinous exudate may become organized (Figure 2.62), with the infiltration of fibrocytes and fibroblasts which leads to intra-alveolar fibrosis (Figure 2.63).

The alveolar walls may also become thickened by macrophages and fibroblasts (interstitial fibrosis). Pulmonary fibrosis may be defined in several different ways, but is probably best described simply as the 'abnormal deposition of collagen in the lungs'[41]. Pulmonary fibrosis is usually a sequel to chronic inflammatory and degenerative conditions, and involves the secretion of an extracellular collagenous matrix by fibroblasts[42]. Increased amounts of laminin and basement membrane reduplication are found in the lungs of rats treated with bleomycin (which subsequently develop fibrosis), but not of those with induced granulomatous inflammation (which do not develop fibrosis)[42]. It may be speculated that abnormal basement membrane accumulation plays a role in the development of pulmonary interstitial fibrosis[42].

The time scale and success of Type II pneumonocyte proliferation following alveolar damage is believed to be critical in determining the development of pulmonary fibrosis[41]. This may be demonstrated experimentally in

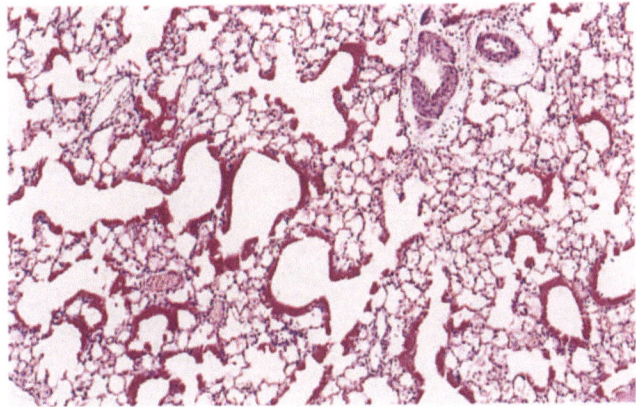

Figure 2.61 Hyaline membranes in a rat lung. Such changes may be found in acute inhalation studies. These structures appear eosinophilic in H & E sections, they line damaged alveolar walls and stain strongly with PAS

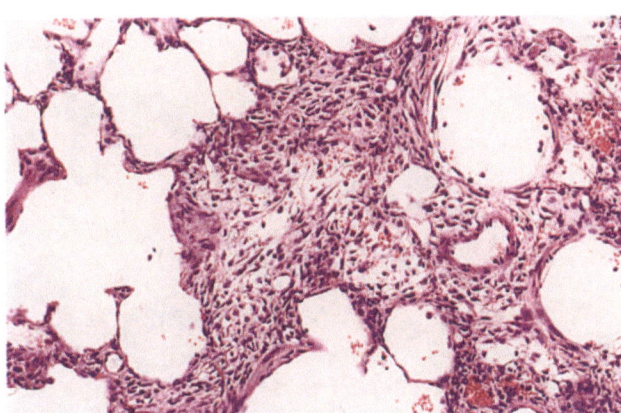

Figure 2.62 Severe diffuse alveolar damage in the lung of a rat after inhalation of an industrial chemical. The intra-alveolar exudate becomes organized with the infiltration of fibroblasts. These cells are usually loosely arranged and although often appearing active little demonstrable collagen is laid down. H & E

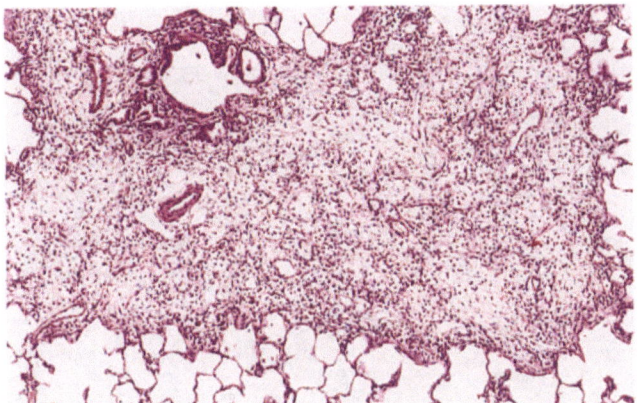

Figure 2.63 Alveolar fibrosis in the lung of a rat following inhalation of an industrial chemical. A large area of the parenchyma is replaced by loosely arranged fibroblasts and inflammatory cells. H & E

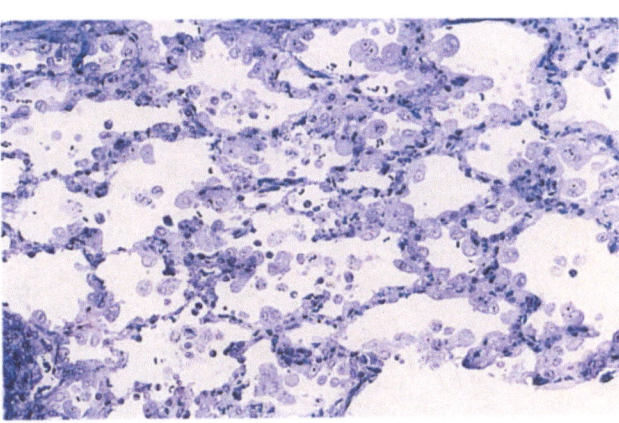

Figure 2.64 Lung from a dog treated with paraquat. Following initial diffuse alveolar damage, the repair process in this case involves proliferation of Type II pneumonocytes. The alveolar epithelialization is often bizarre and the new hypertrophic Type II cells project bulbously into the alveoli. 1 μm resin section. Toluidine Blue

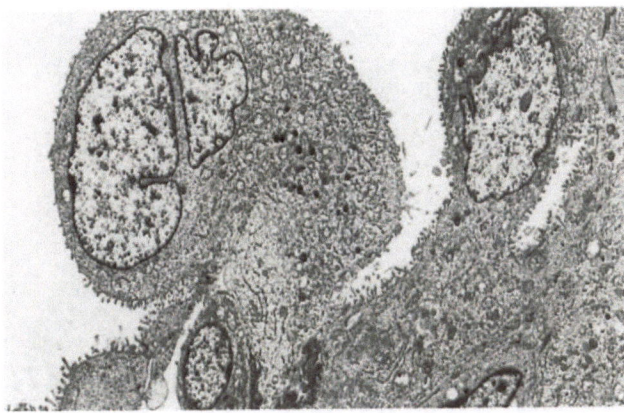

Figure 2.65 Electron micrograph of Type II pneumonocytes from the same animal as Figure 2.64. The thickened alveolar wall is lined by hypertrophic cells which appear primitive, with few recognizable organelles. Electron micrograph

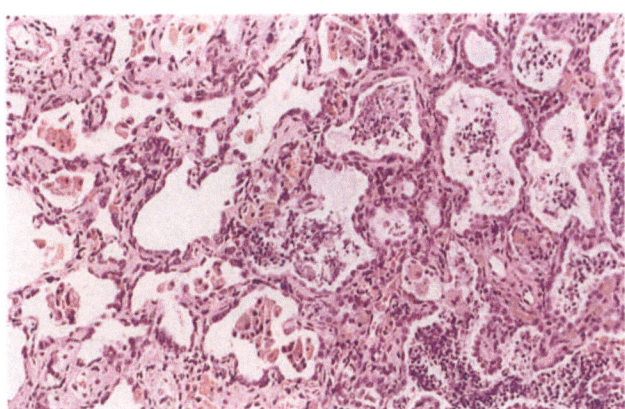

Figure 2.66 Adenomatous hyperplasia in the lung parenchyma from a rat following chronic treatment with a plant extract by dietary administration. The alveolar walls are lined by cuboidal cells imparting an adenomatous pattern. The macrophages contain brown pigment presumably a metabolic product of the test compound. H & E

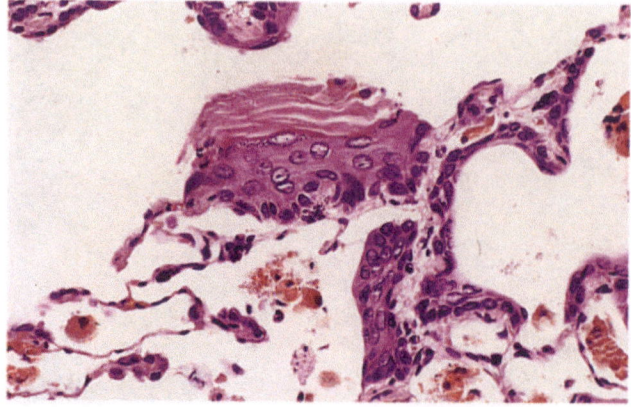

Figure 2.67 Squamous metaplasia of an alveolar wall from a rat. In this case (from the same study as Figure 2.66) a small nest of squamous cells with superficial keratinization has developed on an alveolar wall. Some alveolar walls show epithelialization. In this study the epithelialization developed in the absence of initial diffuse alveolar damage.   H & E

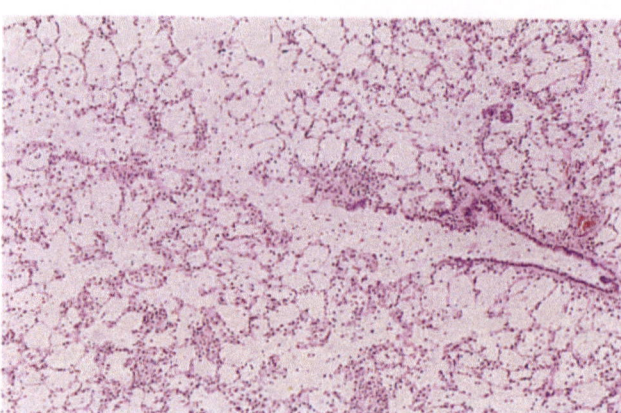

Figure 2.68 Alveolar lipoproteinosis induced in a rat by inhalation of quartz. The alveoli are filled with an amorphous, weakly eosinophilic material with increased numbers of macrophages and focal thickening of the alveolar walls.   H & E

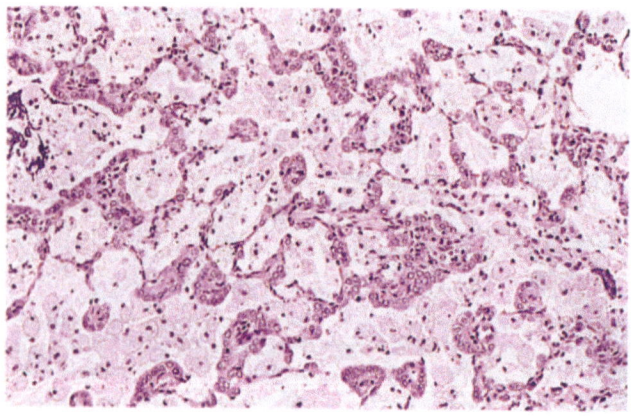

Figure 2.69 Higher magnification of lesion shown in Figure 2.68. The alveolar macrophages are swollen with a slight foamy appearance. The alveolar walls are thickened by proliferation of Type II pneumonocytes.   H & E

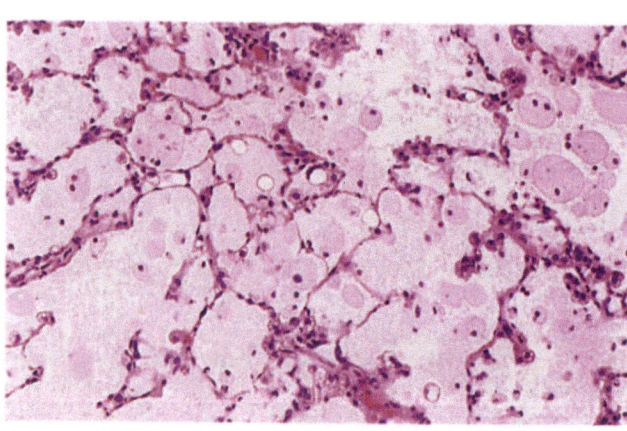

Figure 2.70 Pulmonary phospholipidosis induced in the rat by systemic administration of a cationic amphiphilic compound. The lesion is characterized by eosinophilic intra-alveolar material. Foamy macrophages and focal hypertrophy and proliferation of Type II pneumonocytes. A few Type II cells contain single large vacuoles.   H & E

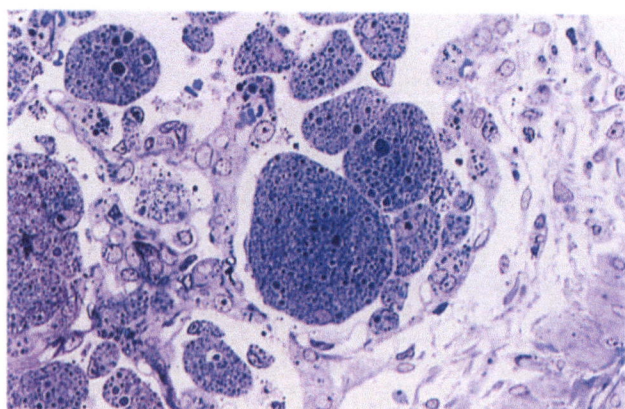

Figure 2.71 Alveolar macrophages from a rat with induced phospholipidosis. These phagocytic cells are distended with tightly packed, round inclusions. 1 µm section. Toluidine Blue

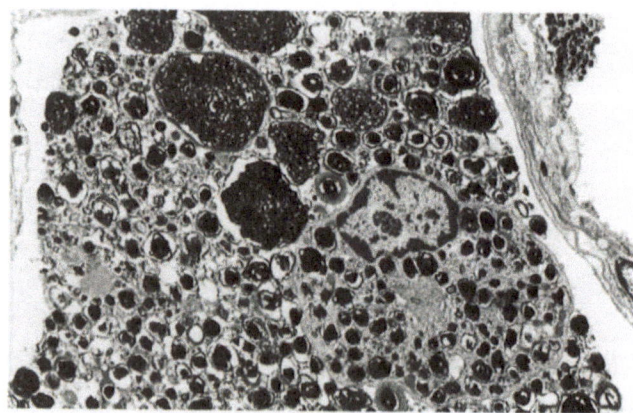

Figure 2.72 Phospholipidosis induced in a rat lung. The alveoli and macrophages contain numerous electron-dense multilamellar bodies which are believed to be produced by the Type II pneumonocytes. Electron micrograph

rats following butylated hydroxytoluene-induced damage, in which inhibition of epithelial cell proliferation (and re-epithelialization) by high oxygen concentration results in fibrosis[41]. In both intra-alveolar and interstitial fibrosis, in spite of the presence of numerous fibroblasts, the amount of collagen, demonstrable with Van Gieson or trichrome stains, is usually surprisingly sparse. However, with a reticulin stain a more dense network of fibres may be detected. The lack of demonstrable collagen is in contrast to the collagenization of alveolar ducts described earlier.

Epithelialization of the walls due to proliferation of Type II pneumonocytes is a common alveolar repair mechanism and may become extensive. Although initially often associated with alveolar wall damage and a variable inflammatory reaction (Figures 2.64 and 2.65) it may subsequently appear as the predominant cellular change in a lesion. The proliferation results in a cuboidal appearance of the alveolar walls. Rarely, epithelialization may be associated with the development of squamous metaplasia. Following intratracheal instillation of silica to rats, both hypertrophy and hyperplasia of Type II pneumonocytes are recorded[43]. The Type II cells are demonstrable by alkaline phosphatase activity. With the light microscope, they appear vacuolated and ultrastructurally there are increased numbers of multilamellar bodies. In some cases proliferation of Type II cells appears to develop without prior damage to the Type I pneumonocytes[25]. In mice, the infiltration of inflammatory cells into the alveoli, through the alveolar walls induces Type II cell proliferation, in the absence of detectable injury to Type I cells[44]. The proliferation is related to the degree and timing of the inflammatory infiltration.

The terms adenomatous hyperplasia and adenomatosis are used synonomously to describe localized, non-neoplastic proliferative lesions of the alveolar walls. This proliferative lesion may sometimes be difficult to distinguish from pulmonary adenomata and frequently develops without prior alveolar change. Adenomatosis is poorly defined, non-circumscribed and does not cause compression of adjacent tissue. The proliferation is generally due to hyperplasia of Type II pneumonocytes which do not show nuclear pleomorphism and have a low mitotic rate. These cuboidal cells form a single layer and use the existing alveolar walls as a framework. Thus, the alveolar architecture is essentially maintained, although the accumulation of macrophages in the alveolar spaces may impart a more solid appearance. The lesion grows by successive cellular replacement of the cells of adjacent alveolar walls. Chronic oral administration of dimethyl hydrogen phosphite to rats, results in a complex of non-neoplastic pulmonary lesions which involve alveolar epithelial hyperplasia, chronic interstitial pneumonia and adenomatous hyperplasia[45]. We have seen a similar complex of lesions following the chronic dietary administration of a plant extract to rats (Figure 2.66). The pigmented compound caused accumulation and aggregation of brown alveolar macrophages, bronchiolization, adenomatous hyperplasia and focal squamous metaplasia of the alveolar walls (Figure 2.67).

Pulmonary lipoproteinosis is described in both experimental animals and in man exposed to dust particles, especially quartz[2]. In man, nearly half the cases in one survey occurred in patients who had been exposed to various dusts including silica, asbestos, cadmium, broken fluorescent tubes and tin[46]. Lipoproteinosis is also described in experimental animals after exposure to aluminium powder, volcanic ash, coal dust, nickel dust, small fibreglass particles and bismuth orthovanadate[30].

The condition is characterized by the accumulation of fine, eosinophilic material in the alveoli; increased numbers of large, often rounded macrophages with a vacuolated or foamy cytoplasm; and proliferation of Type II pneumonocytes (Figures 2.68 and 2.69). It is suggested that the intra-alveolar material is surfactant from the hyperactive Type II cells, which accumulates because alveolar macrophages become overloaded with inhaled material with consequent failure of lung clearance[30]. The intra-alveolar material may be shown, by electron microscopy, to be largely composed of multilamellar structures[47]. The possible role of defective macrophage clearance may be taken further with the suggestion that in man, at least, alveolar proteinosis could in some cases be brought about by immunosuppression manifested as either a recruitment deficiency or an intrinsic malfunction of the phagocytes[48].

A similar if not identical condition to alveolar lipoproteinosis is induced by the systemic administration of a wide range of drugs, such as chlorphentermine, iprindole, triparanol, chlorcyclizine and cloforex[49]. These drugs although having diverse therapeutic and pharmacological properties have a common cationic, amphiphilic structure. This condition, generally known as phospholipidosis, is widely reported in rats and is seen occasionally in dogs and primates. There is some evidence of species differences in the development of phospholipidosis with some drugs[49], but at least one compound (amiodarone) produces the condition in both rats and man[50]. The dual nomenclature for the apparently identical basic lesions of phospholipidosis and lipoproteinosis has some value in that the term alveolar proteinosis is generally ascribed to lesions induced by dust inhalation whereas phospholipidosis is usually restricted to conditions produced via the systemic route. Like lipoproteinosis, phospholipidosis involves the accumulation of eosinophilic, intra-alveolar material, foamy macrophages and Type II pneumonocyte proliferation (Figure 2.70). In 1 μm plastic sections the macrophage cytoplasm is filled with variably sized inclusions (Figure 2.71). Type II pneumonocytes contain increased numbers of large, sometimes multilocular inclusions. Electron microscopy suggests that the inclusions correspond to multilamellar bodies (Figures 2.72 and 2.73). In some cases multilamellar inclusion bodies are found in the Clara cells of the terminal bronchioles and rarely in Type I pneumonocytes of the alveolar walls.

Calcification of alveolar walls may be induced by several mechanisms:

(i) as a metastatic response to severe, chronic induced renal disease with hyperparathyroidism, which may occur in rats with high doses of furosemide;

(ii) with hypervitaminosis-D; and

(iii) in experimental calciphylaxis which involves systemic sensitization with a calcifying factor (e.g. vitamin D compounds) followed by intratracheal challenge by agents such as aluminium chloride or thorium chloride[51].

Pulmonary emphysema is 'a condition characterized by abnormal, permanent enlargement of air spaces distal to the terminal bronchioles accompanied by destruction of their walls and without obvious fibrosis'[52]. It is rarely produced in laboratory animals during inhalation toxicity studies, although NO_2, cadmium chloride aerosol, hexane and also some lathyritic agents such as β-aminopropionitrile, when given to rapidly growing animals are reported to produce positive results[52]. Useful animal

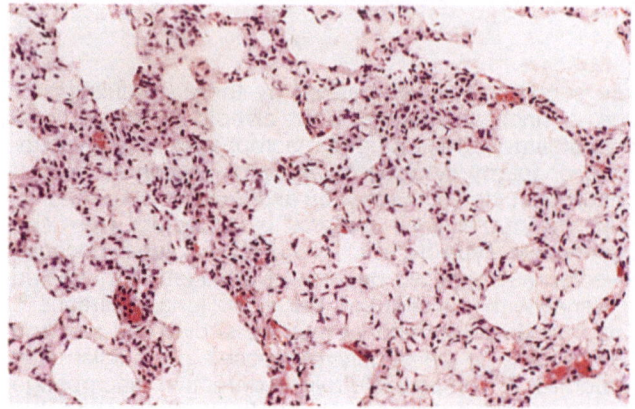

Figure 2.73 Phospholipidosis induced in a rat lung by a cationic amphiphilic drug. The proliferated Type II pneumonocytes are hypertrophic with numerous large, often multilocular, multilamellar bodies. Similar bodies are found free in the alveolar spaces. Electron micrograph

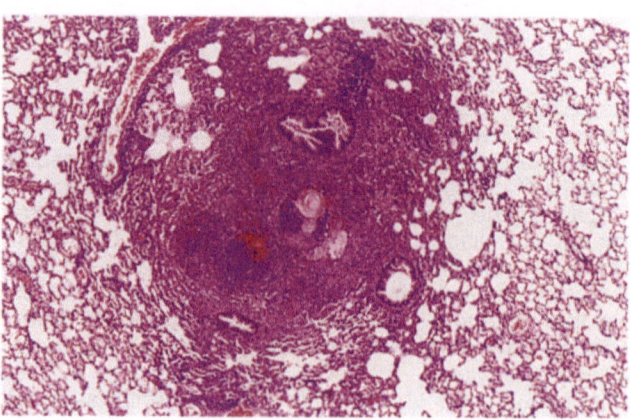

Figure 2.74 Pulmonary granulomatous reaction induced by lodging of a hair-shaft embolus (at centre) following intravascular injection in a rat.   H & E

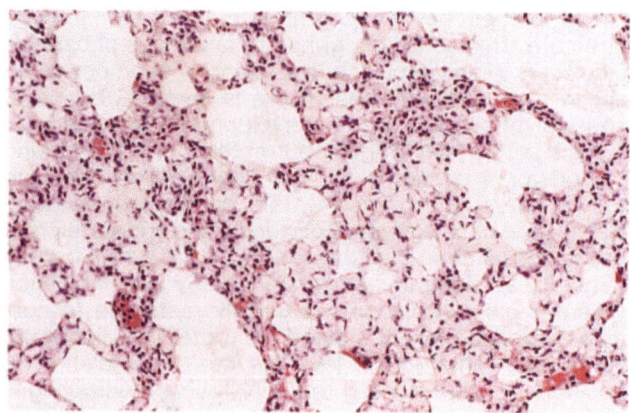

Figure 2.75 Thickening of the alveolar interstitium by foamy histiocytes in a dog treated systemically with a novel 'reticuloendothelial system expander'. No evidence of degenerative changes is detected.   H & E

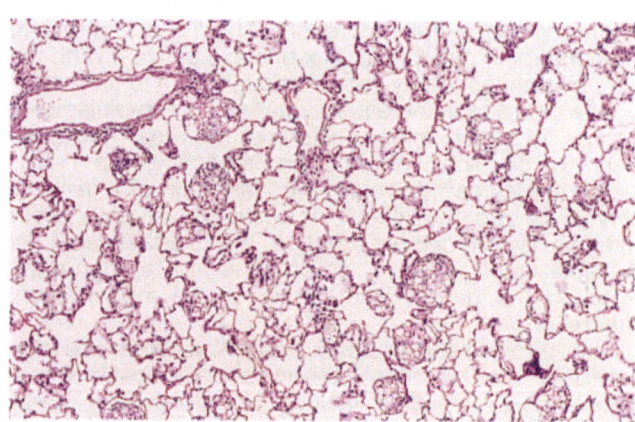

Figure 2.76 Focal accumulation of large vacuolated histiocytes in the alveolar walls of a rat following oral administration of a novel agrochemical. The condition induced a widespread systemic histiocytosis.   H & E

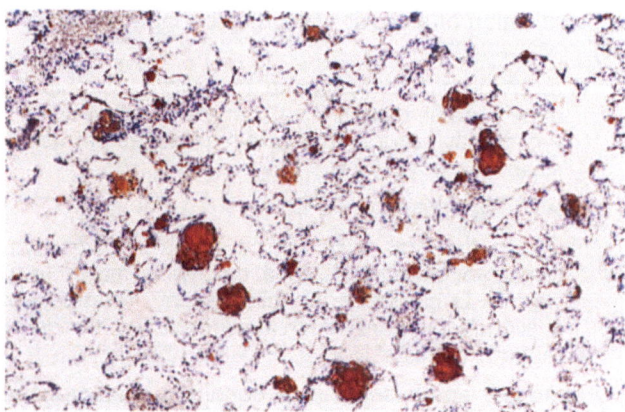

Figure 2.77 Demonstration of neutral lipid in vacuolated histiocytes shown in Figure 2.76. Frozen section. Oil Red O

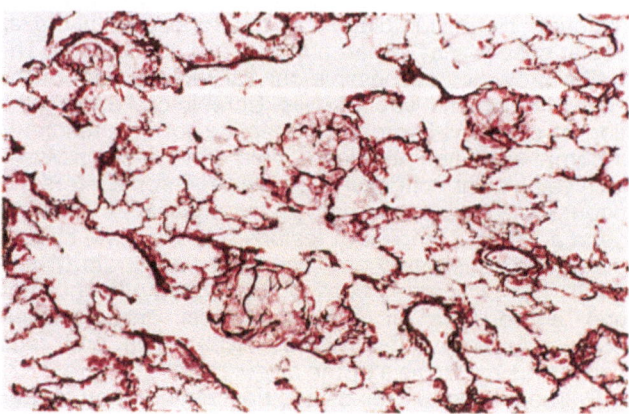

Figure 2.78 Reticulin stain clearly demonstrates the position of vacuolated histiocytes (shown in Figures 2.76 and 2.77) within the alveolar interstitium. Reticulin

models for this chronic debilitating disease involve the inhalation or intratracheal instillation of papain, elastase and other proteolytic enzyme preparations[52].

Pulmonary hypertension is known to be produced in man by some drugs such as Aminorex[35] but it is rarely encountered during routine toxicity studies. Animal models are available and hypertensive vascular disease can be induced in rats by feeding *Crotalaria spectabilis* seeds[53]. The vascular medial hypertrophy is associated with pulmonary haemorrhage, haemosiderosis, fibrinous exudation and interstitial fibrosis. Pulmonary hypertension may also be seen in narcotic addicts. Talcum powder and other foreign body granulomas in the lungs of addicts are common following intravascular injections[35]. Similar vascular conditions may accidentally be induced in the lungs of animals in intravascular toxicity studies. During the injection procedure (which is often repeated daily for considerable periods of time) fragments of hair and tissue may become punched out by the needle and inadvertently introduced into the vein. These emboli become trapped in the pulmonary vasculature, causing thrombosis and subsequent perivascular granulomas (Figure 2.74) and interstitial pneumonitis[54]. A form of fat embolism is produced in dogs and baboons given single intravenous injections of oleic acid[38]. Initially intravenous fat emboli are present in the alveolar capillaries and thrombi with fibrin and platelets form. This leads to disseminated intravascular coagulation. The lesion is suggested as a model for fat embolism in man.

In rats fed a cholesterol and cotton-seed oil supplemented diet, macrophages containing lipid droplets are found in the alveolar septae and in the alveoli. Later, the lipid-laden macrophages aggregate in the subpleural, peribronchiolar and perivascular regions[55]. In dogs and sub-human primates, high doses of some novel 'reticulo-endothelial system expanders' intended as immunomodulators cause the accumulation of foamy histiocytes in the interstitium of the alveolar walls, and in other organs. Focally, these cells cause swelling of the alveolar walls (Figure 2.75) and also accumulate perivascularly. Similar changes are described in rabbits following infusion of perfluorochemicals intended as blood substitutes[56]. In addition to the alveolar interstitium foam cells also accumulate in and around small arterioles and muscular arteries. We have observed accumulation of neutral fat-containing histiocytes in alveolar walls of rats (Figures 2.76–2.78) treated orally with a novel agrochemical. The treatment caused a systemic histocytosis.

Pulmonary lesions may also occasionally be encountered in toxicity studies following the accidental instillation of test solution into the trachea during oral gavage[57]. Even in cases of correct oral dosing a small amount of the compound may be inadvertently deposited at the laryngeal orifice and would be inhaled during inspiration. With many compounds this results in negligible pulmonary lesions but others, although well tolerated orally, may be highly toxic to pulmonary tissue. We observed necrotizing pneumonitis in mice from a study in which methyl cellulose was used as the vehicle. Substitution of another vehicle in subsequent studies did not induce lesions.

An unusual mild form of aspiration pneumonia, characterized by peribronchiolar macrophage aggregates and occasional giant cells, has been found in several studies with different compounds in our laboratory. In all these studies the test compound was administered either intravascularly or by admixture with the diet, thus excluding the form of accidental mis-dosing described above. A common feature in all these studies was markedly excessive salivation. We consider the most likely expla-nation for this pulmonary lesion to be the involuntary inhalation of the excessive saliva, leading to a macrophage reaction more typical of an inhalation study. Aspiration of oropharyngeal secretions is believed to be common in man[1] and does not usually induce significant pulmonary reactions. However, under conditions of increased salivation a macrophage reaction around terminal bronchioles would be expected. Occasionally fragments of plant-like (possibly food) material may also be present in the pulmonary reaction; these probably originate from the oral cavity. It is possible that laryngeal paralysis or laryngospasm such as that known to be induced by barbiturates[58] may contribute to inhalation of the saliva in some cases. Animals and man who are sedated, comatose, debilitated or have oesophageal motility abnormalities all have a greater incidence of aspiration pneumonitis[35].

Another indirect mechanism by which pulmonary lesions may occasionally be produced involves studies with high doses of potent corticosteroids. In these studies atrophy of the lymphoid tissues, with associated lymphopenia and immunosuppression, leads to increased susceptibility to infectious agents and may allow clinical manifestations of latent infections. Examples of these types of condition include: *E. coli*-induced bronchopneumonia in dogs; and severe exacerbation of *Paragonimus* sp. (lung fluke) infestation in wild-caught cynomolgus monkeys.

Inhalation of antigenic dusts may induce both systemic and local immune responses. When subjected to repeated antigenic exposure an allergic alveolitis develops. Inhalation of concanavalin A to non-immunized rabbits produces a diffuse interstitial pneumonitis[59].

It is suspected that mast cells may have a role in regulating connective tissue with degranulation affecting fibroblast proliferation. Parenchymal mast cell hyperplasia is reported in several pulmonary conditions, for example a tenfold increase in rats treated with bleomycin[41].

References

1. Brain, J. D. and Valberg, P. A. (1979): Deposition of aerosol in the respiratory tract. *Am. Rev. Respir. Dis.*, **120**, 1325–1373
2. Lee, K. P. (1985). Lung response to particulates with emphasis on asbestos and other fibrous dusts. *CRC Crit. Rev. Toxicol.*, **14**, 33–85
3. Hannan, S. E., Pratt, D. S., Hannan, J. M. and Brienza, L. T. (1984). Foreign body aspiration associated with the use of an aerosol inhaler. *Am. Rev. Respir. Dis.*, **129**, 1025–1027
4. Kehrer, J. P. and Kacew, S. (1985). Systemically applied chemicals that damage lung tissue. *Toxicology*, **35**, 251–293
5. Cooper, J. A. D., White, D. A. and Matthay, R. A. (1986). Drug-induced pulmonary disease. Part 1. Cytotoxic drugs. *Am. Rev. Respir. Dis.*, **133**, 321–340
6. Cooper, J. A. D., White, D. A. and Matthay, R. A. (1986). Drug-induced pulmonary disease. Part 2. Noncytotoxic drugs. *Am. Rev. Respir. Dis.*, **133**, 488–505
7. Young, J. T. (1981). Histopathologic examination of the rat nasal cavity. *Fundam. Appl. Toxicol.*, **1**, 309–312
8. Buckley, L. A., Morgan, K. T., Swenberg, J. A., James, R. A., Hamm, T. E. and Barrow, C. S. (1985). The toxicity of dimethylamine in F–344 rats and $B_6C_3F_1$ mice following a 1-year inhalation exposure. *Fundam. Appl. Toxicol.*, **5**, 341–352
9. Giddens, W. E. and Fairchild, G. A. (1972). Effects of sulfur dioxide on the nasal mucosa of mice. *Arch. Environ. Health.*, **25**, 166–173
10. Morse, C. C., Boyd, M. R. and Witschi, H. (1984). The effect of 3-methylfuran inhalation exposure on the rat nasal cavity. *Toxicology*, **30**, 195–204
11. Woutersen, R. A., Appelman, L. M., Feron, V. J. and Van der Meijen, C. A. (1984). Inhalation toxicity of acetaldehyde in rats. II carcinogenicity study: interim results after 15 months. *Toxicology*, **31**, 123–133

12. Reznik, G., Stinson, S. F. and Ward, J. M. (1980). Respiratory pathology in rats and mice after inhalation of 1,2-dibromo-3-chloropropane or 1,2-dibromoethane for 13 weeks. *Arch. Toxicol.*, **46**, 233–240

13. Maronpot, R. R., Miller, R. A., Clarke, W. J., Westerberg, R. B., Decker, J. R. and Moss, O. R. (1986). Toxicity of formaldehyde vapor in B₆C₃F₁ mice exposed for 13 weeks. *Toxicology*, **41**, 253–266

14. Turk, M. A. M., Flory, W. and Henk, W. G. (1986). Chemical modulation of 3-methylindole toxicosis in mice: effect on bronchiolar and olfactory mucosal injury. *Vet. Pathol.*, **23**, 563–570

15. Dahl, A. R. and Hadley, W. M. (1983). Formaldehyde production promoted by rat nasal cytochrome P-450-dependent monooxy-genases with nasal decongestants, essences, solvents, air pollutants, nicotine and cocaine as substrates. *Toxicol. Appl. Pharmacol.*, **67**, 200–205

16. Lewis, D. J. (1981). Mitotic indices of rat laryngeal epithelia. *J. Anat.*, **132**, 419–428

17. Lewis, D. J. (1981). Factors affecting the distribution of tobacco smoke-induced lesions in the rodent larynx. *Toxicol. Lett.*, **9**, 189–194

18. Miller, M. L., Vinegar, A. A. A., Adams, W. D., Cibulas, W. and Brooks, S. M. (1986). Morphology of tracheal and bronchial epithelial and type II cells of the peripheral lung of the guinea pig after inhalation of toluene diisocyanate vapors. *Exp. Lung Res.*, **11**, 145–163

19. Lewis, D. J. and Jakins, P. R. (1981). Effect of tobacco smoke exposure on rat tracheal submucosal glands: an ultrastructural study. *Thorax*, **36**, 622–624

20. Jeffery, P. K., Widdicomb, J. G. and Reid, L. (1975). Anatomical and physiological features of irritation of the bronchial tree. In Aharonson, E. F., Ben-David, A. and Klingberg, M. A. (eds) *Air Pollution and the Lung*. pp. 253–267. (New York: Wiley)

21. Sturgess, J. and Reid, L. (1973). The effect of isoprenaline and pilocarpine on (a) bronchial mucus-secreting tissue and (b) pancreas, salivary glands, heart, thymus, liver and spleen. *Br. J. Exp. Pathol.*, **54**, 388–402

22. Jeffery, P. K. and Reid, L. M. (1977). The respiratory mucous membrane. In Brain, J. D., Proctor, D. F. and Reid, L. M. (eds) *Respiratory Defense Mechanisms*. pp. 193–245. (New York: Marcel Dekker)

23. Adamson, I. Y. R. and Bowden, D. H. (1986). Crocidolite-induced pulmonary fibrosis in mice. *Am. J. Pathol.*, **122**, 261–267

24. Rand, G. M., Nees, P. O., Calo, C. J., Clarke, G. C. and Edmondson, N. A. (1982). The Clara cell: an electron microscopy examination of the terminal bronchioles of rats and monkeys following inhalation of hexachlorocyclopentadiene. *J. Toxicol. Environ. Health*, **10**, 59–72

25. Witschi, H. and Côte, M. G. (1977). Primary pulmonary responses to toxic agents. *CRC Crit. Rev. Toxicol.*, **5**, 23–66

26. Doster, A. R., Farrell, R. L. and Wilson, B. J. (1983). An ultrastructural study of bronchiolar lesions in rats induced by 4-ipomeanol, a product from mold-damaged sweet potatoes. *Am. J. Pathol.*, **111**, 56–60

27. Widdicombe, J. G. and Pack, R. J. (1982). The Clara cell. *Eur. J. Respir. Dis.*, **63**, 202–220

28. Johnson, N. F., Wagner, J. C. and Wills, H. A. (1980). Endocrine cell proliferation in the rat lung following asbestos inhalation. *Lung*, **158**, 221–228

29. Tateishi, R. and Ishikawa, O. (1985). The effect of N-Nitrosob-is(2-hydroxypropyl)amine on pulmonary neuroepithelial cells in Syrian golden hamsters. *Am. J. Pathol.*, **119**, 326–335

30. Lee, K. P., Henry, N. W., Trochimowicz, H. J. and Reinhardt, C. F. (1986). Pulmonary responses to impaired lung clearance in rats following excessive TiO₂ dust deposition. *Environ. Res.*, **41**, 144–167

31. Pimental, J. C. (1973). A granulomatous lung disease produced by bakelite. *Am. Rev. Respir. Dis.*, **108**, 1303–1310

32. Netteisheim, P. and Szakal, A. K. (1972). Morphogenesis of alveolar bronchiolisation. *Lab. Invest.*, **26**, 210–216

33. Davis, B. R., Whitehead, J. K., Gill, M. E., Lee, P. N., Butterworth, A. D. and Roe, F. J. C. (1975). Response of rat lung to inhaled tobacco smoke with or without prior exposure to 3,4-benzpyrene given by intratracheal instillation. *Br. J. Cancer*, **31**, 469–475

34. Hammond, T. G. and Mobbs, M. (1984). Lung oedema – microscopic detection. *J. Appl. Toxicol.*, **4**, 219–221

35. Whimster, W. F. and de Poitiers, W. (1982). The lung. In Riddell, R. H. (ed.) *Pathology of Drug-Induced and Toxic Diseases*. pp. 167–200. (New York: Churchill Livingstone)

36. Witschi, H. (1976). Proliferation of type II alveolar cells; a review of common responses in toxic lung injury. *Toxicology*, **5**, 267–277

37. Dinsdale, D., Verschoyle, R. D. and Ingham, J. E. (1984). Ultrastructural changes in rat Clara cells induced by a single dose of O,S,S-trimethylphosphorodithioate. *Arch. Toxicol.*, **56**, 59–65

38. Johanson, W. G., Holcomb, J. R. and Coalson, J. J. (1982). Experimental diffuse alveolar damage in baboons. *Am. Rev. Respir. Dis.*, **126**, 142–151

39. Dinsdale, D., Verschoyle, R. D. and Cabral, J. R. P. (1982). Cellular responses to trialkylphosphorothioate-induced injury in rat lung. *Arch. Toxicol.*, **51**, 79–89

40. de la Monte, S. M., Hutchins, G. M. and Moore, G. W. (1986). Respiratory epithelial cell necrosis is the earliest lesion of hyaline membrane disease of the newborn. *Am. J. Pathol.*, **123**, 155–160

41. Reiser, K. M. and Last, J. A. (1986). Early cellular events in pulmonary fibrosis. *Exp. Lung Res.*, **10**, 331–335

42. Singer, I. I., Kawka, D. W., McNally, S. M., Eiermann, G. J., Metzgen, J. M. and Peterson, L. B. (1986). Extensive laminin and basement membrane accumulation occurs at the onset of bleomycin-induced rodent pulmonary fibrosis. *Am. J. Pathol.*, **125**, 258–268

43. Miller, B. E., Dethloff, L. A. and Hook, G. E. R. (1986). Silica-induced hypertrophy of type II cells in the lungs of rats. *Lab. Invest.*, **55**, 153–163

44. Shami, S. G., Evans, M. J. and Martinez, L. A. (1986). Type II cell proliferation related to migration of inflammatory cells into the lung. *Exp. Mol. Pathol.*, **44**, 344–352

45. Dunnick, J. K., Boormann, G. A., Haseman, J. K., Langloss, J., Cardy, R. H. and Manus, A. G. (1986). Lung neoplasms in rodents after chronic administration of dimethyl hydrogen phosphite. *Cancer Res.*, **46**, 264–270

46. Vijeyaratnam, G. S. and Corrin, B. (1973). Pulmonary alveolar proteinosis developing from desquamative interstitial pneumonia in long term toxicity studies of iprindole in the rat. *Virchows Arch. A: Pathol. Anat.*, **358**, 1–10

47. Hook, G. E. R., Gilmore, L. B. and Talley, F. A. (1986). Dissolution and reassembly of tubular myelin-like multilamellated structures from the lungs of patients with pulmonary alveolar proteinosis. *Lab. Invest.*, **55**, 194–208

48. Bedrossian, C. W. M., Luna, M. A., Conklin, R. H. and Miller, W. C. (1980). Alveolar proteinosis as a consequence of immunosuppression. *Hum. Pathol.*, **11** Suppl., 527–535

49. Reasor, M. J. (1981). Drug-induced lipidosis and the alveolar macrophage. *Toxicology*, **20**, 1–33

50. Costa-Jussa, F. R., Corrin, B. and Jacobs, J. M. (1984). Amiodarone lung toxicity: a human and experimental study. *J. Pathol.*, **143**, 73–79

51. Allegra, L. (1965). Experimental pulmonary calcification. *Exp. Med. Surg.*, **24**, 227–238

52. Snider, G. L., Lucey, E. C. and Stove, P. J. (1986). Animal models of emphysema. *Am. Rev. Respir. Dis.*, **133**, 149–169

53. Smith, P., Kay, J. M. and Heath, D. (1970). Hypertensive pulmonary vascular disease in rats after prolonged feeding with *Crotalaria spectabilis* seeds. *J. Pathol.*, **102**, 97–106

54. Schneider, P. and Pappritz, G. (1976). Hairs causing pulmonary emboli. *Vet. Pathol.*, **13**, 394–400

55. Bernick, S. and Patek, P. R. (1961). Effect of cholesterol feeding in rat reticuloendothelial system. *Arch. Pathol.*, **72**, 78–88

56. Nanney, L., Fink, L. M. and Virmani, R. (1984). Perfluorochemicals. *Arch. Pathol. Lab. Med.*, **108**, 631–637

57. Leslie, G. B., Noakes, D. N., Pollitt, F. D., Roe, F. J. C. and Walker, T. F. (1981). A two-year study with cimetidine in the rat: assessment for chronic toxicity and carcinogenicity. *Toxicol. Appl. Pharmacol.*, **61**, 119–137

58. van Haeringen, J. R., Hilvering, C. and Sluiter, H. J. (1972). Diseases of the respiratory tract due to drugs. In Meyler, L. and Peck, H. M. (eds) *Drug-Induced Diseases*. Vol. 4, pp. 498–523. (Amsterdam: Excerpta Medica)

59. Willoughby, W. F., Willoughby, J. B., Cantrell, B. B. and Wheelis, R. (1979). *In vivo* responses to inhaled proteins. *Lab. Invest.*, **40**, 399–405

The Liver

3

By virtue of its anatomical location and its metabolic role, the liver is uniquely exposed to a wide variety of exogenous and endogenous products. These include environmental toxins, therapeutic agents, chemicals present in food or drinking water either as additives or as contaminants, various hormones and other endogenous products. Many of these substances evoke injurious or adaptive responses in the liver.

Hepatotoxic agents vary in the way in which they exert their effect on the liver. Some produce liver cell injury directly by their specific affinity for hepatocellular organelles or subcellular constituents. Other chemicals exert their effects by being metabolically biotransformed into more toxic radicals. Agents which are known to evoke injury to the liver of several species in a predictable manner are classified as intrinsic hepatotoxins[1]. The intrinsic hepatotoxins can be subdivided, according to the means by which they exert their injurious responses, into direct or indirect. Direct hepatotoxins produce the primary injury which then leads to metabolic derangements. Hepatotoxic effects produced by phosphorus and tannic acid come under this classification[2]. Indirect hepatotoxins exert their injurious effect on the cells by interfering with some of the metabolic pathways essential for cell integrity. Responses produced in liver cells by ethionine and some anabolic steroids are examples of indirect hepatotoxins[1]. Cholestatic indirect hepatotoxins such as certain contraceptive steroids and lithocholic acid are also included in this group. Some hepatotoxic agents which do not fall into the above categories produce injury as a result of host idiosyncracy; hepatic injury occurs only in a limited proportion of the exposed population and in an unpredictable manner. The cause may be hypersensitivity or, in some cases, the hepatotoxic agent may be metabolized in the host by an aberrant metabolic pathway[1,3].

A classification based on mechanism alone is occasionally insufficient; there are instances where the factual information needed for classifying a specific toxicity is inadequate and mechanistic classification has to be based on presumptions. Classifications of toxic hepatic injury based instead on morphological changes have been reported by several workers[1,3-5]. A combination of mechanistic and morphological factors as the basis for classification can be more meaningful. Details of the mechanistic stages in the action of different hepatotoxic agents are beyond the scope of this text; the theme of this chapter is the assessment of the responses of the liver to toxic agents from the morphological point of view.

Most hepatotoxicities encountered in routine toxicity studies come under predictable dose and time related liver injuries. Toxic effects are exerted either directly by the agent itself or by its metabolites. Secondary host factors, such as nutritional status, levels of drug handling enzymes, of glutathione, acetyl coenzyme A and other essential metabolites can influence the hepatotoxic manifestation[6]. Whilst some of the metallic poisons are examples of direct injury, halocarbons are examples of hepatotoxic agents which cause direct toxicity by way of intermediary metabolites. Halocarbons cause liver cell injury by biotransformation to reactive radicals which interact with vulnerable sites on cell macromolecules resulting in changes in macromolecular configuration or hepatocellular function[7]. Impaired blood flow, cell membrane injury, organelle damage and sometimes mesenchymal cell alterations can occur in hepatotoxicity. These structural alterations may be accompanied by reduced protein synthesis, altered lipid metabolism, enzyme leakage, altered excretory and secretory functions and histological changes. The toxic changes can usually be monitored or detected by various non-invasive or invasive tests, whose results often reflect the degree of hepatotoxicity. The histological changes following exposure to a hepatotoxic agent are usually represented by a series of degenerative changes and cell death.

Other agents may cause 'adaptive changes'. These are usually cellular responses to foreign compounds and result in alterations to organelles. Such changes are not by themselves necessarily injurious in nature, they are often a proliferative accommodating response of organelles. Several compounds induce a series of organelle alterations which are accompanied by compound-related liver weight increases. These reactions are reversible. Such responses are considered to be a sequel to metabolic overload and an expression of the liver's ability to cope with this. For example, lipid-soluble xenobiotics are processed by non-specific enzyme systems in the liver. However, during the process of metabolism by the liver some of these reactions induce modification of these enzyme systems resulting in their enhancement or neutralization. This in turn has the consequence of potentiating or inhibiting toxic responses to other foreign chemicals. For example, repeated administration of DDT and hexachlorobenzene leads to proliferation of smooth endoplasmic reticulum along with induction of mixed function oxidase components[8]. The capacity of these biologically persistent haloaromatics to induce drug metabolizing enzyme systems, including cytochrome P-450, can be significant in the generation of unstable intermediate radicals potentially capable of cytotoxic or mutagenic effects, from several chemicals[7].

Agents which induce drug metabolizing enzyme systems tend to potentiate hepatic injury produced by compounds such as chloroform, carbon tetrachloride or halothane. On the other hand pretreatment with compounds which inhibit drug metabolizing enzyme systems tends to protect the liver from these hepatotoxins[9].

Morphological Lesions in the Liver

In routine toxicological testing of pharmaceuticals and agrochemicals, histo-morphological examination provides excellent evidence of hepatotoxicity. Toxic injuries occur most frequently as zonal lesions in the liver. The concept of a hexagonal lobule arranged around a central vein is now outdated, although classical terminologies such as centrilobular, mid-zonal and periportal locations are still in vogue. This terminology is restrictive, however. The dynamics of liver pathology can only be fully understood in terms of the micro-circulatory physio-anatomical basis of a liver acinus[10]. The zonal location of injury is attributable in part to the availability of handling enzymes which are required for the synthesis of toxic metabolites. Other factors such as circulatory predisposition, specific affinity due to compound-binding sites, relative anoxia or hypercarbia may also play a role in the zonal distribution of lesions.

The response of the liver to acute toxic injury is in the form of a series of degenerative changes which may lead to cell death depending on the dose and potency of the agent. These changes are represented in the cytoplasm by increased cytoplasmic granularity, cell swelling, change in staining features such as eosinophilia, rarefaction, vacuolation and fatty change. Such cytoplasmic alterations tend to be grouped together loosely under the heading of degeneration. Although the various changes are separate entities, and as such are reversible, in practice cellular degeneration, fatty change and necrosis tend to appear concurrently, albeit in varying proportions, following administration of a hepatotoxic compound. Induced hepatic lesions are listed in Table 3.1.

Table 3.1 Induced lesions

Liver
  Hydropic degeneration
  Fatty change
  Necrosis
  Apoptosis
  Cholestasis
  Sinusoidal leukocytosis
  Nuclear changes
  Glycogen infiltration
  Intracytoplasmic inclusions
  Pigmentation
  Hepatocyte hypertrophy
  Hepatocyte atrophy
  Foci of altered hepatocytes
  Cystic degeneration
  Fibrosis
  Diffuse nodular hyperplasia
  Cholangitis
  Bile duct hyperplasia
  Cholangiofibrosis
  Oval cell proliferation
  Sinusoidal cell vacuolation and distension
  Focal sinusoidal dilation
  Peliosis hepatis

Gallbladder
  Epithelial pigmentation
  Cystic mucinous hyperplasia
  Cholecystitis

Hydropic degeneration

A frequent and easily recognizable degenerative lesion seen in the liver is hydropic degeneration, where the cells are swollen and often enlarged with cytoplasmic vacuolation and, in extreme cases, the cells appear ballooned (Figure 3.1). Hydropic degeneration is a reversible lesion. Vacuolation and ballooning occur due to intracytoplasmic accumulation of fluid because of disturbed integrity of the cell membrane. Ballooned cells are observed in the centrilobular lesion produced by carbon tetrachloride in laboratory animals. Carbon disulphide, when given to experimental animals pretreated with phenobarbitone sodium, causes marked hydropic degeneration of cells (Figure 3.2) around the central hepatic vein and those from the mid-zone[11,12]. High doses of certain radio-opaque agents used for contrast media purposes can also result in marked liver cell vacuolation, apparently due to hydropic degeneration.

Fatty change

Fatty change (steatosis) is a common lesion in the liver and this term is used when there is morphological evidence of excess intracytoplasmic fat, which appears as intracytoplasmic vacuolation (Figure 3.3). The mechanism of this change is complex. Intracytoplasmic fat can be due to a number of factors, e.g. organelle injury at different subcellular loci, metabolic disorders, deficiency of essential lipotrophic factors, excessive mobilization of fat from extrahepatic sources or varying combinations of any of these factors. Fat can appear in the hepatocyte cytoplasm in macrovesicular or microvesicular patterns. Tetracyclin and aflatoxin produce microvesicular, and methotrexate macrovesicular steatosis[1]. Fatty change may occur as a zonal lesion or as a diffuse change. Carbon tetrachloride produces centrilobular (periacinar) fatty change (Figures 3.4 and 3.5); phosphorus produces periportal (centriacinar) fatty change and certain amino acid deficiencies such as choline result in midzonal fatty change (Figures 3.6 and 3.7). Diffuse fatty change is seen in ethionine overdose. Fatty change is reversible except in cases when the initiating injury is so severe as to cause cell death or when the lesion is so persistent as to result in other hepatic compensatory responses such as fibrosis and regenerative hyperplasia.

Necrosis

Morphological changes associated with death of liver cells whilst still part of viable liver tissue are described as necrosis. Toxic liver cell necrosis is viewed as a disorder in the control of intracellular calcium homeostasis involving disturbance of cell membrane integrity with loss of a relative impermeability to calcium ions[13]. Centrilobular (periacinar) coagulative necrosis with scant inflammatory response is a frequent acute response (Figure 3.8) to several hepatotoxic agents such as carbon tetrachloride, chloroform, copper salts and tannic acid[5]. In acute carbon tetrachloride and chloroform toxicity the necrosis is associated with hydropic degeneration and fatty change. The necrotic lesion is accompanied by depletion of glycogen (Figure 3.9) and loss of liver-specific enzymes from the affected zone (Figure 3.10). On the other hand, histochemically, the necrotic zone reveals increased alkaline phosphatase activity (Figure 3.11). In some instances centrilobular liver necrosis is not associated with any inflammatory reaction (Figure 3.12). The centrilobular reticulin is usually intact favouring rapid recovery in a short time without any scar or lobular distortion. In certain toxicities such as dimethylnitrosamine, the necrotic lesion is associated with a haemorrhagic component due to superimposed vascular endothelial damage[14]. In this haemorrhagic lesion destruction of the reticulin framework is apparent.

Periportal (centriacinar) necrosis may be induced by white phosphorus, ferrous sulphate and allyl formate[1]. Mid-zonal necrosis is noted in toxicities due to ngaione,

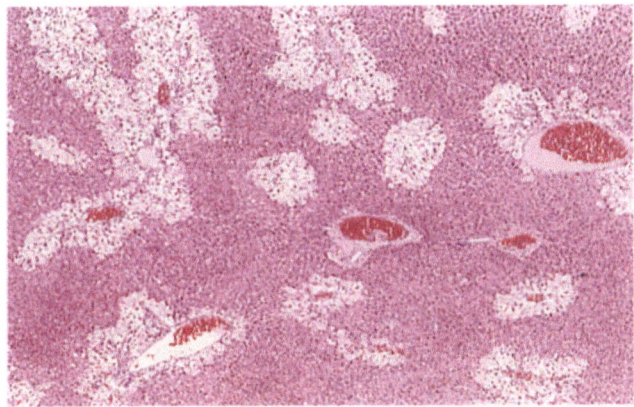

Figure 3.1 Hydropic degeneration in the liver of a rat treated with high doses of paracetamol. The condition is characterized by ballooning and vacuolation of centrilobular liver cells.   H & E

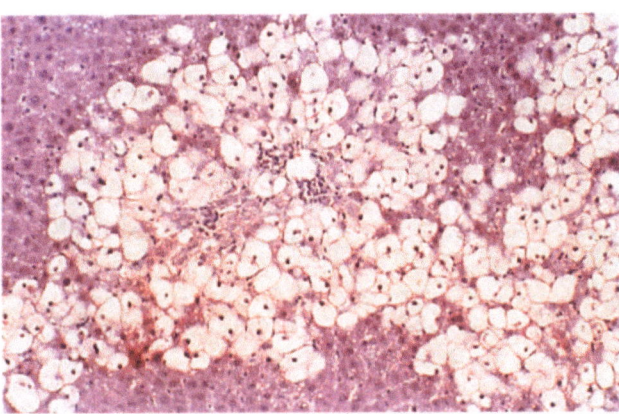

Figure 3.2 Pronounced hydropic degeneration of centrilobular and mid-zonal cells in the liver of a rat. The ballooned cells show loss of cytoplasmic staining. Note the central position of the nuclei in the affected cells. This type of lesion can be induced by carbon disulphide in rats pretreated with phenobarbitone. Compare with fatty change shown in Figure 3.3.   H & E

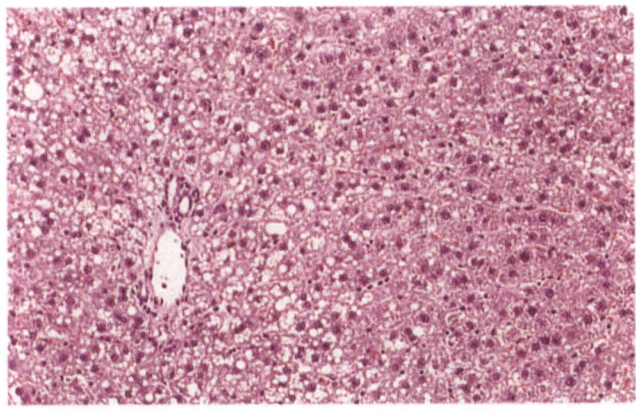

Figure 3.3 Periportal fatty change in the liver of a rat. Note the intracytoplasmic vacuolation is more prominent in the liver cells around the portal structures. In the cells with larger vacuoles the nuclei are peripherally displaced.   H & E

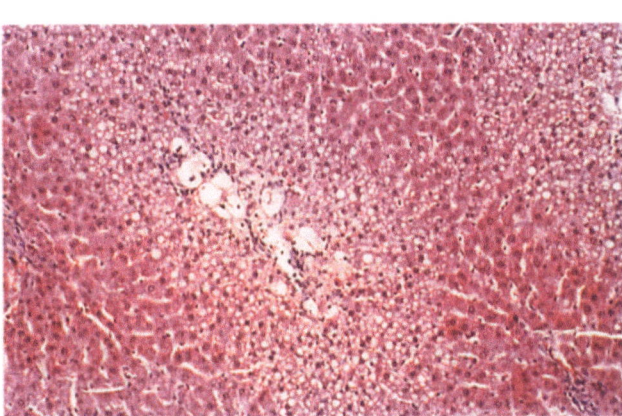

Figure 3.4 Fatty change in the liver of a rat induced by carbon tetrachloride. Centrilobular (periacinar) cells show fine vacuolation. A few ballooned cells are also encountered.   H & E

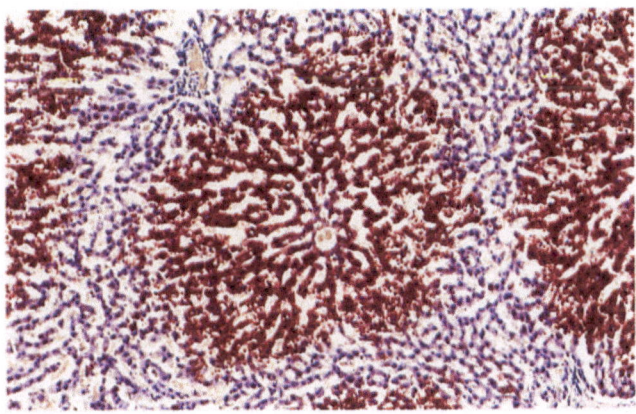

Figure 3.5 Centrilobular fat deposition in the liver of a mouse treated with a novel pharmaceutical compound. Frozen section. Oil Red O

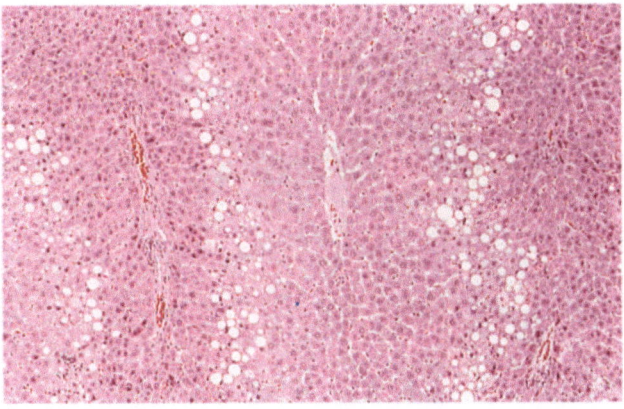

Figure 3.6 Mid-zonal hepatocyte vacuolation due to fatty change in the liver of a mouse induced by choline deficiency.   H & E

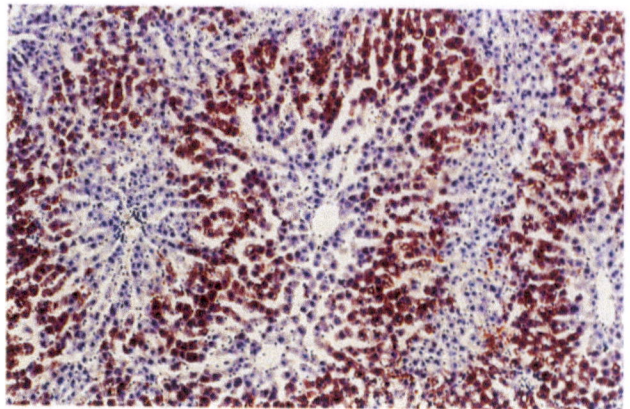

Figure 3.7 Mid-zonal fat deposition in the liver of the mouse in Figure 3.6. Frozen section. Oil Red O

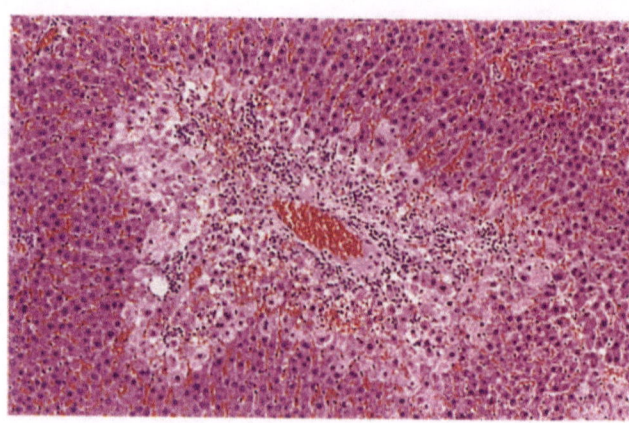

Figure 3.8 Centrilobular (periacinar) necrosis of liver in a rat treated with carbon tetrachloride. Note the perivenous area of coagulative necrosis and occasional cells with cytoplasmic vacuolation and ballooning. The affected area reveals a minimal inflammatory reaction.   H & E

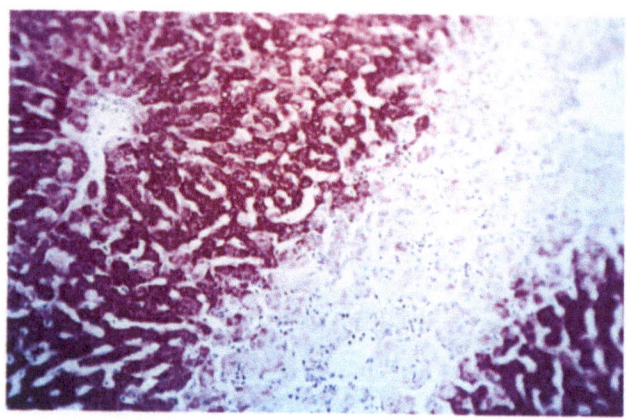

Figure 3.9 Centrilobular area of necrosis and degeneration showing depletion of glycogen staining in the liver of a calf given a single oral dose of chloroform. PAS

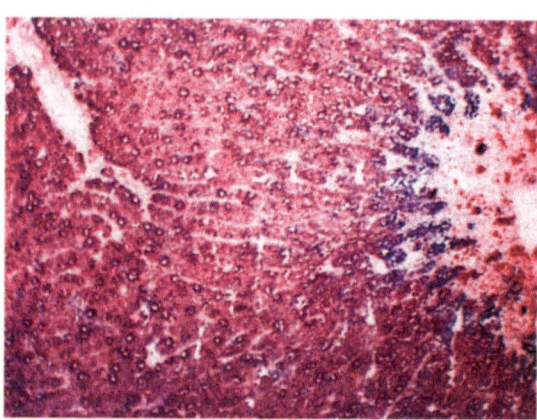

Figure 3.10 Centrilobular area of necrosis showing histochemical loss of liver specific enzyme in the liver of a horse treated with a single dose of chloroform. Glutamic dehydrogenase

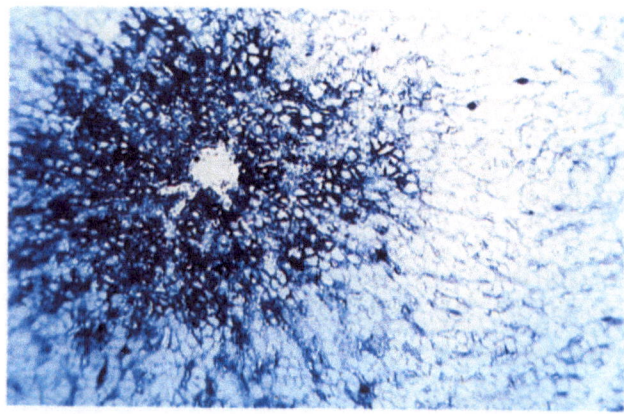

Figure 3.11 Centrilobular area of necrosis showing increased activity of non-specific alkaline phosphatase in the liver of a horse treated with a single oral dose of chloroform. Non-specific alkaline phosphatase

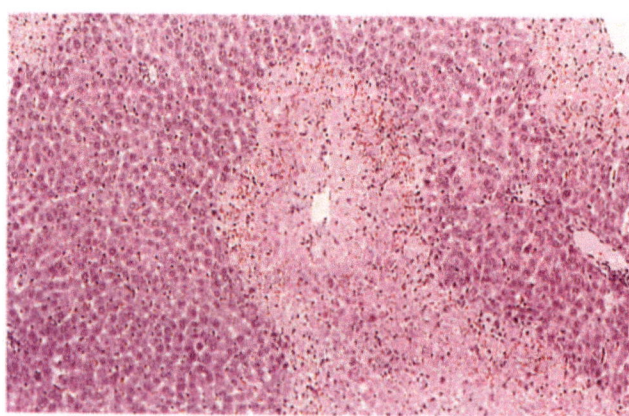

Figure 3.12 Coagulative necrosis of centrilobular hepatocytes of a rat treated with an industrial chemical. Note the absence of an inflammatory response.   H & E

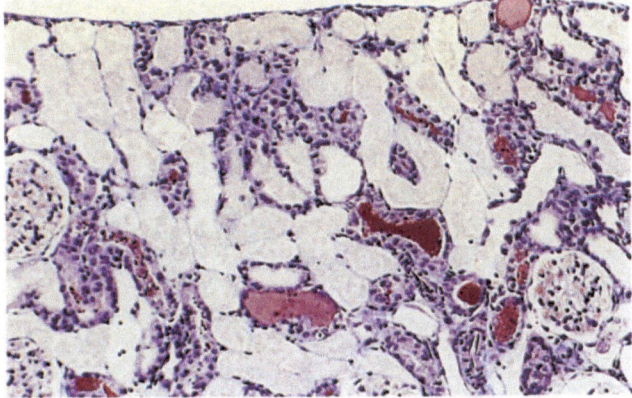

Figure 3.13 Diffuse necrosis affecting cells from all zones of the lobule in the liver of a rat. The lesion was induced by potentiating the hepatotoxicity of chloroform by pretreating the rat with phenobarbitone sodium. H & E

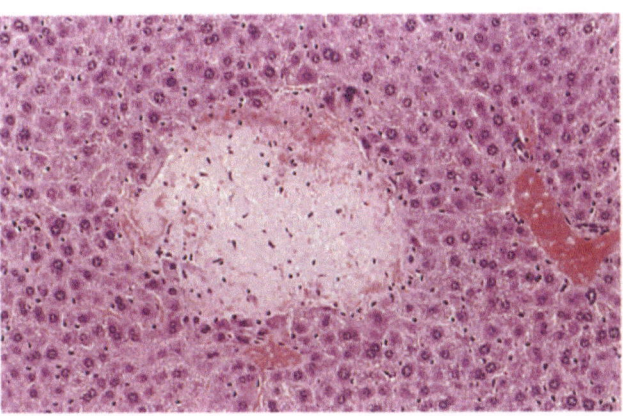

Figure 3.14 Focal necrosis on the liver of a rat following surgical ligation of the bile duct. The foci of necrosis occur irrespective of zones. H & E

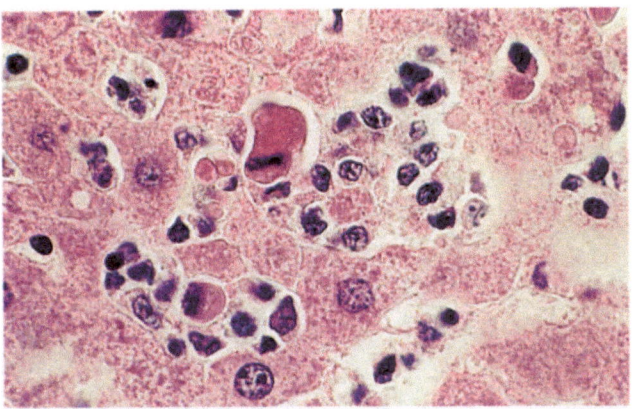

Figure 3.15 Single cell necrosis in the liver of a rat treated with a pharmaceutical. Large eosinophilic necrotic cells with scattered pyknotic nuclei. The necrotic cells are surrounded by inflammatory cells. H & E

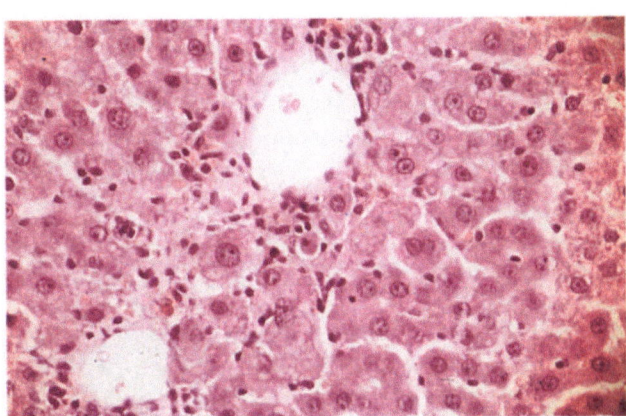

Figure 3.16 Single cell necrosis adjacent to the central vein in the liver of a rat treated with high doses of paracetamol. The necrotic cells are associated with an inflammatory cell reaction. H & E

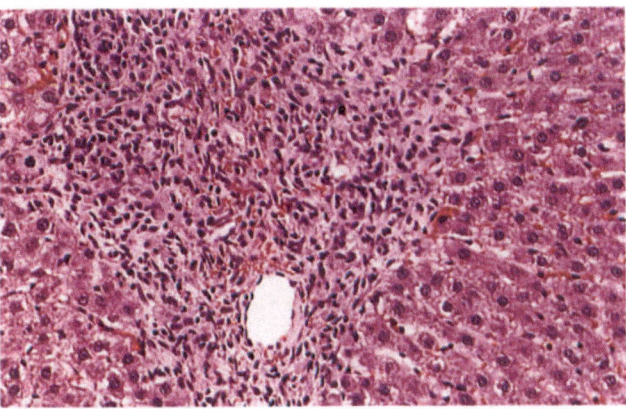

Figure 3.17 Centrilobular area of collapse, fibrosis and inflammatory cell infiltration in the liver of a rat treated with high doses of paracetamol. H & E

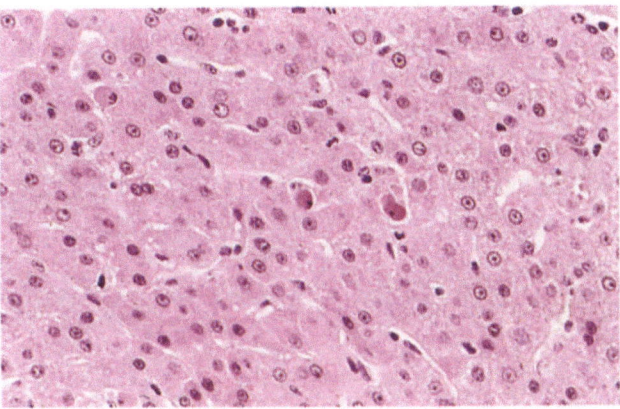

Figure 3.18 Apoptotic bodies in the liver of a monkey induced by a novel pharmaceutical compound. Note the intracytoplasmic eosinophilic, spherical bodies with pyknotic nuclear remnants and the absence of any inflammatory response. H & E

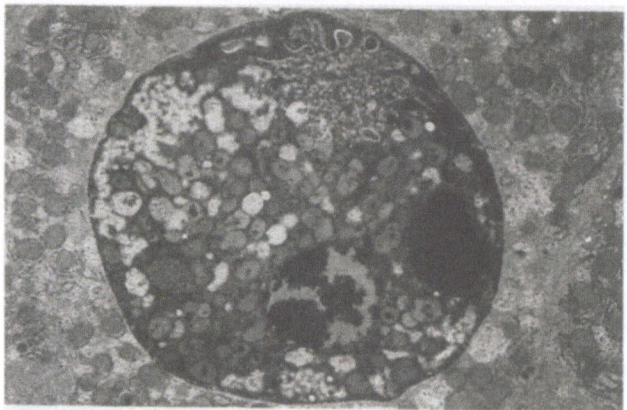

Figure 3.19 Apoptotic body in the liver of a rat treated with xylidine. Membrane-bound cell fragments with organelles and nuclear chromatin within the cytoplasm of a hepatocyte. Electron micrograph

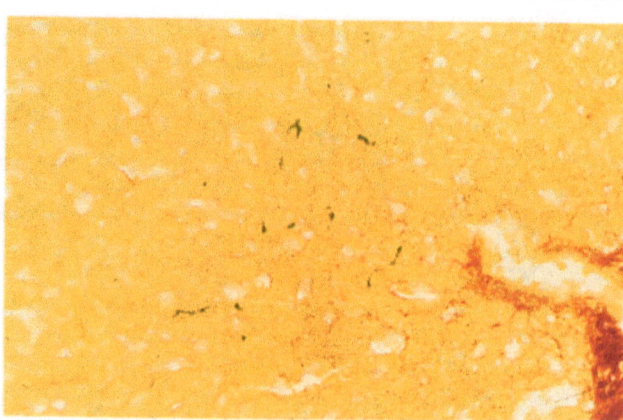

Figure 3.20 Cholestasis in the liver of a dog treated with a novel antidepressive pharmaceutical compound. Intracanalicular bile pigment appearing as olive green plugs. Hall-Fouchet

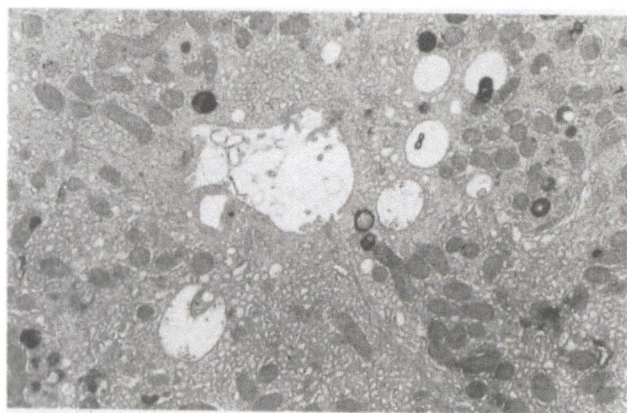

Figure 3.21 Dilation of bile canaliculus with blunting and loss of microvilli in the liver of a rat with manganese chloride-induced cholestasis. Electron micrograph

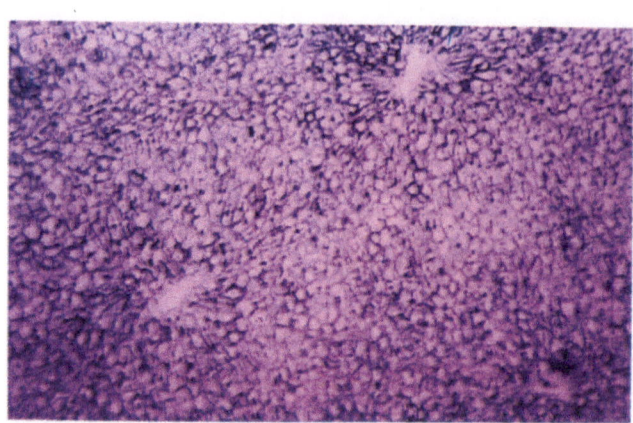

Figure 3.22 Increased cytoplasmic and canalicular alkaline phosphatase activity in the rat liver in surgically induced biliary obstruction. Non-specific alkaline phosphatase

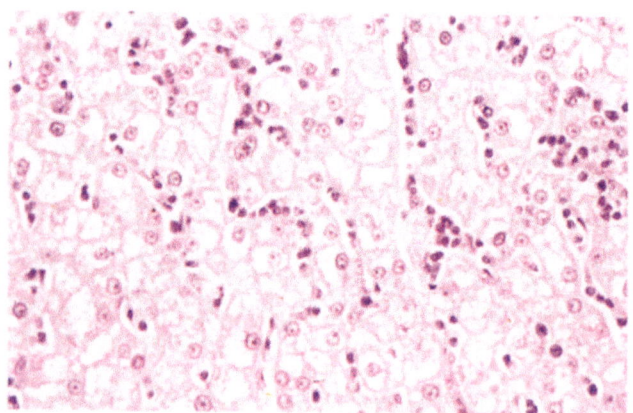

Figure 3.23 Sinusoidal leukocytosis giving a 'beaded' appearance in the liver of a monkey from a toxicity study with an immunostimulant drug. H & E

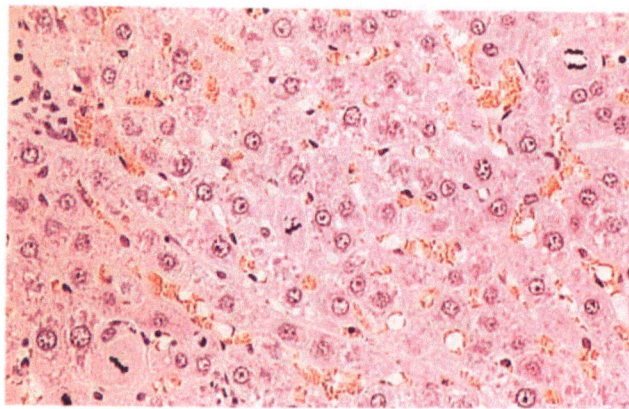

Figure 3.24 Several mitotic figures in the liver of a rat induced by treatment with a pyridine derivative. H & E

beryllium and frusemide. Galactosamine produces diffuse necrosis (Figure 3.13) in experimental animals[3]. Focal necrosis irrespective of zonal location (Figure 3.14), although uncommon in toxic injury, occurs with manganese chloride[15]. In addition, occasional single cell necrosis or piecemeal necrosis associated with an inflammatory cell infiltration (Figures 3.15 and 3.16) may be encountered in safety studies as in some cases of paracetamol toxicity. Recovery following a minimal or moderate zonal coagulative necrosis is rapid. However, when the necrosis is massive, or in instances associated with reticulin collapse or sinusoidal injury, recovery is slow and is mediated through inflammation, fibrosis and scarring (Figure 3.17). Repeated administration of certain hepatotoxic agents like chloroform does not necessarily produce cumulative necrosis; sometimes hepatotoxic effects gradually diminish after the first dose[16].

Although not restricted to the liver, the term apoptosis must be discussed in connection with necrosis. Apoptosis is an active process of cellular self-destruction, occurring as a growth and regression regulatory response and thus controlling the cell population[17]. This type of change may also be found in atrophy and in retardation of growth caused by radiation or cytotoxic drugs. Increased rate of apoptosis is also seen during the regression of hepatic hyperplasia induced in rats by compounds or by promoting agents. High doses of cyproterone acetate administered to rats cause liver enlargement and cessation of dosing is accompanied by the appearance of numerous apoptotic bodies in the liver associated with a rapid decline of the increased liver weight[18]. Increased apoptosis is also reported in ischaemic injury following ligation of portal venous supply[19]. The presence of a moderate number of apoptotic bodies is an index of increased cell deletion[17]. Apoptosis is often inconspicuous and occurs in scattered cells within the parenchyma. The affected cells assume spherical or ovoid shapes and appear as eosinophilic bodies of varying size often containing specks of pyknotic chromatin (Figure 3.18). Apoptotic bodies may be detected either in intracytoplasmic or extracellular locations. Apoptotic bodies appear as membrane-bound cell fragments under the electron microscope, often containing intact organelles and fragments of nuclear chromatin (Figure 3.19).

Confusion can arise in the differential diagnosis of single cell necrosis and apoptosis. The latter, which is often an inconspicuous histological change, does not excite any inflammatory response. Apoptotic bodies are small in size, have rounded contours and possess pyknotic nuclear fragments. Organelles in apoptosis are frequently intact within the limiting membrane.

Cholestasis

Cholestasis is a rare morphological entity in experimental toxicity but not so in man where it is known to occur as a toxic response to chlorpromazine, anabolic and contraceptive steroids[1]. When it occurs, bile is retained in the hepatocytes, Kupffer cells and canaliculi. Bile pigment can be visualized within the canaliculi using special stains (Figure 3.20). Lipofuscin pigment is present in excess in Kupffer cells. Electron microscopy shows dilatation of canaliculi with blunting of microvilli (Figure 3.21), prominent pericanalicular lysosomes and vacuoles in the cytoplasm[15]. The lesion is often associated with cholestatic jaundice. During experimentally induced biliary stasis, increased canalicular and cytoplasmic activity of alkaline phosphatase (Figure 3.22) can be demonstrated histochemically[15].

Sinusoidal leukocytosis

Inflammatory lesions of the liver are also rare in experimental hepatotoxicities. However, recent toxicity tests with high doses of certain compounds with immunostimulant properties have resulted in induced portal, perivascular and sinusoidal leukocytosis in the liver (personal observations) (Figure 3.23).

Nuclear changes

Increased mitotic activity follows several acute necrogenic injuries to the liver including those produced by dimethylnitrosamine. Mitotic activity and binucleated liver cells increase (Figure 3.24) with toxic doses of some pyridine derivatives. However, in this case, the change is not preceded by any necrotic or degenerative lesions. Acute injury due to aflatoxin or pyrrolizidine alkaloids is not followed by increased mitotic activity[20,21]. These compounds, however, cause enlargement initially of liver cell nuclei (karyomegaly) with hyperchromatosis which then progresses to megalocytosis (Figures 3.25 and 3.26). Formation of multinucleated liver cells is also known to occur (Figure 3.27) in the hepatic injury of rats following administration of 2,3,7,8-tetrachloro-dibenzo-p-dioxin[14]. The multinucleated cells are reported to arise by cell fusion rather than by cell division[22].

Glycogen infiltration

The appearance of hepatocyte cytoplasm may alter during experimental toxicity studies. Administration of certain glucocorticoids causes glycogen infiltration in centrilobular (periacinar) or periportal (centriacinar) cells of some species. The affected cells are often enlarged and show a characteristic cytoplasmic rarefaction in conventional preparations (Figures 3.28 and 3.29). Glycogen infiltration can also occur in other zones, resulting sometimes in a characteristic 'clumping' appearance of the stainable cytoplasm (Figure 3.30). This is a result of partial displacement of the normal cytoplasmic organelles by a glycogen 'lake' (Figure 3.31). This change has been observed as a reversible reaction in a few toxicity studies using high doses of certain novel antibiotics (personal observations). Changes in staining affinity such as diffuse basophilia or eosinophilia of the hepatocyte cytoplasm are not uncommon in toxicity studies. These features usually reflect the status of rough and smooth endoplasmic reticulum and the glycogen content of the liver cells.

Intracytoplasmic inclusions

Intracytoplasmic inclusions, sometimes pale hyaline droplets, eosinophilic inclusions or multilamellar bodies (Figures 3.32 and 3.33), are seen in subacute toxicity studies with certain xenobiotic treatments and with amphiphilic cationic compounds[23]. Some of the eosinophilic and hyaline inclusions reveal ultrastructural concentric whorls of smooth endoplasmic reticulum (Figure 3.34). Mallory bodies are seen as intracytoplasmic inclusions in liver cells of mice given prolonged treatment with dieldrin[24]. Many of these have a deeply stained central core surrounded by a pale intermediate zone and an eosinophilic periphery. Other inclusions are irregular and reveal amphiphilic staining. Electron microscopy shows these inclusions as concentric whorls of rough endoplasmic reticulum.

Pigmentation

Endogenous pigmentation is occasionally observed in the liver as a non-specific response to repeated admini-

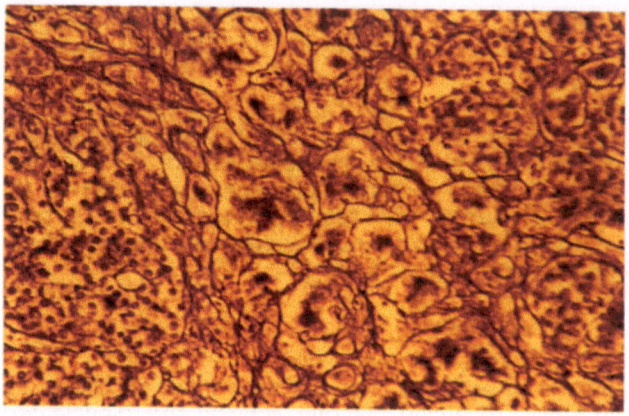

Figure 3.25 Megalocytosis in the liver of a chick in ragwort (*Senecio jacobea*) toxicity. A few unusually enlarged cells within a pleomorphic population of liver cells. Reticulin

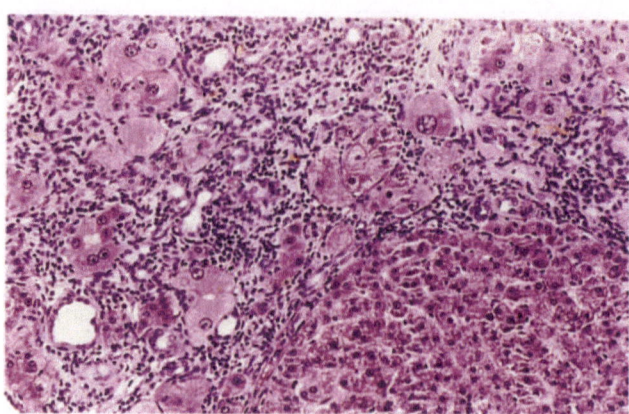

Figure 3.26 Megalocytosis in the liver of a rat from a chronic feeding study with 2-AAF. A few enlarged hepatocytes with abundant eosinophilic cytoplasm and large vesicular nuclei. Megalocytes adjacent to the portal area.   H & E

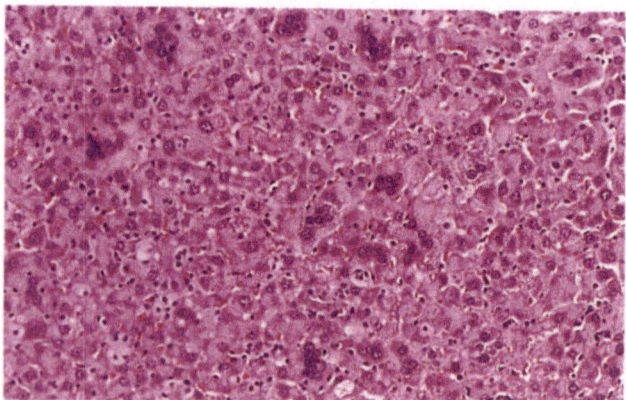

Figure 3.27 Numerous multinucleated hepatocytes in the liver of a rat treated with an industrial chemical. Some cells have up to eight nuclei.   H & E

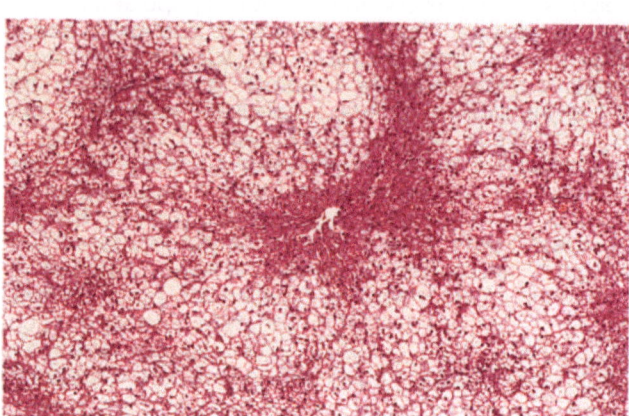

Figure 3.28 Widespread rarefaction of cytoplasmic staining and enlargement of periportal (centriacinar) and mid-zonal hepatocytes in a dog following treatment with a glucocorticosteroid. The centrilobular cells (periacinar cells) reveal normal cytoplasmic staining.   H & E

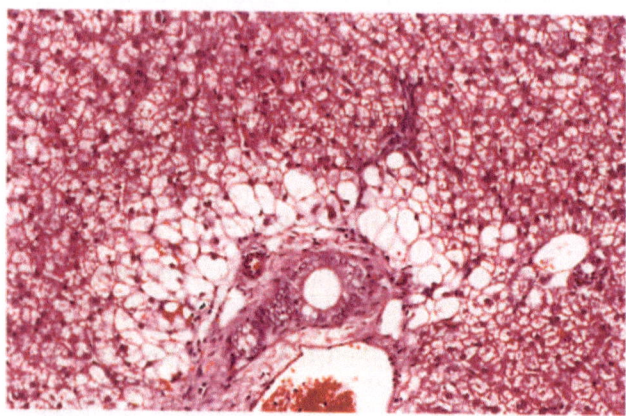

Figure 3.29 Rarefaction of cytoplasmic staining and distension of periportal hepatocytes in the liver of a dog from a toxicity study with a glucocorticosteroid. In this case the changes are confined to periportal cells.   H & E

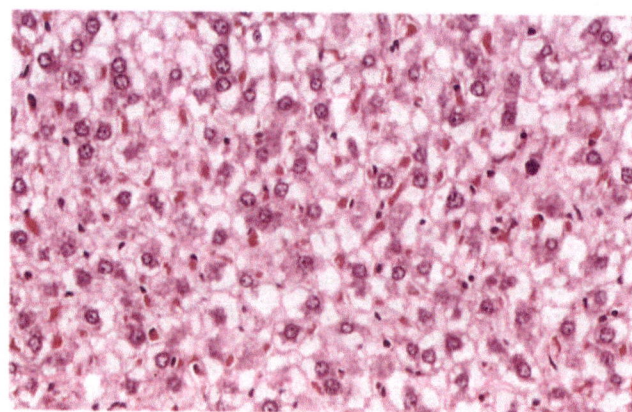

Figure 3.30 'Clumping' of stainable cytoplasm in hepatocytes of a rat from a toxicity study with a novel antibiotic. The clear areas are due to displacement of normal cytoplasm by glycogen. H & E

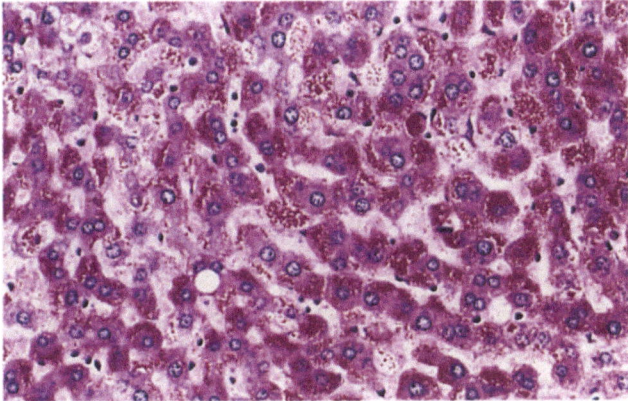

Figure 3.31 'Glycogen lakes' in the hepatocyte cytoplasm of a rat causing displacement of normal cytoplasmic staining, resulting in clumping. This case is taken from the same study as Figure 3.30. PAS

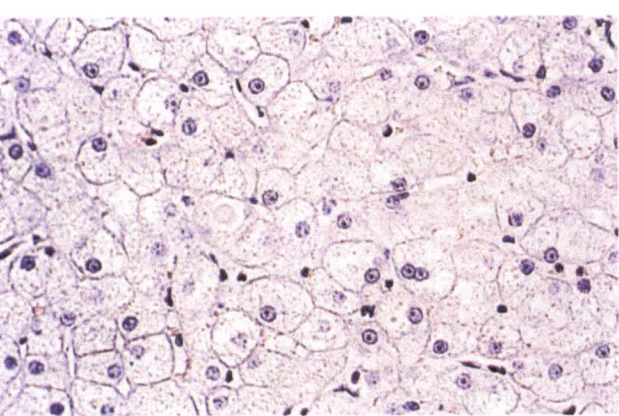

Figure 3.32 Intracytoplasmic hyalin droplets in the liver cells of a rat treated with a novel antimycotic compound in a chronic toxicity study. H & E

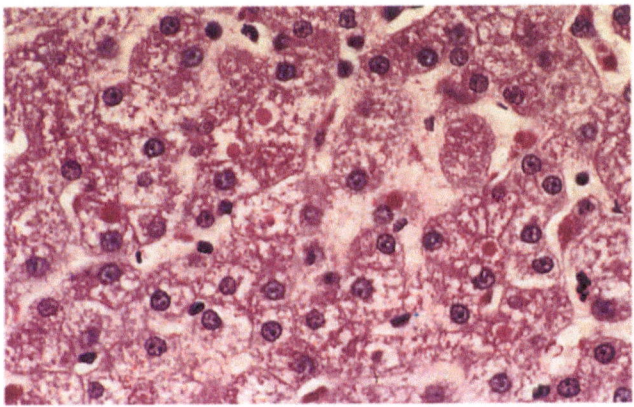

Figure 3.33 Intracytoplasmic eosinophilic spheroidal inclusions in the hepatocytes of a dog from a toxicity study with a novel pharmaceutical. These inclusions are PAS-positive and diastase resistant. H & E

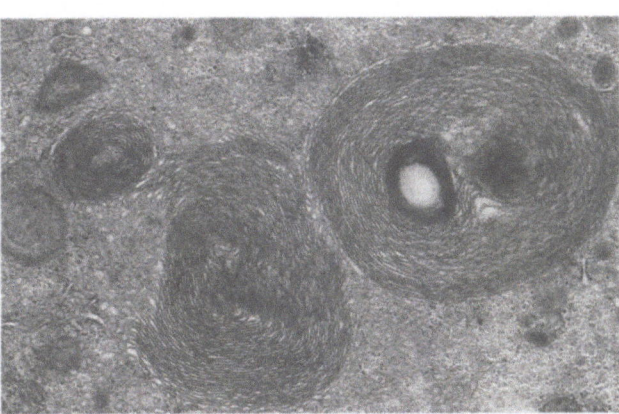

Figure 3.34 Multilamellar inclusions, consisting of concentric whorls of endoplasmic reticulum, are present in a hepatocyte of a rat treated with an insecticide. Electron micrograph

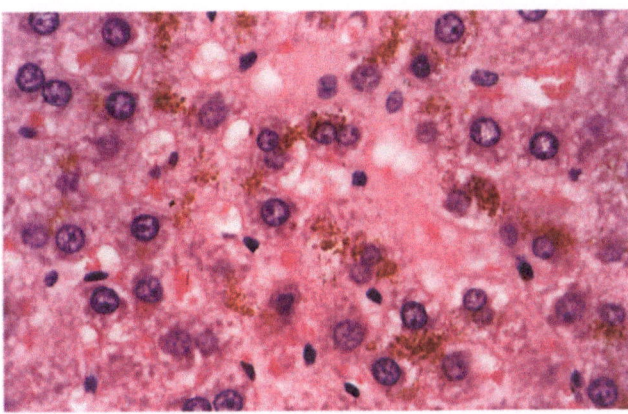

Figure 3.35 Yellowish-brown granular pigment deposition in the cytoplasm of liver cells in a dog treated with a vincamine alkaloid. Similar pigment deposition was seen in the epithelium of gall bladder and in thyroid follicular cells. H & E

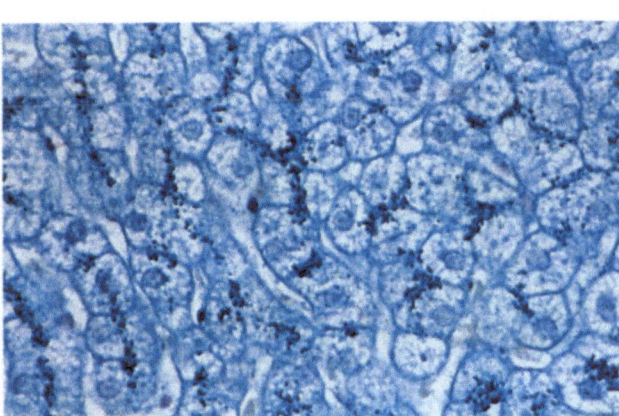

Figure 3.36 Pericanalicular deposition of lipofuscin in hepatocytes of a dog. This type of change is found particularly in dogs as a non-specific reaction. Schmorl's stain

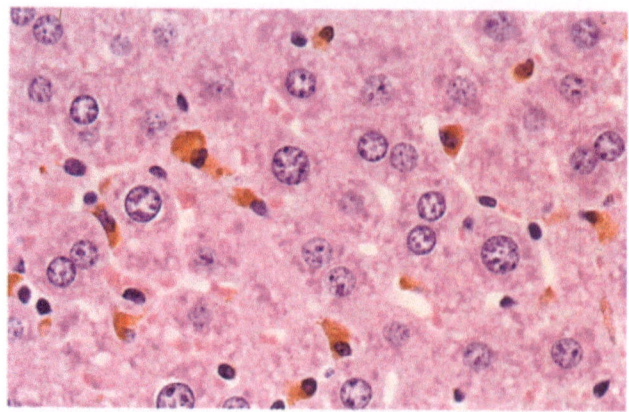

Figure 3.37 Yellow pigment in Kupffer cells in the liver of a dog. In this case, the pigment was not identified by special staining and most probably represented the test compound and/or a metabolite. H & E

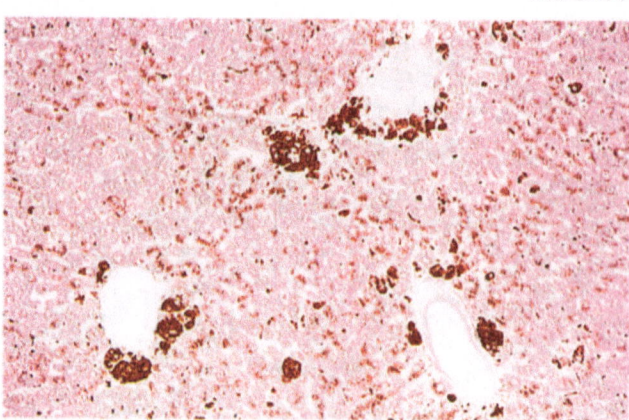

Figure 3.38 Brown pigment deposition in Kupffer cells and macrophages, some in perivascular locations, in the liver of a dog treated with a neuroleptic-type compound. The pigment stains positively for lipofuscin. H & E

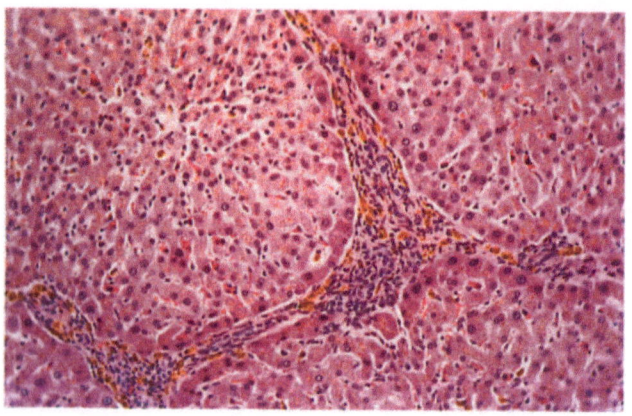

Figure 3.39 Brown pigment deposition in Kupffer cells and macrophages, with interlobular fibrosis, in the liver of a dog from a chronic toxicity study with a novel cardiovascular compound. H & E

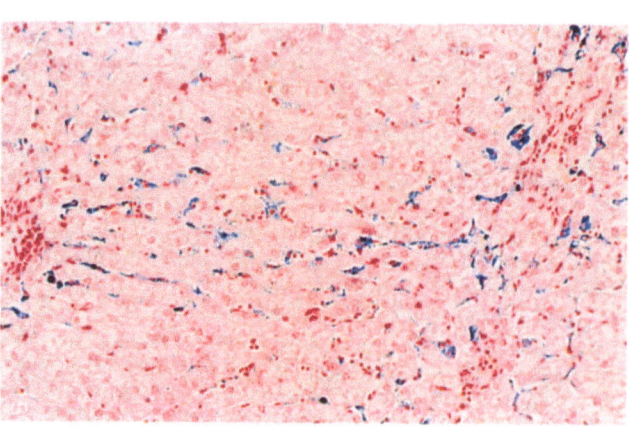

Figure 3.40 Haemosiderin deposition in the liver of a dog with haemolytic anaemia from a toxicity study. Note the iron pigment in Kupffer cells and macrophages. Perl's stain

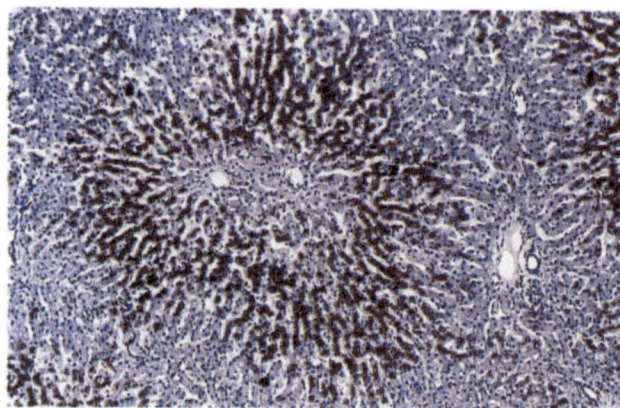

Figure 3.41 Brown pigment deposition in the mid-zonal liver cells in a rat from a chronic feeding study. The pigment (probably test compound) was not detected in the paraffin sections, suggesting removal by lipid solvents during histological processing. Frozen section. Oil Red O

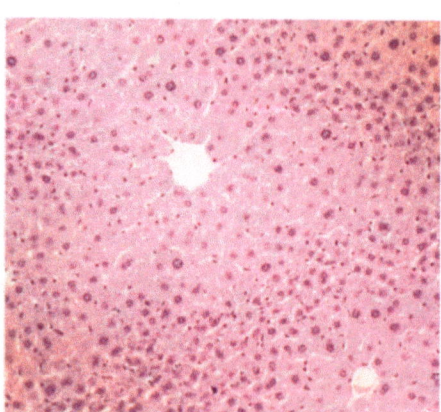

Figure 3.42 Centrilobular hypertrophy of the hepatocytes in a rat. The enlarged cells appear eosinophilic. Several xenobiotic compounds are known to induce this type of response. H & E

stration of a number of unrelated compounds. The pigment appears as intracytoplasmic brownish granules usually with a centrilobular predisposition and sometimes with pericanalicular orientation (Figures 3.35 and 3.36). Pigments occur more frequently in the livers of dogs and primates than in other species. These pigments stain for lipofuscins and are also found in the Kupffer cells. A lipofuscin-like pigment is found in hepatocytes and Kupffer cells of dogs treated with certain vincamine compounds. An autofluorescing lipofuscin pigment is known to accumulate in rodent liver (hepatocytes and Kupffer cells) exposed to prolonged administration of hypolipidaemic agents[25]. Pigment deposition may be encountered in Kupffer cells and occasionally also in macrophages (Figures 3.37–3.39) in dogs from toxicity studies with a variety of compounds. Iron-containing pigments are seen in the liver cells and Kupffer cells in haemolytic conditions (Figure 3.40). Copper bound to protein is demonstrable in liver cells and Kupffer cells in experimental copper toxicities[26,27]. Lipid-soluble pigments are often obscured in routine histological preparations and examination of frozen sections is more useful in such instances (Figure 3.41).

Hypertrophy

A number of unrelated compounds induce liver enlargement associated with liver weight increase and in many instances there is histological evidence of hepatocyte hypertrophy. Hypertrophy occurs most commonly in xenobiotic treatment as centrilobular (periacinar) enlargement of hepatocytes (Figure 3.42). Hypertrophy can be found in periportal (centriacinar) hepatocytes as in *Lantana camara* poisoning in sheep[28] or as a diffuse change. When the hypertrophy is slight and diffuse, involving all zones (Figure 3.43), the detection of this change without the aid of a comparison head microscope may be difficult. The affected cells usually assume a pale, ground glass appearance (Figure 3.44), or in some cases a more eosinophilic staining. Electron microscopy may reveal a specific organelle proliferation or alteration. Some xenobiotic treatment induces proliferation of smooth endoplasmic reticulum (Figure 3.45) associated with microsomal enzyme induction. Several hypolipidaemic agents and certain industrial plasticizers result in proliferation of microbodies (peroxisomes) with a significant increase in peroxisome-associated enzymes, e.g. catalase (Figure 3.46) in rodent livers[25]. The hypolipidaemic compound ciprofibrate induces peroxisome proliferation in the liver (Figure 3.47) of several species including primates[29].

Liver weight increase may not be accompanied by definite histological changes in conventional preparations, as in short term treatment of rodent liver with ethinyl oestradiol. However, enzyme histochemistry reveals the induction of canalicular alkaline phosphatase (Figure 3.48)[30].

Atrophy

Hepatocyte atrophy appearing as increased basophilia and loss of cytoplasmic volume is a rare phenomenon in routine toxicity studies, although it may be associated with inanition in some chronic toxicity studies. The mechanism of hepatocyte atrophy is poorly understood.

Foci or areas of altered hepatocytes

A variety of cellular alterations arise during long-term exposure of rodent liver to hepatotoxins. Foci of altered cells occur in rodents in the early stages of carcinogenesis following administration of different chemicals.

The alterations appear as distinct groups of liver cells showing certain characteristic cytoplasmic features embedded amongst otherwise normal parenchyma within the lobular configuration. These altered foci display numerous phenotypic variations and appear as groups of eosinophilic, clear, basophilic or mixed cells (Figures 3.49–3.51). Within the basophilic population a subdivision of tigroid cells with a striped pattern has recently been described[31]. The altered foci may be associated with cytoplasmic vacuolation and also with dilated sinusoids. The cell size is frequently larger or smaller in comparison with the surrounding parenchyma. Various markers, based on the altered biochemical profiles, are used to demonstrate these foci (Figure 3.52). Enzymes like γ-glutamyl transpeptidase, glucose-6-phosphatase, adenosine triphosphatase, and glucose-6-phosphatase dehydrogenase are among those used as markers. However, their general use as markers of cellular alterations frequently meets with practical difficulties as the foci themselves are a heterogeneous group with differing biochemical features. The clear cell and eosinophilic cell foci are glycogen-rich, the mixed cell and basophilic cell foci are glycogen-deficient[32]. Eosinophilic foci are usually γ-glutamyl transpeptidase positive whilst some basophilic foci are γ-glutamyl transpeptidase negative. In some situations the glycogen-rich clear cell and acidophilic foci progress to mixed and basophilic cell populations which are deficient in glycogen and rich in ribosomes[32]. Foci of cellular alterations are proliferative lesions possessing an increased mitotic index and they appear regularly in the early stages of hepatocarcinogenesis[32]. They may increase in size, undergo remodelling, disappear or persist, but a small proportion may progress to neoplasia[33]. The γ-glutamyl transpeptidase-positive altered foci of liver cells are known to occur spontaneously in rats[34]. A higher incidence of these foci of cellular alterations are encountered in the liver of rodents given long term treatment with a number of non-genotoxic compounds; γ-glutamyl transferase positive foci are encountered in mice given prolonged phenobarbitone treatment[35]. They are also reported to occur in the changes associated with diffuse nodular hyperplasia induced by portocaval anastamosis in rats[36]. Foci of altered liver cells have been described in a number of other species including primates[37].

Another lesion encountered during prolonged toxicity studies in rodent liver is cystic degeneration or spongiosis hepatis (Figure 3.53). This change is characterized by the appearance of markedly distended or ballooned cells, or multilocular cyst-like formations within the parenchyma, and it may also be encountered within altered areas or even within liver tumours. Flattened nuclei are discernible within the walls of the cystic spaces. More recently it was suggested that spongiosis hepatis arises from altered perisinusoidal fat-storing cells[38].

Fibrosis

Fibrosis in the liver may be a sequel to liver cell necrosis and collapse of the reticulin framework. If the damage is slight then fibrosis is minimal and transient with little residual effects. However, if the damage is severe or persistent, as with repeated insults, then the ensuing fibrosis can be extensive leaving scar tissue with distortion of the lobular architecture. The fibrosis can appear as zonal fibrosis, interlobular bridging, perilobular fibrosis (Figure 3.54) or in some cases pericellular fibrosis.

In extensive liver damage involving loss of liver cells, as in massive necrosis, adjacent areas of regenerative hyperplasia can be seen as poorly demarcated areas of

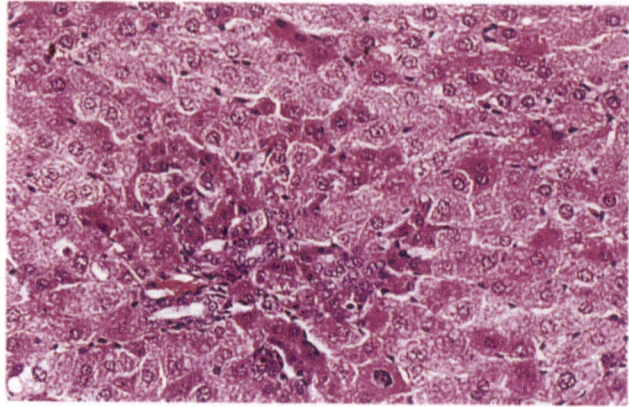

Figure 3.43 Diffuse enlargement of hepatocytes affecting cells from all the zones of the lobules in a rat treated with xylidine. H & E

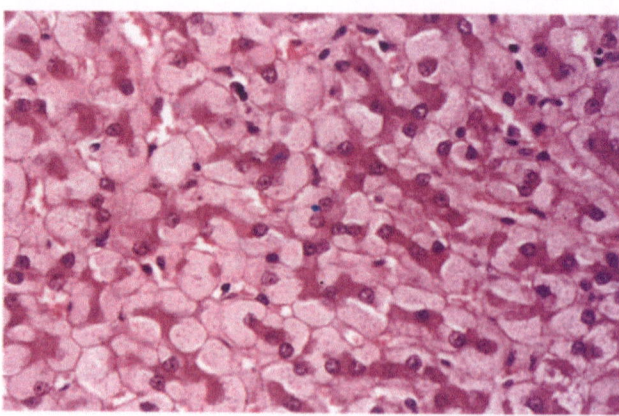

Figure 3.44 Ground glass appearance of cytoplasm of hepatocytes in the liver of a dog from a toxicity study with a xenobiotic. H & E

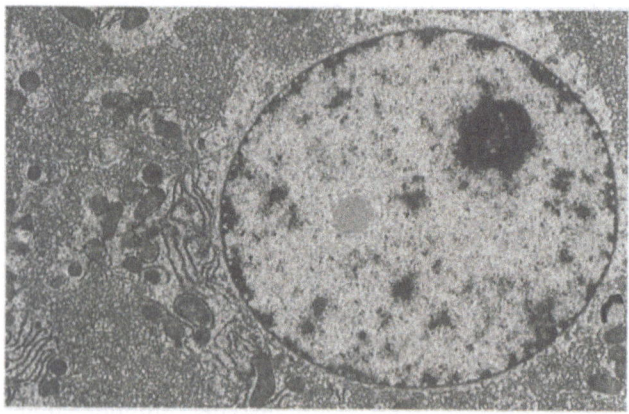

Figure 3.45 Liver cells showing proliferation of smooth endoplasmic reticulum from a rat given phenobarbitone sodium. Electron micrograph

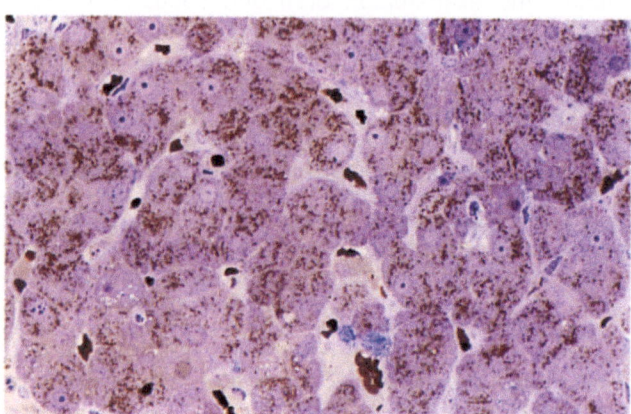

Figure 3.46 Increased catalase activity in peroxisomes in the liver of a monkey from a toxicity study with a hypolipidaemic drug. Note the brown particulate deposits in the hepatocyte cytoplasm. 1 μm resin section. Catalase

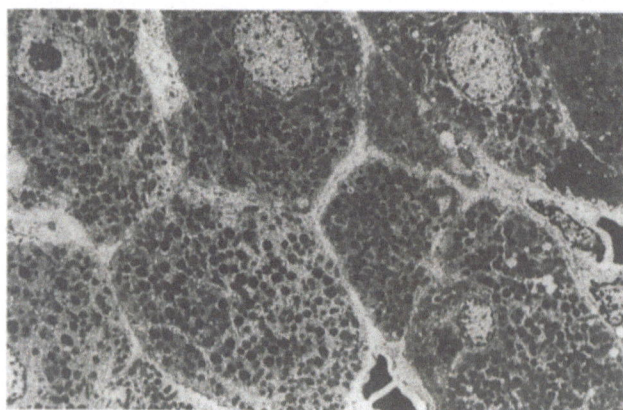

Figure 3.47 Prominent increase in microbodies (peroxisomes) in the liver of a rat from a toxicity study with a hypolipidaemic drug. Electron micrograph

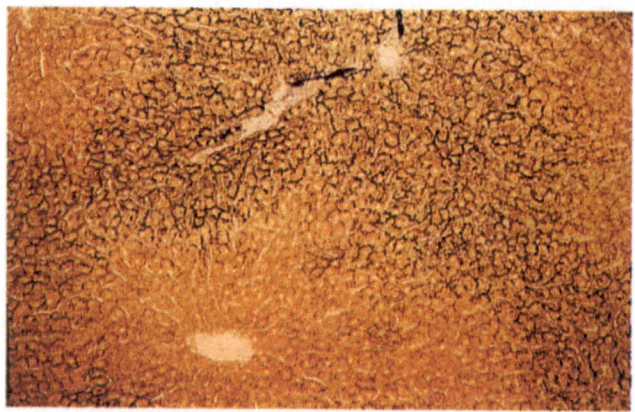

Figure 3.48 Strong canalicular alkaline phosphatase activity in the periportal hepatocytes in the liver of a rat treated with ethinyl oestradiol. Alkaline phosphatase

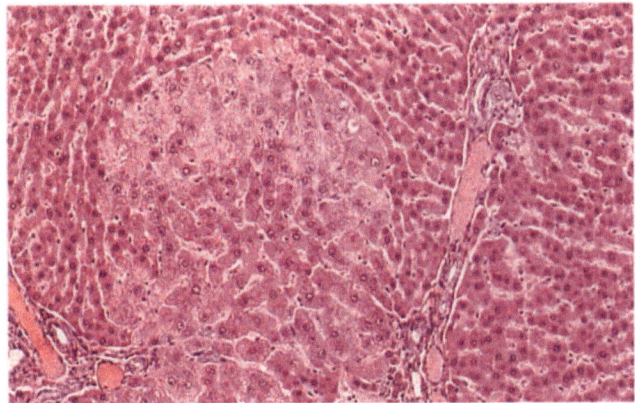

Figure 3.49 A focus of altered eosinophilic hepatocytes in the liver of a rat from a chronic toxicity study. A group of enlarged cells with eosinophilic cytoplasm is embedded within the normal parenchyma. H & E

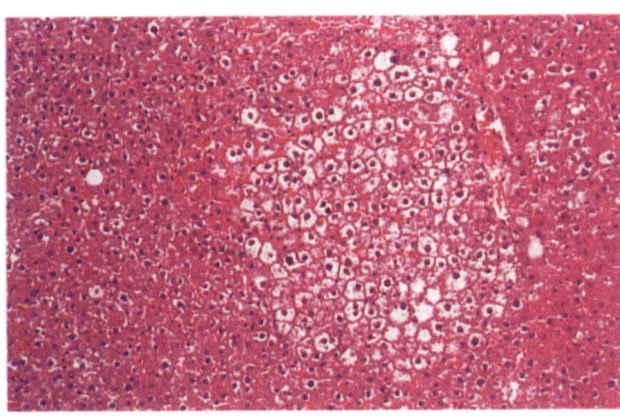

Figure 3.50 A focus of altered clear cells in the liver of a rat from a chronic toxicity study. A group of liver cells with rarefied cytoplasmic staining are embedded within the normal parenchyma. H & E

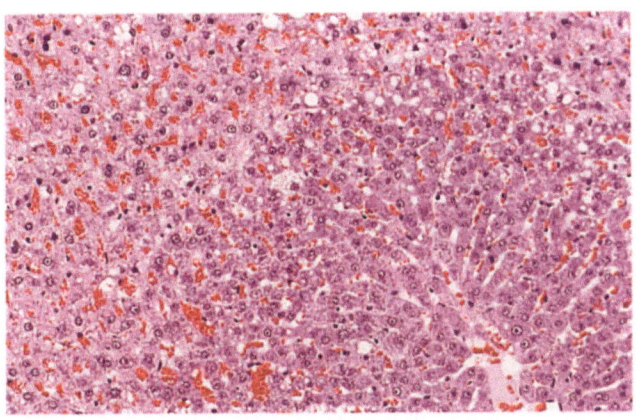

Figure 3.51 A focus of altered basophilic hepatocytes in the liver of a rat from a chronic toxicity study. A group of smaller cells with more basophilic cytoplasm is embedded within the normal parenchyma. H & E

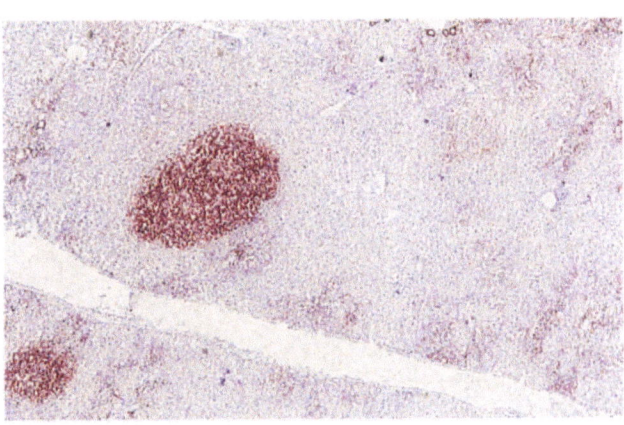

Figure 3.52 Foci of altered hepatocytes in a rat showing positive γ-glutamyltranspeptidase staining. γ-Glutamyltranspeptidase

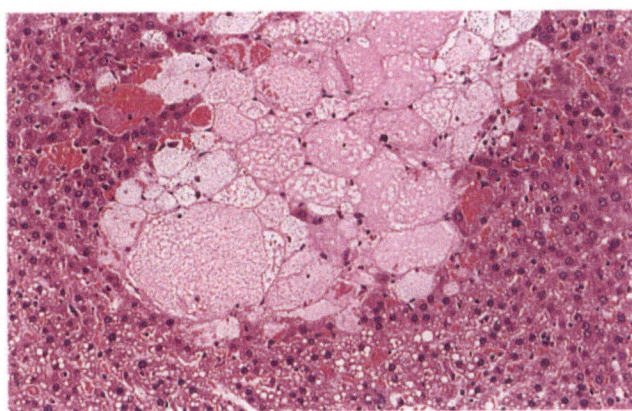

Figure 3.53 An area of cystic degeneration (spongiosis hepatis) in the liver of a rat from a chronic toxicity study. Markedly distended cells and multilocular cystic spaces containing pale homogeneous pink material. Flattened nuclei are present on the lining of the cystic structures. H & E

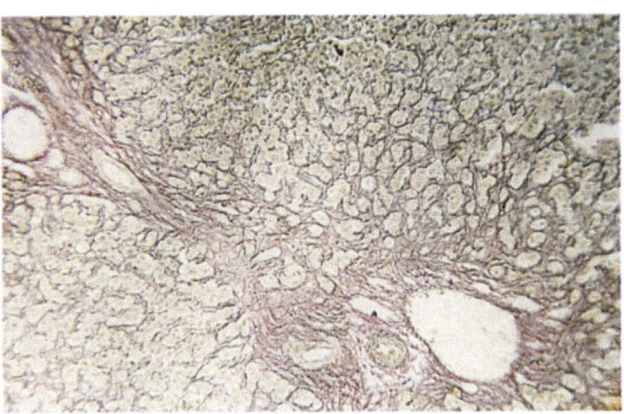

Figure 3.54 Periportal and perilobular fibrosis and reticulin duplication in the liver of a rat from a chronic toxicity study. Reticulin

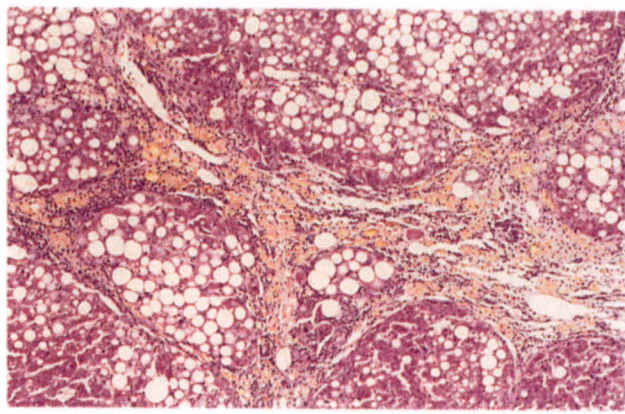

Figure 3.55 Fatty change, diffuse nodular hyperplasia and inter-lobular fibrosis in the liver of a rat maintained for prolonged periods on a choline-deficient diet.   H & E

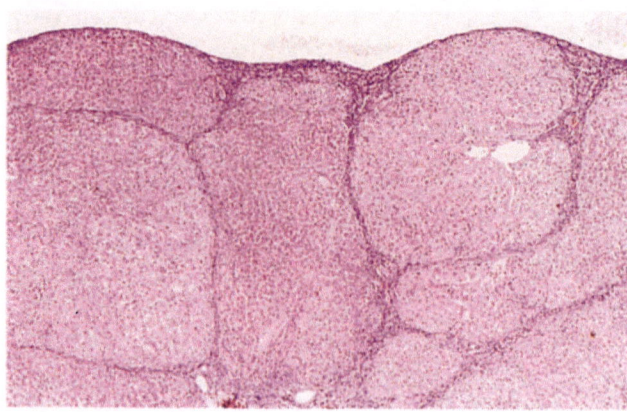

Figure 3.56 Diffuse nodular hyperplasia in the liver of a rat treated with 2-AAF. Normal lobular architecture is replaced by multiple groups of hyperplastic liver cells separated by strands of fibrous tissue.   H & E

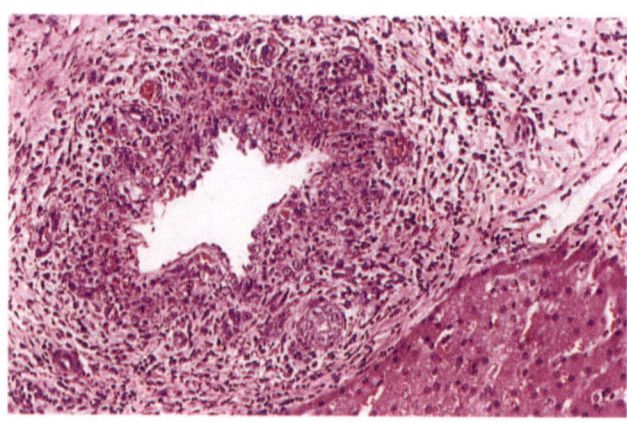

Figure 3.57 Necrotizing cholangitis and pericholangitis in the liver of a dog from a toxicity study with an anti-hypertensive. Necrosis and loss of the epithelium of bile ducts. Inflammation affecting the wall of the duct and periductular connective tissue.   H & E

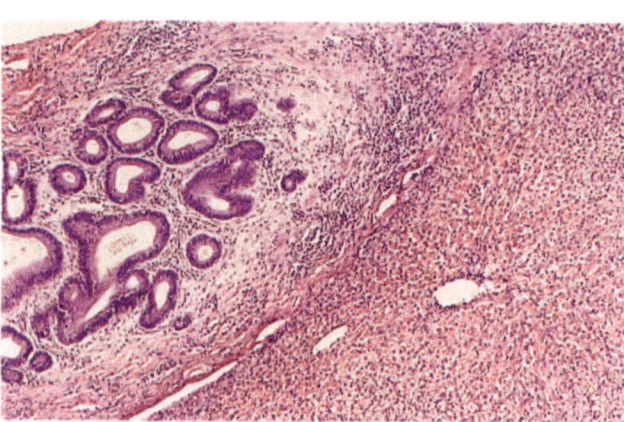

Figure 3.58 Bile duct hyperplasia, periductular inflammation and fibrosis affecting major intrahepatic ducts in the liver of a dog from a toxicity study with a novel antidepressant. This form of intrahepatic bile duct proliferation with fibrosis is, in our experience, extremely rare in the dog.   H & E

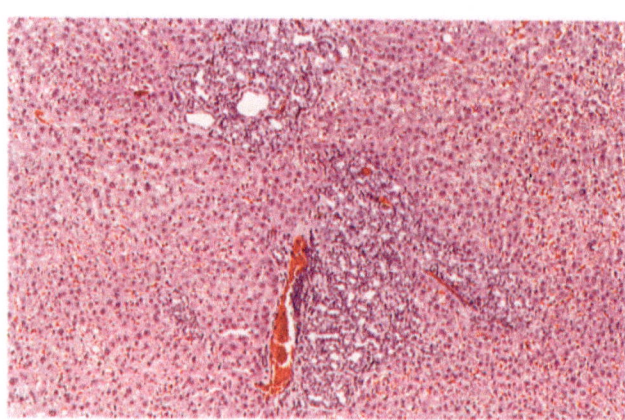

Figure 3.59 Bile duct hyperplasia in the liver of a rat from a chronic toxicity study. Intrahepatic biliary proliferation is a relatively common toxic response in the rat.   H & E

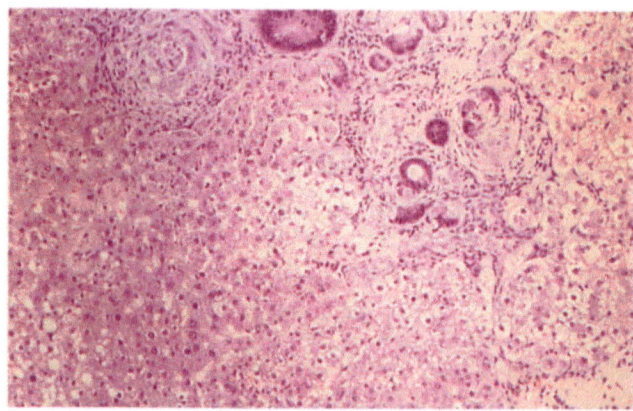

Figure 3.60 Cholangiofibrosis in the liver of a rat from a chronic toxicity study. The portal area reveals proliferation of bile ducts with abnormal epithelium and dense collagenous tissue.   H & E

basophilic liver cells with vesicular nuclei. Prolonged experimental choline deficiency leads to extensive fatty change, fibrosis, diffuse nodular hyperplasia and cirrhosis (Figure 3.55). Experimentally repeated administration of the hepatotoxin carbon tetrachloride can also cause fibrosis, diffuse nodular hyperplasia (Figure 3.56) and cirrhosis[39]. Cirrhosis may be described as a progressive condition where there is evidence of destruction of the parenchyma, with fibrosis and nodular hyperplasia. This is associated with distortion of the normal architecture and circulatory disorientation due to repeated reconstruction. Diffuse nodular hyperplasia of rodent liver can be induced by both carcinogenic and non-carcinogenic chemicals and by dietary factors[14].

Bile duct lesions

Necrosis of bile duct epithelium, cholangitis, pericholangitis and hyperplasia are some of the toxic responses which may be encountered (Figures 3.57–3.59). The epithelial damage and inflammation represent the acute reaction and prolonged or delayed reaction is expressed as bile duct hyperplasia. Chemicals such as α-naphthyl isothiocyanate in rodents, and phytotoxins and mycotoxins in several species are known to produce biliary lesions. Ulcerative inflammation of the common bile duct is induced in rats given high doses of bis-(tri-*n*-butyltin)oxide[40], obstructive cholangitis with necrosis of the epithelium is reported in sporidesmin toxicity of sheep[41].

Cholangiofibrosis is a rare lesion seen in the rat liver under certain chronic hepatotoxic conditions. The lesion is characterized by marked proliferation of bile ducts within a dense fibrous tissue and the epithelium often shows metaplastic changes including goblet cell differentiation (Figures 3.60 and 3.61). The ductular lumina are distended with mucus. Cholangiofibrosis in rats is found in chronic feeding studies with carcinogens like 4-dimethyl-aminoazobenzine (DAB) or 2-acetylaminofluorine (2-AAF)[14].

Oval cell proliferation

The term oval cell proliferation is used to describe groups of proliferating cells usually in periportal (centriacinar) areas. The cells are small with pale-staining oval nuclei and scanty basophilic cytoplasm usually seen in rodent studies with carcinogens like DAB (Figure 3.62). The origin of oval cells is a much discussed subject, with some reports proposing bile ducts[42] while others suggest stem cells, with the ability to differentiate into transitional forms and hepatocytes[43]. However, the ability of oval cells to convert into hepatocytes has recently been disputed[44].

Glandular cells resembling exocrine pancreas tissue are reported in the liver of rats fed polycholorinated biphenyls for 6 months[45].

Sinusoidal cell changes

Changes affecting sinusoidal lining cells are rare in toxicity studies. Sinusoidal cells and Kupffer cells distended with foamy cytoplasm are seen in drug-induced systemic phospholipidosis. Vacuolation or distension of cytoplasm of sinusoidal cells due to storage of lipoid and other components have been recorded in chronic feeding studies (Figures 3.63 and 3.64). Increased prominence of Ito cells (fat storing cells) is seen in dogs and other laboratory animals given high and prolonged dosages with carotenoid compounds (Figure 3.65). Groups of macrophages with foamy and vacuolated cytoplasm, some of which contain lipoid substances, have been encountered in the liver sinusoids of dogs and rats in prolonged dietary studies (Figures 3.66–3.68). Prolonged dosing with nitrate salts or certain contraceptive steroids containing oestrogens produces focal sinusoidal dilation (Figure 3.69). Focal sinusoidal dilation and peliosis hepatis are induced in rodent liver by agents such as nitrosamines and pyrrolizidine alkaloids[46,47]. Peliosis hepatis is a vascular lesion of the liver appearing as multiple cystic spaces forming blood lakes, associated with loss of hepatic cell cords (Figure 3.70). Plant toxins containing pyrrolizidine alkaloids are known to cause vascular endothelial damage and veno-occlusion of the branches of hepatic veins (centrilobular) in several species including man[14].

Gallbladder Lesions

Gallbladder lesions are uncommon in routine toxicity studies (Table 3.1). Some of the vincamine derivatives cause brown granular pigmentation of the epithelium at high doses in dogs. Prolonged administration of synthetic progestogens to dogs results in cystic mucinous hyperplasia (Figure 3.71) of the gallbladder mucosa[48]. Gallstones can be induced by lincomycin in guinea pigs, by dihydrocholesterol in rabbits and with a high cholesterol diet in squirrel monkeys[49–51]. The lincomycin-induced gallstones in guinea pigs are associated with mucosal change, including cholecystitis and development of tubulo-alveolar glands[50]. Epithelial hyperplasia and hypertrophy with cystic dilation are induced in the gallbladder of monkeys treated with polychlorinated biphenyl[52]. Dogs given high doses of clindamycin develop ulceration of gallbladder mucosa[53]. Subepithelial oedema and inflammation has been noticed in certain acute toxicity studies with a novel pharmaceutical in the canine gallbladder in our laboratories (Figure 3.72).

References

1. Zimmerman, H. J. and Ishak, K. G. (1979). Hepatotoxic injury due to drugs and toxins. In MacSween, R. N. M., Anthony, P. P. and Scheur, P. J. (eds.) *Pathology of Liver.* p. 335. (London: Churchill Livingstone)
2. Plaa, G. L. (1980). Toxic responses of the liver. In Doull, J., Klaassen, C. D. and Amdur, M. O. (eds) *Casarett and Doull's Toxicology.* 2nd Edn, p. 206. (London: Macmillan Publishing Co. Inc.)
3. Zimmerman, H. J. (1982). Chemical injury and its detection. In Plaa, G. L. and Hewitt, W. R. P. L. (eds.) *Toxicology of the Liver.* (New York: Raven Press)
4. Popper, H. and Schaffner, F. (1959). Drug-induced hepatic injury. *Ann. Intern. Med.,* **51**, 1230–1252
5. Rouiller, C. (1964). Experimental toxic injury of the liver. In Rouiller, C. (ed.) *The Liver.* Vol. 2, p. 335. (New York: Academic Press)
6. Jollow, D. J., Mitchell, J. R., Zampaglione, N. and Gillette, J. R. (1974). Bromobenzene-induced liver necrosis. Protective role of glutathione and evidence for 3,4-bromobenzene oxide as hepatotoxic metabolite. *Pharmacology,* **11**, 151–169
7. Reynolds, E. S. and Moslen, M. T. (1980). Environmental liver injury. Halogenated hydrocarbons. In Part B. Farber, E. and Fisher, M. M. (eds.) *Toxic Injury of the Liver,* p. 541. (New York: Marcel Dekker)
8. Ortega, P. (1966). Light and electron microscopy of dichloro-diphenyl trichloroethane (DDT) poisoning in the rat liver. *Lab. Invest.,* **15**, 657–679
9. Gopinath, C. and Ford, E. J. H. (1975). The role of microsomal hydroxylases in the modification of chloroform hepatotoxicity in rats. *Br. J. Exp. Pathol.,* **56**, 412–422
10. Rappaport, A. M. (1979). Physicochemical basis of toxic injury. In Farber, E. and Fisher, M. M. (eds.) *Toxic Injury of the Liver.* Part A, p. 2. (New York: Marcel Dekker Inc.)
11. Magos, L. and Butler, W. H. (1972). Effect of phenobarbitone

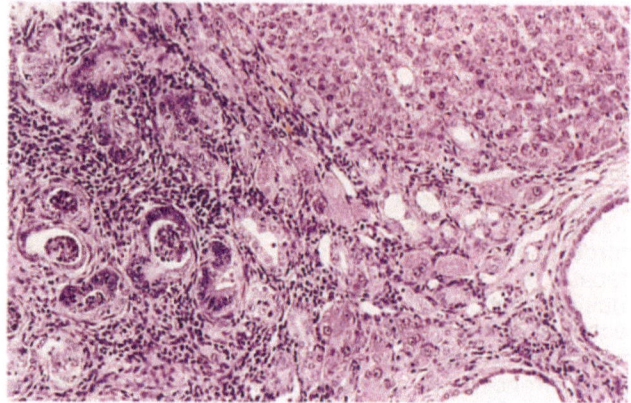

Figure 3.61 Cholangiofibrosis in a rat treated with 2-AAF. Hyperplasia of bile ducts, metaplasia of the bile duct epithelium, fibrosis and inflammation in portal areas.   H & E

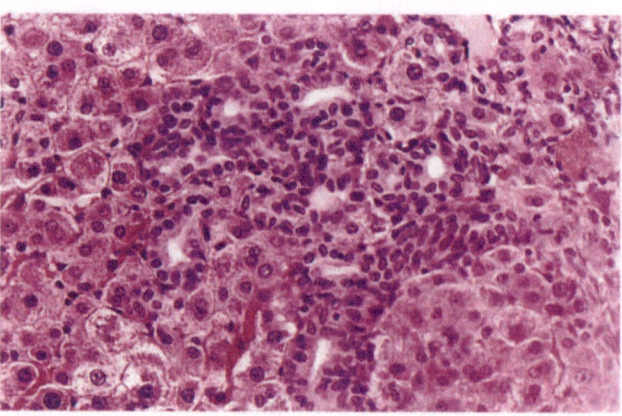

Figure 3.62 Oval cell proliferation in the liver of a rat from a chronic toxicity study with 2-AAF. Groups of basophilic, oval shaped, undifferentiated cells around proliferating bile ducts. The origin of these cells remains uncertain.   H & E

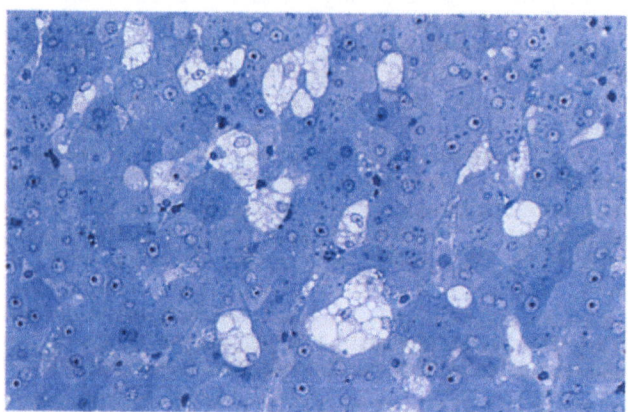

Figure 3.63 Vacuolated and distended Kupffer cells in the liver of a monkey from a toxicity study with a novel antineoplastic drug. 1 μm resin section. Toluidine Blue

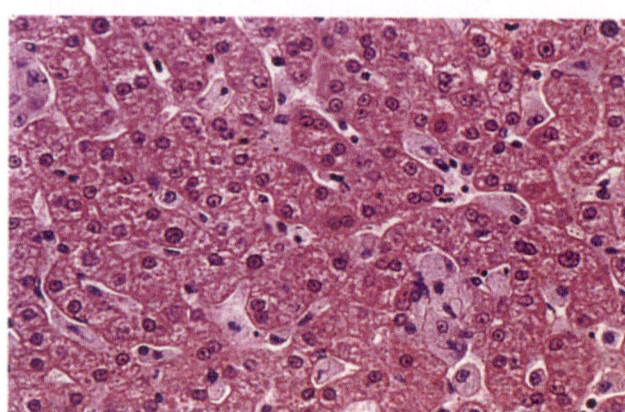

Figure 3.64 Distended cells with pale ground glass appearance of the cytoplasm in the hepatic sinusoids in a dog from a toxicity study using an antineoplastic compound. Similar changes were present in glomeruli.   H & E

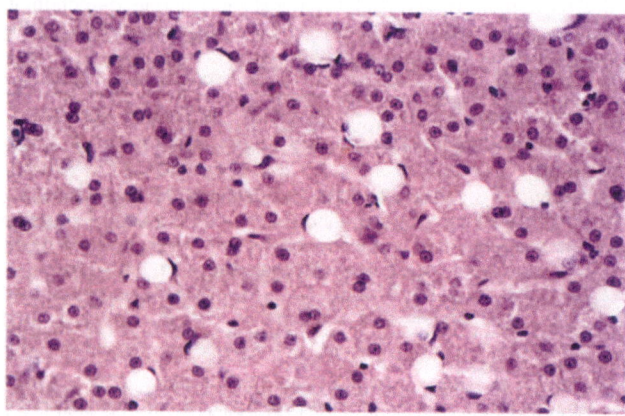

Figure 3.65 Prominent vacuolated Ito cells (fat storing cells) with clear cytoplasm and flattened nuclei in the hepatic sinusoids of a dog treated with a carotenoid compound.   H & E

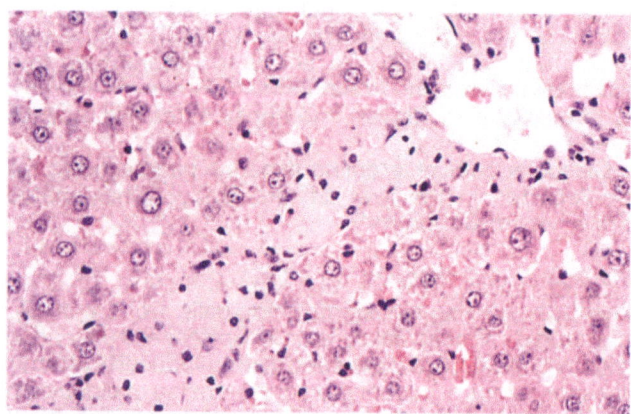

Figure 3.66 Groups of macrophages with foamy cytoplasm in the hepatic sinusoids of a mouse from a chronic toxicity study. H & E

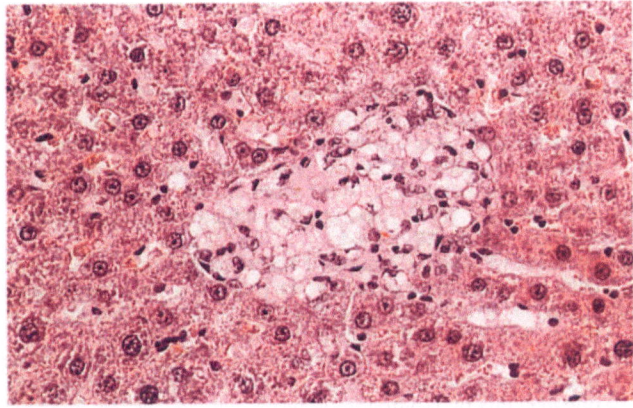

Figure 3.67 Lipoid granuloma ('fatty cysts') in the liver of a dog from a long-term toxicity study with chloroform. Note the group of macrophages with vacuolated cytoplasm.   H & E

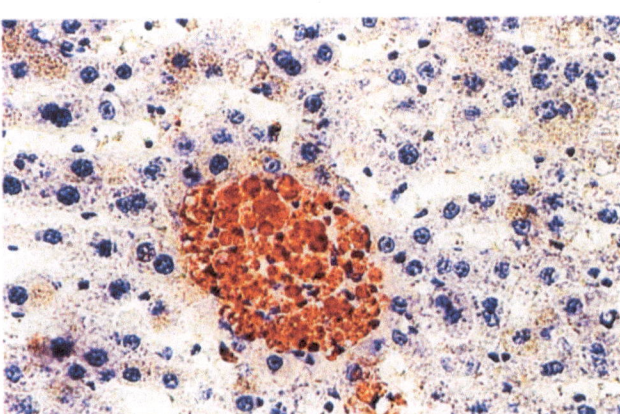

Figure 3.68 Group of macrophages ('fatty cysts') with fat in the cytoplasm in the liver of a rat from a chronic feeding study with a novel agrochemical. Frozen section. Oil Red O

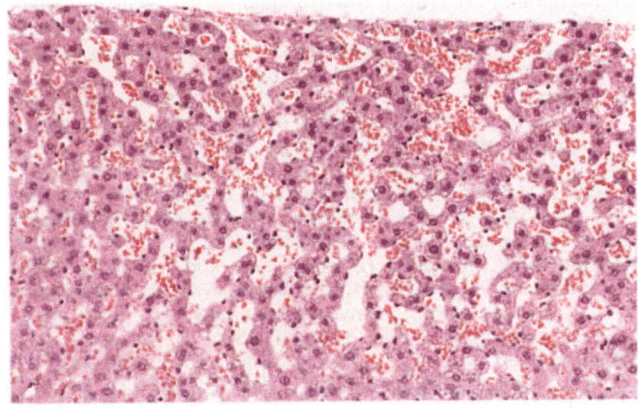

Figure 3.69 Focal sinusoidal dilation in the liver of a rat from a chronic toxicity study. Note the area of subcapsular sinusoids showing abnormal distension. These changes are recorded with nitrate salts and oestrogenic steroids.   H & E

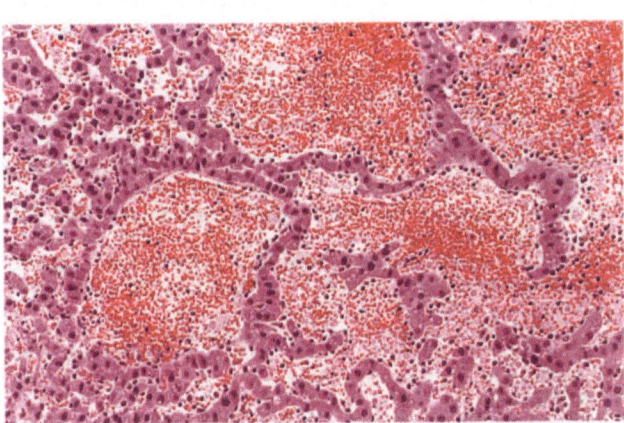

Figure 3.70 Peliosis hepatis in a rat liver. Cystic sinusoidal spaces containing blood with loss of hepatic cords. Agents such as nitrosamines and pyrrolizidine alkaloids induce such changes.   H & E

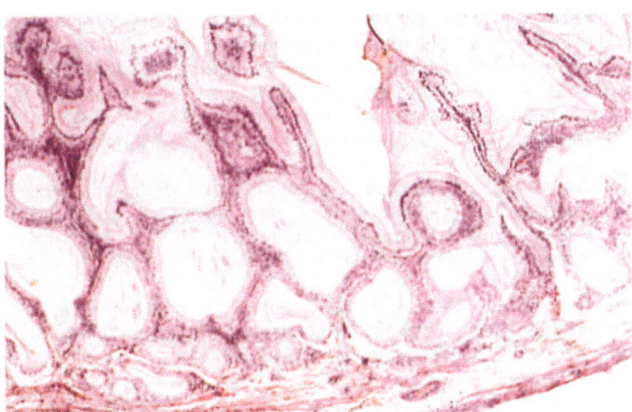

Figure 3.71 Cystic mucinous hyperplasia of the gall bladder in a dog from a long-term toxicity study with a contraceptive steroid.   H & E

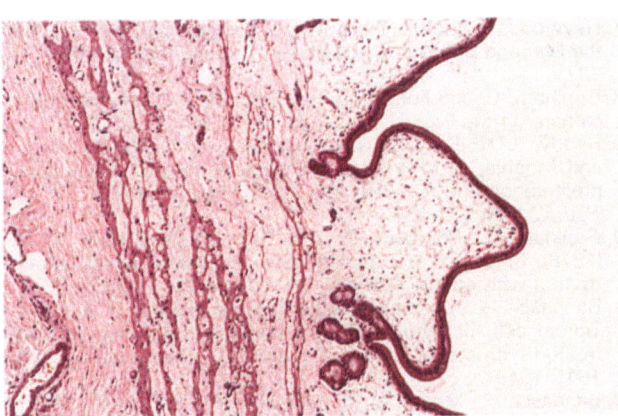

Figure 3.72 Subepithelial oedema and inflammatory cells induced in the gall bladder of a dog by an industrial chemical. H & E

and starvation on hepatotoxicity in rats exposed to carbon disulfide. *Br. J. Ind. Med.*, **29**, 95–98

12. Gopinath, C. and Ford, E. J. H. (1976). The effect of induced hepatic microsomal amidopyrine demethylase activity on the susceptibility of the liver of the calf and horse to carbon disulphide. *J. Comp. Pathol.*, **86**, 251–258

13. Farber, J. L. (1979). Reaction of the liver to injury. In Farber, E. and Fisher, M. M. (eds.) *Toxic Injury of the Liver*. Part A, p. 215. (New York: Marcel Dekker Inc.)

14. Butler, W. H. (1979). Experimental liver injury. In MacSween, R. N. M., Anthony P. P. and Scheur, P. (eds.) *Pathology of the Liver*. p. 55. (London: Churchill Livingstone)

15. Gopinath, C., Prentice, D. E., Street, A. E. and Crook, D. (1980). Serum bile acid concentration in some experimental liver lesions of rat. *Toxicology*, **15**, 113–127

16. Thorpe, E., Gopinath, C., Jones, R. S. and Ford, E. J. H. (1969). The effect of chloroform on the liver and the activity of serum enzymes in the horse. *J. Pathol.*, **97**, 241–251

17. Kerr, J. F. R., Bishop, C. J. and Searle, J. (1986). Apoptosis. In Anthony, P. P. and MacSween, R. N. M. (eds.) *Recent Advances in Histopathology 12*. p. 1. (London: Churchill Livingstone)

18. Bursch, W., Lauer, B., Timmermann-Trosiener, I., Barthel, G., Schuppler, J. and Schulte-Herman, R. (1984). Controlled death (apoptosis) of normal and putative preneoplastic cells in rat liver following withdrawal of tumour promoters. *Carcinogenesis*, **5**, 453–458

19. Kerr, J. F. R. (1971). Shrinkage necrosis: a distinct mode of cellular death. *J. Pathol.*, **105**, 13–20

20. Butler, W. H. (1964). Acute toxicity of aflatoxin, B₁ in rats. *Br. J. Cancer*, **18**, 756–762

21. Schoental, R. and Magee, P. N. (1959). Further observations on the sub acute and chronic liver changes in rats after a single dose of various pyrrolizidine (senecio) alkaloids. *J. Pathol. Bacteriol.*, **78**, 471–482

22. Jones, G. and Butler, W. H. (1974). A morphological study of the liver lesion induced by 2,3,7,8-tetrachloro-dibenzo-p-dioxin in rats. *J. Pathol.*, **112**, 93–97

23. Lüllmann, H., Lüllmann-Rauch, R. and Wassermann, O. (1975). Drug induced phospholipidosis. II. Tissue distribution of the amphophilic drug chlorphentermine. *CRC. Crit. Rev. Toxicol.*, **4**, 185–218

24. Meierhenry, E. F., Ruebner, B. H., Greshuin, M. E., Hsieh, L. S. and French, S. W. (1981). Mallory body formation in hepatic nodules of mice ingesting dieldrin. *Lab. Invest.*, **44**, 392–396

25. Reddy, J. K., Lalwani, N. D., Reddy, M. K. and Qureshi, S. A. (1982). Excessive accumulation of autofluorescent lipofuscin in the liver during hepatocarcinogenesis by methylclofinapate and other hypolipidaemic peroxisome proliferators. *Cancer Res.*, **42**, 259–266

26. Ishmael, J., Gopinath, C. and McHowell, J. (1971). Experimental chronic copper toxicity in sheep. Histological and histochemical changes during the development of the lesions in the liver. *Res. Vet. Sci.*, **12**, 358–366

27. Heywood, S. (1980). The effect of excess dietary copper on the liver and kidney of the male rat. *J. Comp. Pathol.*, **90**, 217–232

28. Gopinath, C. and Ford, E. J. H. (1969). The effect of Lantana camara on the liver of sheep. *J. Pathol.*, **99**, 75–85

29. Reddy, J. K., Lalwani, N. D., Qureshi, S. A., Reddy, M. K. and Moehle, C. M. (1984). Induction of hepatic peroxisome proliferation in non-rodent species including primates. *Am. J. Pathol.*, **114**, 171–183

30. Gopinath, C., Rombout, P. J. A. and van Versendaal, R. G. (1978). Serum alkaline phosphatase elevation in female rats treated with ethinyl estradiol. *Toxicology*, **10**, 91–102

31. Bannasch, P., Benner, V., Enzmann, H. and Hacker, H. J. (1985). Tigroid cell foci and neoplastic nodules in the liver of rats treated with a single dose of aflatoxin B₁. *Carcinogenesis*, **6**, 1641–1648

32. Bannasch, P., Moore, M. A., Klimek, F. and Zerban, H. (1982). Biological markers of pre-neoplastic foci and neoplastic nodules in rodent liver. *Toxicol. Pathol.*, **10**, 19–36

33. William, G. M. and Watanabe, K. (1978). Quantitative kinetics of development of N-2-fluo-renyl acetamide induced altered foci. *J. Natl. Cancer Inst.*, **61**, 113–121

34. Ogawa, K., Onoe, T. and Takeuchi, M. (1981). Spontaneous occurrence of γ–glutamyl transpeptidase-positive hepatocyte foci in 105-week old Wistar and 72-week old Fischer 344 male rats. *J. Nat. Cancer Inst.*, **67**, 407–412

35. Ohmori, T., Rice, J. M. and Williams, G. M. (1981). Histochemical characteristics of spontaneous and chemically induced hepatocellular neoplasms in mice and the development of neoplasms with γ-glutamyl transpeptidase activity during phenobarbital exposure. *Histochem. J.*, **13**, 85–99

36. Weinbren, K. (1982). Experimental diffuse nodular hyperplasia. *Toxicol. Pathol.*, **10**, 81–94

37. Bannasch, P. (1983). Strain and species differences in susceptibility to liver tumour induction. In Turusov, V. and Montesana, R. (eds.) *Modulators of Experimental Carcinogenesis*. p. 9. (Lyon: IARC Scientific Publications 51)

38. Bannasch, P., Bloch, M. and Zarban, H. (1981). Spongiosis hepatis: specific changes of the perisinusoidal liver cells induced in rats by N-nitrosomorphiline. *Lab. Invest.*, **44**, 252–264

39. McLean, E. K., McLean, A. E. M. and Sutton, P. M. (1969). 'Instant Cirrhosis'. An improved method of producing cirrhosis of the liver in rats by simultaneous administration of carbon tetrachloride and phenobarbitone. *Br. J. Exp. Pathol.*, **50**, 502–506

40. Krajnc, E. J., Wester, P. W., Loeber, J. G., van Leeuwen, F. X. R., Vos, J. G., Vaessen, H. A. M. G. and van der Heijden, C. A. (1984). Toxicity of Bis-(tri-n-butyl tin) oxide in the rat. 1. Short term effects of general parameters and on the endocrine and lymphoid systems. *Toxicol. Appl. Pharmacol.*, **75**, 363–383

41. Mortimer, P. H. (1963). The experimental intoxication of sheep with sporidesmin, a metabolic product of Pathomyces chartarum IV. Histological and histochemical examinations of orally dosed sheep. *Res. Vet. Sci.*, **4**, 166–185

42. Grisham, J. W. and Hartroft, W. S. (1961). Morphological identification by electron microscopy of 'oval' cells in experimental hepatic degeneration. *Lab. Invest.*, **10**, 317–332

43. Dempo, K., Chisaka, N., Yoshida, Y., Kaneko, A. and Onoe, T. (1975). Immunofluorescent study on α-fetoprotein producing cells in early stage of 3'-methyl-4-dimethylamino-azobenzene carcinogenesis. *Cancer. Res.*, **35**, 1282–1287

44. Tatematsu, M., Kaku, T., Ekem, J. K. and Farber, E. (1984). Studies on the proliferation and fate of oval cells in the liver of rats treated with 2-acetylaminofluorene and partial hepatectomy. *Am. J. Pathol.*, **114**, 418–430

45. Kimbrough, R. D. (1973). Pancreatic type tissue in livers of rats fed polychlorinated biphenyls. *J. Natl. Cancer Inst.*, **51**, 679–681

46. Ruebner, B. H., Watanabe, K. and Ward, J. S. (1970). Lytic necrosis resembling peliosis hepatis produced by lasiocarpine in mouse liver. A light and electron microscopic study. *Am J. Pathol.*, **60**, 247–270

47. Ungar, H. (1986). Veno-occlusive disease of the liver and phlebectatic peliosis in golden hamsters exposed to dimethyl nitrosamine. *Pathol. Res. Pract.*, **181**, 180–187

48. Neilson, L. W. and Kelly, W. A. (1976). Progestogen-induced gross and microscopic changes in female dogs. *Vet. Pathol.*, **13**, 143–156

49. Lee, S. P. and Scott, A. J. (1979). Dihydrocholesterol-induced gall stones in the rabbit: evidence that bile acids cause gall bladder epithelial injury. *Br. J. Exp. Pathol.*, **60**, 231–238

50. Scott, A. J. (1976). Lincomycin-induced cholecystitis and gallstones in guinea pigs. *Gastroenterology*, **11**, 814–820

51. Lofland, H. B. (1975). Cholelithiasis. *Am. J. Pathol.*, **79**, 619–622

52. Tryphonas, L., Truelove, J., Zawidzka, Z., Wong, J., Mes, J., Charbonneau, S., Grant, D. L. and Campbell, J. S. (1984). Polychlorinated biphenyl (PCB) toxicity in adult cynomolgus monkeys (*M. fascicularis*): A pilot study. *Toxicol. Pathol.*, **12**, 10–25

53. Gray, J. E., Weaver, R. N., Bollert, J. A. and Feenstra, E. S. (1972). The oral toxicity of clindamycin in laboratory animals. *Toxicol. Appl. Pharmacol.*, **21**, 516–531

There are several features which might be expected to make the alimentary system a prime target for induced lesions:

(i) Like the skin and lung the alimentary system is directly exposed to environmental chemicals and is the first organ in contact with test substances in toxicity studies where, as is common, they are administered orally.

(ii) The alimentary system is inevitably exposed to high concentrations of orally administered substances and exposure to substances excreted in the bile may be repeated and the effects thus compounded.

(iii) The vulnerability of the critical balance between constant cell division and cell loss leaves obvious scope for erosion or hyperplasia[1].

However, if the gastric ulceration induced by non-steroidal anti-inflammatory compounds is excluded, toxicological changes are not commonly encountered in the alimentary system.

Oral Cavity

Lesions of the oral cavity in general, and dental lesions in particular, are only rarely observed in toxicity studies. Induced lesions are listed in Table 4.1.

However, lesions may be occasionally observed, particularly in studies involving dietary modification and manipulation including sugars and sugar substitutes. When a basic cariogenic diet containing 46% sucrose is used, it is found that replacement of 20% of the sucrose by the substitute xylitol (or by wheat starch) reduces the amount of caries[2].

Table 4.1 Induced lesions of the oral cavity, oesophagus and salivary glands

---

Oral Cavity
 Caries
 Odontogenic lesions
 Gingival hyperplasia

Oesophagus
 Oesophagitis
 Megaoesophagus

Salivary glands
 Acinar hypertrophy
 Acinar atrophy
 Acinar degeneration
 Ductal changes

Odontogenic lesions are reported following single intraperitoneal injections of cyclophosphamide to rats[3]. These lesions include broken, absent, elongated and supernumerary teeth. Single intraperitoneal doses of N-nitroso-N-methylurea also induce odontogenic lesions in rats[4]. The predominant lesion is the development of supernumerary lower incisors which develop adjacent to the apical proliferative part of these continually erupting teeth.

In one study in our laboratories, broken incisors were a frequent finding in rats treated with a compound with chelating properties. The shortened incisors were composed of a thin, hollow tube of enamel and dentine but the central pulp cavity was congested, haemorrhagic and necrotic with disorientation and loss of odontoblasts (Figure 4.1). In man, the chelating action of tetracyclines is believed to cause binding to calcium ions with complex formation in teeth and subsequent hypoplasia[5].

Gingival hyperplasia, with a prominent plasma cell infiltration, is reported in several species, including man, following administration of some compounds[5]. With cyclosporin A, gingivitis with atrophy of periodontal tissue and divergent incisor teeth are reported in rats, and hypertrophic gingivitis (Figure 4.2) and periodontitis in dogs[6]. Gingival hyperplasia appears to be a common side-effect of calcium channel blockers. In our laboratories this lesion has been detected in dogs in several studies and is described in man with nifedipine[7], and in *Macaca arctoides*, cats and man with diphenylhydantoin[5,8]. Histologically, the lesion is characterized by pronounced epithelial hyperplasia, parakeratosis, proliferation, reticulation and elongation of rete pegs with oedema and infiltration of plasma cells and lymphocytes.

Gingival erosions and ulcerations are reported in monkeys treated with a polychlorinated biphenyl[9]. The lesions are associated with epithelial hyperplasia, collagen deposition, necrosis and oedema.

The hamster cheek pouch is a widely used model for oral carcinogenesis and may also be used to assess irritancy. Repeated applications of calcium hydroxide produce hyperplasia with focal epithelial atypia; and betel nut extract and slaked lime induce hyperplastic and hyperkeratotic lesions[10].

Oesophagus

Induced oesophageal lesions are extremely rare (Table 4.1). One of the few treatment-induced lesions we have observed involved necrotizing oesophagitis in dogs (Figure 4.3). This was probably caused by the reflux of gastric contents due to relaxation of the oesophageal sphincter.

Megaoesophagus is reported in dogs exposed to di-isopropyl fluorophosphate and acrylamide[11]. Both these compounds produce peripheral neuropathies and it is considered likely that the oesophageal lesion is secondary to damage to the vagal afferent nerve fibres.

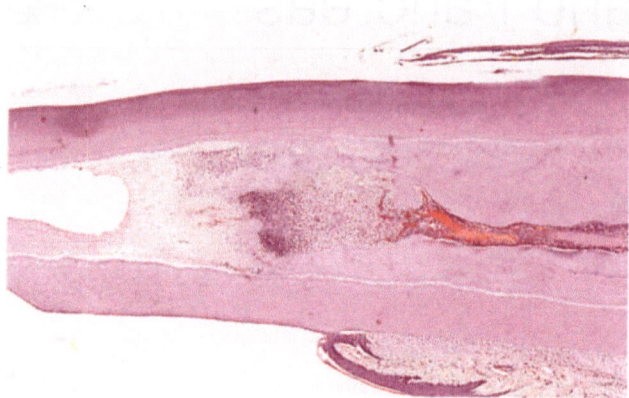

Figure 4.1 Incisor from a rat treated with a compound with chelating properties. The tooth consists of a hollow tube due to necrosis of the pulp cavity. H & E

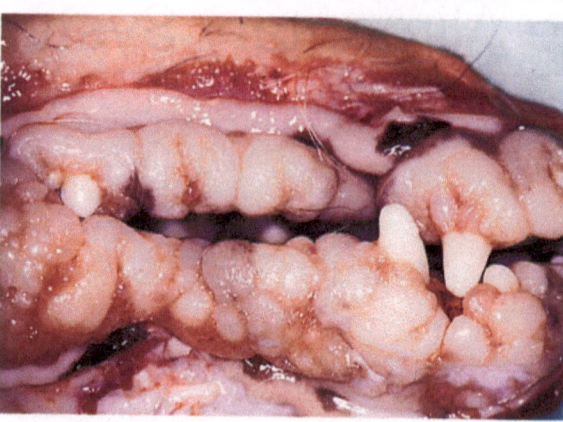

Figure 4.2 Hypertrophic gingivitis in a dog. This type of lesion is encountered following administration of cyclosporin A and calcium channel blockers. Histologically, it consists of a hyperplastic epithelium with subepithelial oedema and inflammation

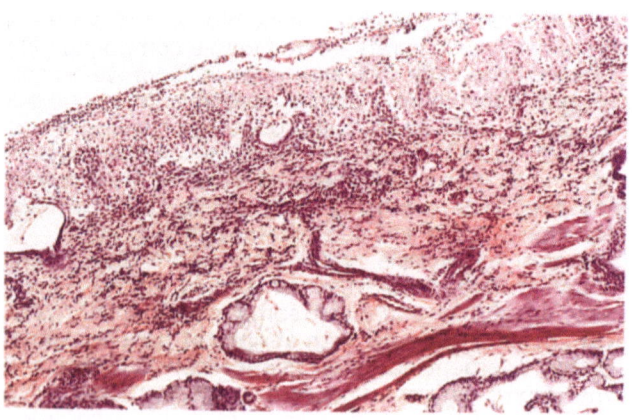

Figure 4.3 Necrotizing oesophagitis in a dog, probably due to gastric reflux following oral administration of a test compound. H & E

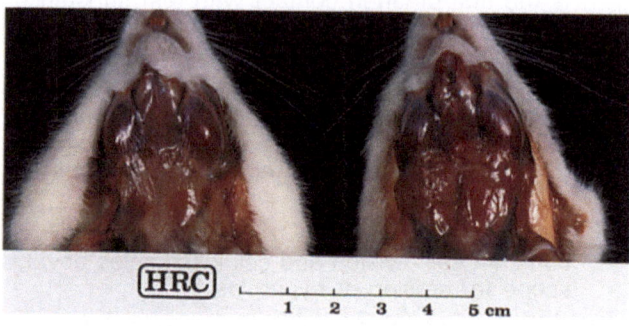

Figure 4.4 Hypertrophy of the rat submandibular salivary glands following administration of a β-sympathomimetic agonist. In comparison with the untreated animal the glands are grossly enlarged

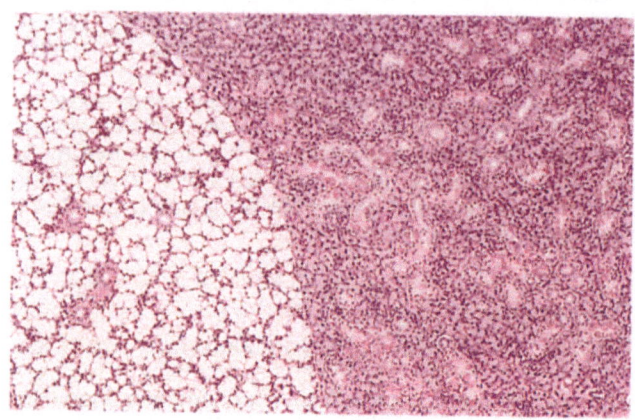

Figure 4.5 Submandibular salivary gland from a control rat. Note size of acinar cells and presence of mucus and serous acini. H & E

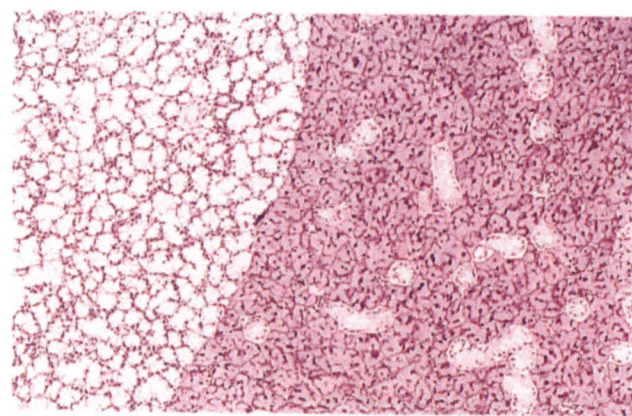

Figure 4.6 Submandibular salivary gland from a rat treated with a β-sympathomimetic agonist. In comparison with Figure 4.5, the individual serous acinar cells appear distended and enlarged. The mucus-secreting acini appear unaffected. H & E

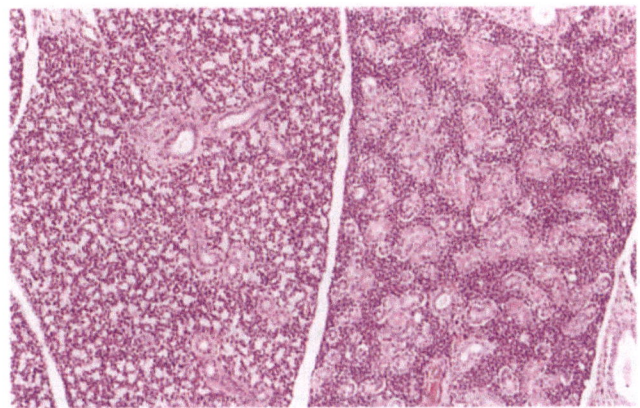

Figure 4.7 Submandibular salivary gland from a rat treated with a β-blocker. Both the serous and mucus acini are atrophic. Ducts appear more numerous due to the atrophy of acinar tissue. Compare with Figure 4.5. H & E

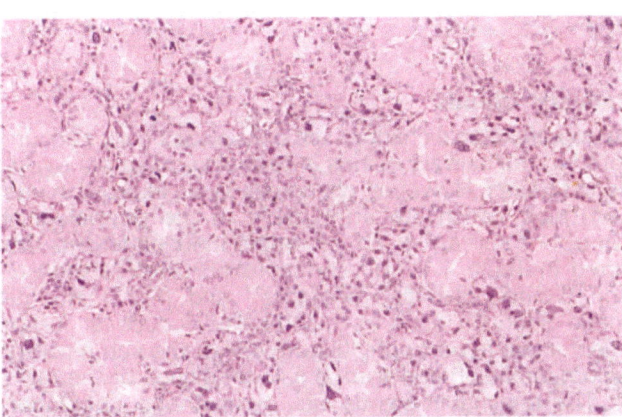

Figure 4.8 Submandibular salivary gland from a rat treated with an industrial chemical. High magnification showing atrophic acinar cells. H & E

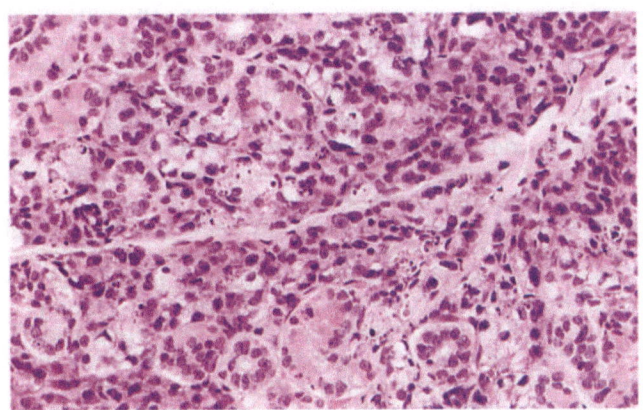

Figure 4.9 Single cell degeneration and atrophy of serous acini from submandibular salivary gland of a rat treated with a novel antibiotic, antineoplastic agent. H & E

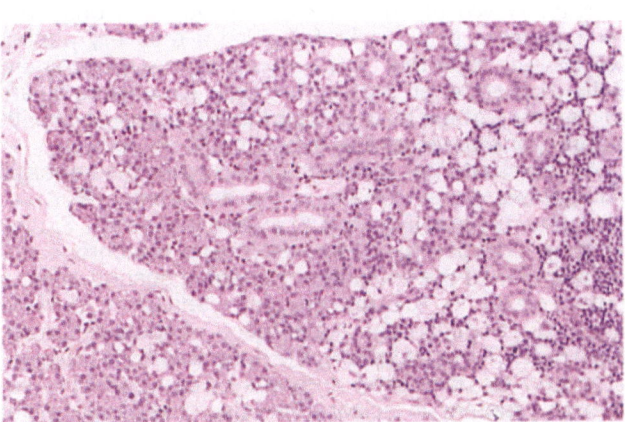

Figure 4.10 Submandibular salivary gland from a monkey following administration of a novel antineoplastic agent. The coarse acinar vacuolation is associated with mononuclear cell infiltrates. H & E

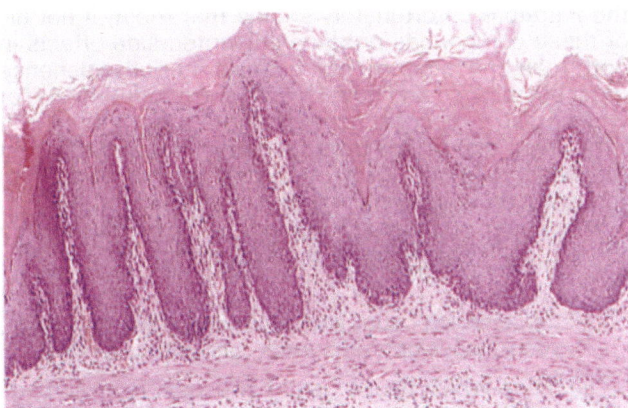

Figure 4.11 Marked hyperplasia and hyperkeratosis of the forestomach of a rat from a feeding study with an industrial chemical. H & E

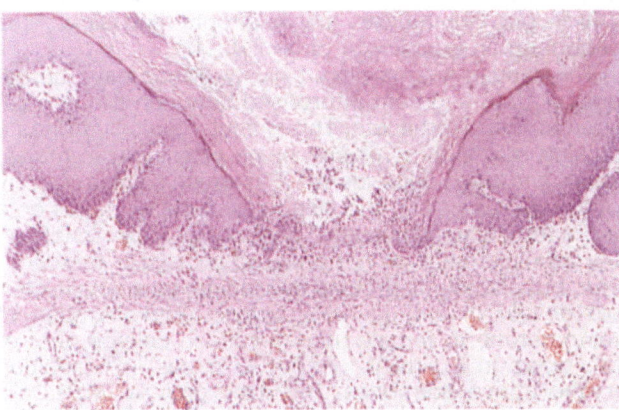

Figure 4.12 Focal ulceration of the forestomach of a rat treated orally with an industrial chemical. The adjacent epithelium shows hyperplasia and hyperkeratosis. A moderate degree of subepithelial oedema, congestion and inflammatory cell infiltration is present. H & E

Salivary Glands

Histopathological changes are only occasionally encountered in the salivary glands in toxicological safety evaluation studies. However, changes may be induced in rats and mice which are attributable to the physiological control of salivary gland secretion. Induced lesions are listed in Table 4.1. Salivary secretion involves both α- and β-catecholamine receptors[12] and β-sympathomimetic agonists such as isoprenaline induce an often spectacular hypertrophy (Figure 4.4) of the submaxillary (submandibular) and parotid salivary glands of the rat[12–14]. The sublingual glands lack sympathetic innervation and do not demonstrate this response[13]. The hypertrophic change in the salivary glands is primarily due to the increase in size of the acinar cells (Figures 4.5 and 4.6) with prominent secretion granules but an increased mitotic activity may also be detected.

Pilocarpine and chronic stimulation of the sympathetic innervation also induce hypertrophy[13,14]. The hypertrophic changes are usually readily reversible and may be regarded as an exacerbation of normal physiological activity. However, in some cases we have observed multinucleate acinar cells following a recovery period. Necrosis is reported[14] with more prolonged treatment with isoproterenol. Not surprisingly simultaneous administration of the β-adrenergic blocker propranolol with isoprenaline prevents the hypertrophic response[12].

Administration of propranolol and other β-adrenergic antagonists alone, results in the converse effect, i.e. atrophic changes (Figure 4.7) in acinar tissue[12]. Similar atrophic changes may also result from the chronic administration of the anti-adrenergic agent guanethidine; a potent α-adrenergic blocking agent, dibenamine; denervation; duct ligation and substitution of liquid ration for solid diet[12,15]. Histologically, the atrophic glands are characterized by decreased numbers of demonstrable secretion granules in acinar cells, decreased cell height and vacuolation of acinar cells. Drug-induced atrophy is also usually reversible, but after prolonged administration, necrosis and inflammatory changes develop in the mouse[16].

In rats given a DL-ethionine supplemented diet, degenerative changes are detected in the salivary glands[17]. The glands appear shrunken with nuclear pyknosis and karyorrhexis, cytoplasmic vacuolation and ductal dilatation. In rats treated with an industrial chemical (Figure 4.8) and a novel antibiotic antineoplastic agent (Figure 4.9) in our laboratories, acinar atrophy and single cell degeneration (apoptosis) were induced.

The mouse submaxillary salivary glands have an additional duct segment interposed between the intercalated and striated ducts. This granular duct illustrates a striking sexual dimorphism, being prominent in males, and is androgen-dependent[13]. Castration causes atrophy of the duct cells and the gland consequently takes on a more female appearance[13]. This change is reversible on the administration of not only the androgen, testosterone, but also of nandrolone decanoate, an anabolic steroid devoid of androgenic activity[18]. Administration of testosterone to female mice results in enlargement of the ducts in a similar manner to males[19]. In addition to the above hormones, the male granular ducts are trophically influenced by thyroxine and adrenocortical hormones[20]. Conversely, absence of thyroid hormone causes severe atrophy of the duct cells[20] and adrenalectomy produces a minor tubular atrophy which is reversible by cortisone administration[21]. Atrophic changes in salivary acinar cells are detected in rats treated with high doses of the diuretic furosemide.

Following administration of a novel antineoplastic compound to cynomolgus monkeys, acinar vacuolation with an associated inflammatory cell infiltration was detected in the salivary glands (Figure 4.10).

Stomach

The stomach of laboratory rodents such as rat, mouse and hamster is anatomically unusual in that the fore–stomach is non-glandular and serves as a food reservoir. Induced gastric lesions are classified in Table 4.2.

Table 4.2 Induced gastric lesions

Proliferative lesions of the forestomach
Ulcerative changes
ECL-cell proliferation
Hyperplastic gastropathy
Parietal cell degeneration
Parietal cell hyperplasia

Proliferative lesions of the rodent non-glandular region (Figure 4.11) are relatively common in gavage and feeding studies, ranging from mild hyperplasia of the keratinized stratified squamous epithelium to extensive papillomatous hyperplasia. Degenerative lesions involve erosion, necrosis, ulceration (Figures 4.12 and 4.13) and occasionally complete perforation with associated peritonitis (Figure 4.14). Other changes which may also be seen include hyperkeratosis, prominent rete pegs and papillae, variable degrees of inflammatory cell infiltration, oedema, haemorrhage, and intra- and subepithelial vesiculation. Following withdrawal of the causal agent regression of most of these lesions may occur. These changes are described following feeding of sodium metabisulphate[22]; dietary deficiency of vitamin A; the antioxidant BHA[23] and a range of phenols and acids[23].

Gastric ulceration is probably the most commonly encountered induced lesion in the alimentary tract. It is usually associated with oral administration of compounds but occasionally occurs via the systemic route. Ulcerative changes may be seen with a range of compounds including both pharmaceuticals and industrial chemicals but especially with non-steroidal anti-inflammatory (NSAI) drugs.

Ulceration may be extensive or extremely focal and careful macroscopic inspection is important for the detection of small lesions (Figure 4.15). NSAI compounds are amongst the most widely used drugs[24]. A review of the literature unfortunately shows that most, if not all, of these compounds produce unwanted side-effects in both man and experimental animals. In our experience most established and novel NSAIs show side-effects, of which gastric mucosal damage is the most frequent. It is believed that NSAIs produce lesions by two different mechanisms: direct contact on the mucosa; and a systemic action which only manifests after absorption.

It has been suggested[25] that drugs can be divided into three groups according to their gastrointestinal toxicity in rats:

(i) those which cause gastric mucosal haemorrhage, such as cyclophosphamide and penicillamine;

(ii) those which cause gastric mucosal haemorrhage and gastric submucosal lesions, such as acetaminophen and aspirin; and

(iii) those which cause gastric mucosal and submucosal lesions and perforations and/or adhesions of the small intestine, such as ibuprofen, indomethacin and phenylbutazone.

The development of haemorrhage, erosion or ulcerations in the gastric mucosa (Figures 4.16 and 4.17) with aspirin and other NSAI agents is frequently demonstrated in laboratory species including dog, rat, guinea-pig, mouse and cat[24]. However, there is some evidence of species differences; the dog and rat being more susceptible than the guinea-pig or mouse[26]. The ulcerogenic activity of NSAI drugs is not directly related to anti-inflammatory potency[26]. However, the degree of reduction of prostaglandin synthesis is a factor[27].

Some induced gastric lesions may be found to be reversible, even with continued administration of the test substance. This cytoprotection is believed to be due to the action of increased levels of prostaglandins[28]. Pretreatment of rats with a series of prostaglandins prevents the extensive necrosis of the gastric mucosa produced in untreated animals by absolute ethanol, hydrochloric acid, sodium hydroxide or 25% sodium chloride[28].

In man, an association between gastric ulceration and glucocorticosteroids is established[1,5], but in our experience gastric changes are not widely seen in safety evaluation studies with these compounds in rats, dogs and monkeys. However, in dogs treated with prednisone, multiple gastric fundic and pyloric ulcers and haemorrhage are reported[29]. Ethanol readily induces gastric mucosal necrosis and ulceration in rats[30]. Investigations into the involvement of hyperosmolarity in the development of this lesion[31] have shown that hyperosmotic glucose and choline chloride solutions both produce similar lesions. Gastric ulceration may also be induced, in rats, by stress, and hypothyroidism exacerbates this lesion[32].

In recent years the development and clinical success of selective histamine H_2-receptor blocking drugs has focused considerable attention on the gastric mucosa. With the competitive, surmountable H_2-antagonists such as ranitidine and cimetidine few serious adverse effects are reported in toxicity studies. In these cases inhibition of gastric acid secretion is associated with the expected physiological response – a parietal cell morphological appearance consistent with cellular resting (i.e. no secretory activity) characterized by large numbers of cytoplasmic tubulovesicles and small canalicular surface area[33].

However, with some other H_2-antagonists, particularly the unsurmountable blockers, more severe adverse toxic side effects are described. With SK & F 93479 trihydrochloride, pronounced epithelial hyperplasia and hyperkeratosis, with focal penetration through the muscularis mucosae into the submucosa of the forestomach, are reported in rats treated for 1 year[34]. Another H_2-blocker, tiotidine, produces glandular proliferation with subsequent development of glandular atypia, penetration into the submucosa and adenocarcinoma[35].

An unusual lesion produced by some H_2-blockers is a hyperplastic gastropathy with associated entero-chromaffin-like (ECL) cell proliferation (and eventual carcinoid tumour development). This lesion is reported in studies with the insurmountable blockers loxtidine[36] and omeprazole[37], but not with ranitidine. The ECL cell hyperplasia may be identified by the presence of neurone-specific enolase or anti-chromogranin (Figure 4.18) and the characteristic dense granules with the electron microscope[36,37]. The mechanism behind the ECL cell proliferation is suggested to be the chronic achlorhydria and associated hypergastrinaemia produced by these drugs. It is believed that the achlorhydria removes an important feedback mechanism[36], the release of gastrin normally being inhibited by gastric acid. With H_2-blockers, the consequent hypergastrinaemia might be expected to cause increased stimulation and hyperplasia of ECL cells.

Proliferation of cells lining the basal areas of gastric glands and characterized by strongly eosinophilic granules is found with the unsurmountable H_2-blockers loxtidine[36] omeprazole[37] and with SKF 93479, but not with ranitidine[36]. The cell type of origin is uncertain, but they may be chief cells[37]. Similar cells are found in rats treated with sulphite, and it is suggested they might represent metaplastic atypical Paneth cells[22] or hyperplastic chief cells[38].

Selective degeneration of parietal cells may rarely occur. This effect, in rats, was observed as an acute lesion in our laboratory and was associated with the subsequent development of atrophic and ulcerative changes and the eventual development of foveolar hyperplasia (Figure 4.19). Single cell degeneration in the fundic region of dogs (Figure 4.20) has also been observed in our laboratories following high doses of some novel H_2-antagonists. The degenerative changes were characterized by shrinkage, condensation and pyknosis. In some cases, groups of these apoptotic cell bodies had apparently been extruded into the gland lumina (Figure 4.21). Although it was difficult to determine if the apoptotic degeneration involved a specific cell type, numbers of parietal cells (and the known site of action of the compounds) suggested a predilection. In addition, in studies of longer duration, no evidence of apoptosis was detected and parietal cells were virtually completely depleted.

Decreased numbers of parietal cells are observed in cynomolgus monkeys treated with polychlorinated biphenyls[9]. In this case the lesion is associated with a diffuse hypertrophy and hyperplasia of the mucinous gastric mucosa. With novel 'reticulo-endothelial system expanders' in monkeys, vacuolation of the gastric mucosa may occur. This is associated with prominent cell deletion by apoptosis. The apoptotic cells or bodies were distributed in all levels of the glands and led to a marked atrophy of the gastric mucosoa (Figure 4.22). In addition to the vacuolation and apoptosis variable numbers of multivacuolated histocytes are present in the lamina propria.

Hyperplasia of parietal cells is reported[39] to occur in rats following administration of pentagastrin (but not with histamine). Some prostaglandins are known to have a trophic effect on gastric, duodenal and colonic mucosae, both by systemic and local administration[40]. Proliferation of the foveolar surface epithelium of the pylorus is described[41] in dogs and monkeys treated with a synthetic analogue of prostaglandin E_1.

Small Intestine

Induced small intestinal lesions are listed in Table 4.3.

Table 4.3 Induced lesions of the small intestine

Villus atrophy
Villus stunting
Villus hypertrophy
Ulcerative changes
'Accumulation enteropathies'
Intussusception
Lacteal dilatation

Atrophy of the intestinal villi may be induced experimentally, and fasting of rats results in decreased villus size, decreased crypt size and a decreased mitotic pool[42]. In rats, although apparently not in the dog, atrophy of the villi of the small intestine is induced by hypophysectomy.

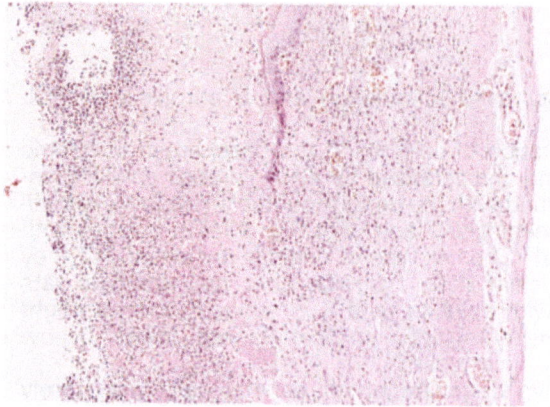

Figure 4.13 Severe ulceration of the rat forestomach with a pronounced inflammatory reaction in the underlying musculature. H & E

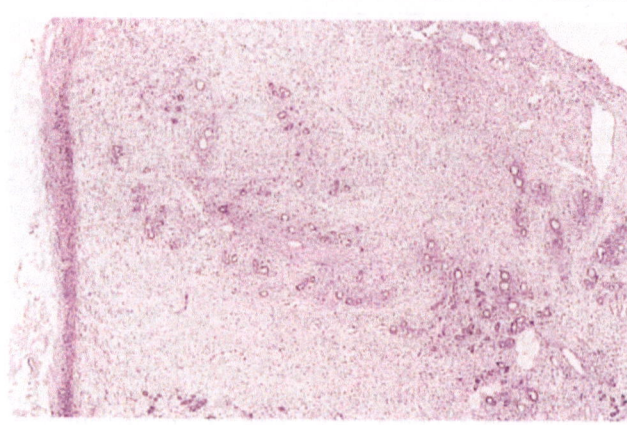

Figure 4.14 Pancreas from a rat with perforated gastric ulcer induced by a non-steroidal anti-inflammatory drug. The pancreatic acinar tissue is replaced by fibrous tissue. H & E

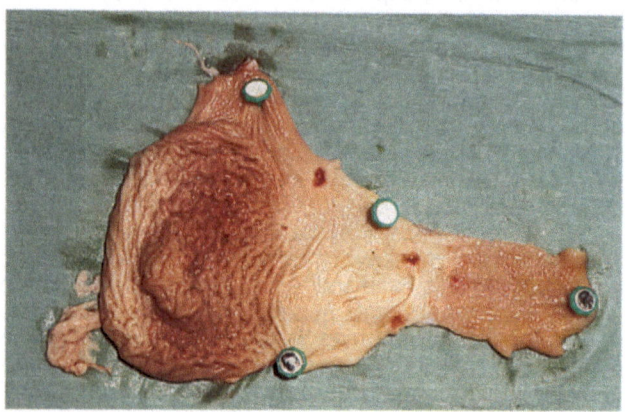

Figure 4.15 Dog stomach showing punctate ulcers in the antral region

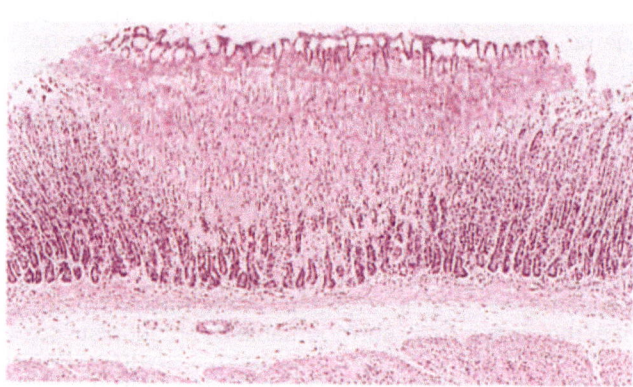

Figure 4.16 A focus of superficial mucosal congestion, haemorrhage and necrosis in the glandular stomach of a rat treated orally with a non-steroidal anti-inflammatory drug. H & E

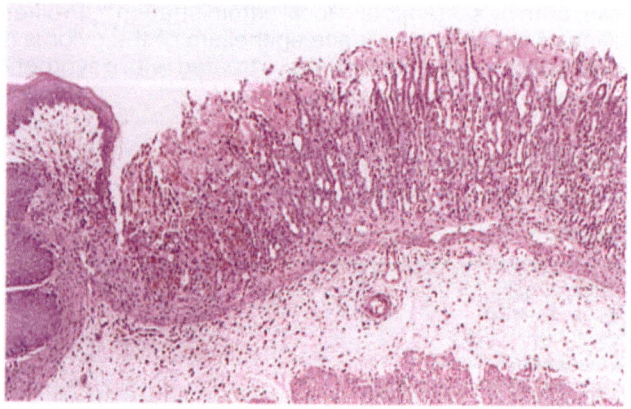

Figure 4.17 Superficial mucosal necrosis in the glandular stomach of a rat. The submucosa is oedematous. H & E

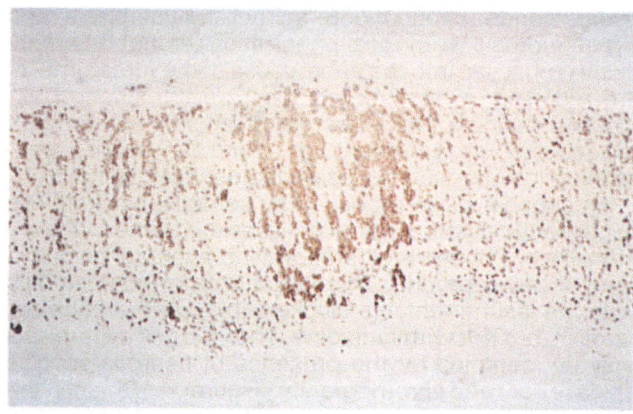

Figure 4.18 Increased numbers of enterochromaffin-like cells in the antral mucosa of a rat treated with an unsurmountable H_2 antagonist. Anti–chromogranin–PAP (Photomicrograph by courtesy of Dr G. R. Betton, Smith Kline and French Research Ltd.)

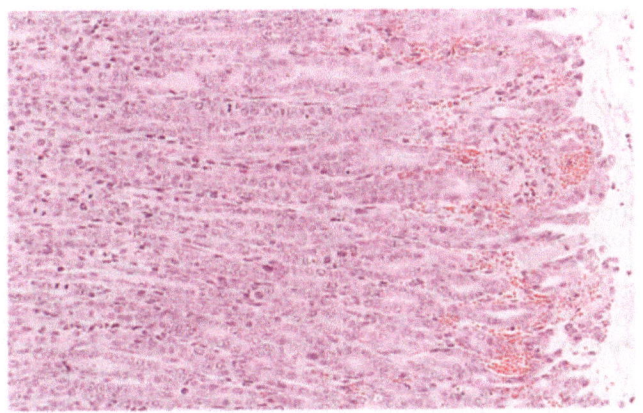

Figure 4.19 Foveolar hyperplasia of the glandular gastric mucosa of a rat. This lesion developed following ulcerative changes and indicates attempted repair. The mucosal cells appear basophilic and generally undifferentiated. H & E

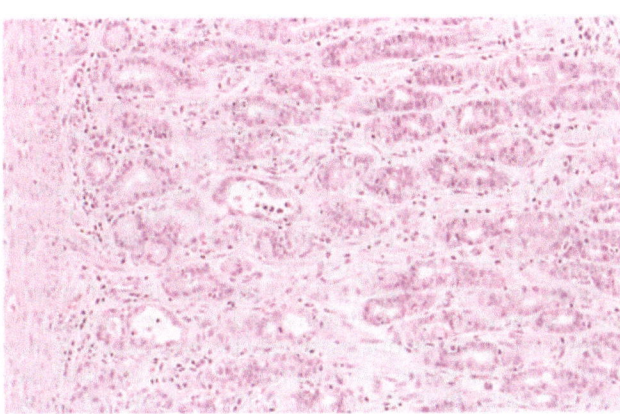

Figure 4.20 Fundic mucosa of a dog treated with a novel H_2 antagonist. Single degenerate cells illustrate features typical of apoptosis i.e. rounded and shrunken with nuclear pyknosis and fragmentation. Note the absence of parietal cells. H & E

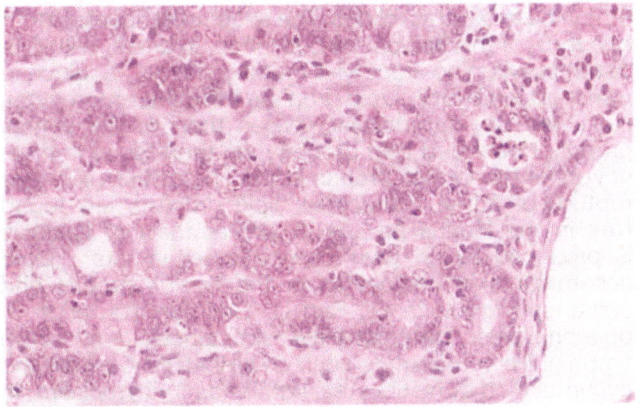

Figure 4.21 Higher power view of dog from Figure 4.20 showing extrusion of apoptotic bodies into glandular lumina. H & E

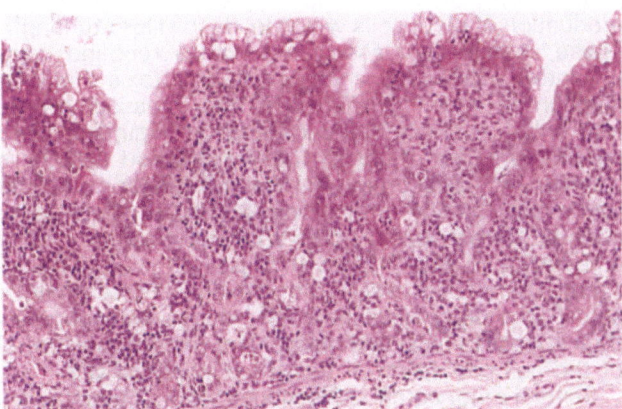

Figure 4.22 Mucosal atrophy in the stomach of a monkey given a novel 'reticuloendothelial system expander'. The lesion begins with extensive vacuolation and apoptosis, inflammatory cell infiltrates and leads to atrophy of the gastric glands. H & E

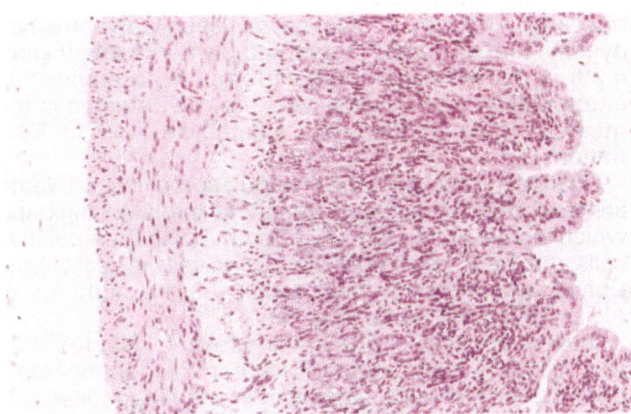

Figure 4.23 Villus 'stunting' of the small intestine in a mouse treated with a cytostatic drug. The villi are broader and shorter than normal and show loss of cellular differentiation. H & E

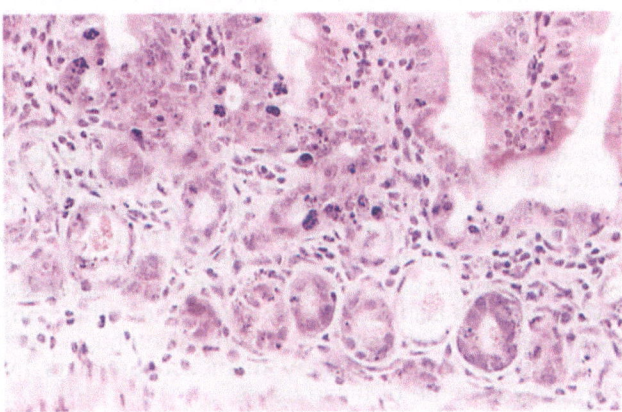

Figure 4.24 Prominent apoptosis in the crypts of the small intestine of a mouse treated with a cytostatic drug. Note also the absence of mitoses. H & E

This is associated with a reduction in the number of enterocytes, defects in the maturation of goblet cells, by hypertrophy and hyperplasia of Paneth cells[43]. The possibility that the atrophy is in fact related to the associated decreased food intake in the hypophysectomized animals was countered in this work by matching the dietary ration of the control rats.

Villus 'stunting' (Figure 4.23) may be regarded as a more severe form of atrophy and can be induced by several compounds but especially by cytostatics. It may be induced by either (or a combination of both) of two mechanisms: (i) inhibition of mitosis in the precursor cells of the crypts, thus preventing the normal replacement of exfoliated villus cells; and (ii) an increased loss of the villus enterocytes occurring at a rate in excess of that at which they can be replaced by the crypts. This results in an increased crypt height (due to increased mitotic activity) but a decrease in that of the villi.

Cytotoxic drugs such as anticancer agents are designed to destroy rapidly dividing tissues. Stunting of the intestinal villi[1] is an obvious side effect of these compounds. Cis-platinum, in the mouse, causes decreased production of crypt cells which leads to villus stunting[44]. These changes are associated with a rebound compensatory increase in crypt height. Cytotoxic drugs, in addition to inhibiting mitosis in the intestinal crypts, also enhance single cell degeneration (Figure 4.24) or apoptosis[45]. The effect of these combined actions is inevitably a reduction in villus height. Apoptosis occurs remarkably quickly after administration of these compounds, for example 2 hours after injection of cytosine arabinoside to mice[45]. On withdrawal of the drug, mucosal regeneration is associated with an increased mitotic activity and decreased apoptosis. Mitosis and apoptosis thus appear to have complementary roles in the control of the cell population of the small intestinal villi.

Several other compounds induce similar changes. Triparanol results in a reversible flattening of the villi in rats[46]. Calcium ethylenediamine tetraacetate causes congestion, haemorrhage and destruction of the epithelium with sloughing. The intestinal glands are decreased in size with obliteration of the lumina and the villi shrunken beyond recognition[47]. The authors suggest that inhibition of DNA synthesis was responsible. A form of enteropathy induced by an antibacterial compound described in rats is characterized by vacuolation of duodenal enterocytes and villus stunting and is associated with a marked decrease in mitotic activity in the crypts[48].

The converse of villus atrophy, that is villus hypertrophy, may also be enountered. This probable physiological response is detected in lactating rats[49] and three possible causes are suggested: (i) 'work hypertrophy' due to hyperphagia; (ii) stimulation of the gut wall by lactogenic hormones; and (iii) functional adaptation due to increased demands by the body. The condition may be induced in the rat by hyperthyroidism[50] and also by thyromimetic compounds. The villus height and total submucosal thickness are both found to be increased. Hypertrophy is also found with a variety of other compounds and conditions which involve hyperphagia, such as alloxan-diabetes[50]. Dietary restriction prevents hypertrophy in some of these cases[50].

Treatment-induced erosion, ulceration and haemorrhage in the small intestine (Figure 4.25) are far less frequently encountered than in the stomach. An animal model has been developed with cysteamine in rats[51]. Ulceration in dogs with intravascular cinchophen or oral indomethacin is found to be associated with Peyer's patches[52]. Necrosis and haemorrhage of the intestinal mucosa are induced in dogs by chromomycin[53]. It is

suggested that the lesions result from a combination of generalized systemic necrosis of lymphoid nodules, including gut-associated lymphoid tissue, and inhibition of nucleic acid synthesis. A similar explanation for the induction of intestinal pathology is suggested for ochratoxin A[54]. In this case most of the mucosal lesions are located directly above necrotic lymphoid nodules.

The administration of enteric-coated potassium chloride tablets as a precaution against diuretic-induced hypokalaemia in man is associated with gastrointestinal ulceration[1]. The effect of potassium chloride tablets is described in monkeys[55]. Lesions are produced predominantly in the small intestine which range from hyperaemia to perforated ulcers. These lesions are believed to be due to the local release of a high concentration of potassium chloride which would be expected to exert a strong caustic effect on the mucosa[5].

Several types of 'accumulation enteropathy' are described which involve the absorption and accumulation in the small intestine of a variety of orally administered compounds or their products. Vacuolation of the enterocytes due to lipid accumulation is seen with puromycin, ethionine and tetracyclines. The sequential development of a form of this lipidosis is described, in detail, with 2,6-di-tert-butylamino-3-acetyl-4-methylpyridine; a glucose transport inhibitor[56]. Lipid droplets from the enterocytes pass into the intercellular spaces then to the lamina propria. Coalesced lipid droplets are then found in histiocytes of the lamina propria at the tips of the villi. After rupture of some histiocytes, lipid droplets are found free in the lamina propria. A similar form of lipidosis is produced by an erythromycin ester in rats[57]. Lipid accumulates in histiocytes in the lamina propria and stains strongly with Oil Red O. Oral administration of phospholipids, detergent-like substances and some amphiphilic compounds such as amiodarone cause the accumulation of histiocytes, with a foamy cytoplasm, in the lamina propria (Figure 4.26). This foamy appearance may be seen with the electron microscope to be due to the presence of numerous, large multilamellar bodies. Another form of 'accumulation enteropathy' is induced in marmosets fed a high cholesterol and coconut oil diet[58]. This jejunal lipodystrophy is associated with steatorrhea and characterized by fat-positive vacuoles in the absorptive cells. Following the administration of some pigmented compounds, accumulation of the test substance within the histiocytes of the lamina propria may be observed. This type of reaction was seen with some hair dyes (Figure 4.27) and pigmented plant extracts (Figure 4.28) in our laboratories. In all forms of 'accumulation enteropathy', similar histiocytes may be detected in the mesenteric lymph nodes (see lymphoid system for illustrations).

Changes in the goblet cell population of the rat ileum are reported with ergocryptine (a prolactin-inhibitor) which increases the number of both Alcian Blue-positive cells and the total number of mucous cells in ileal crypts. Conversely, prolactin itself decreases the numbers of Alcian Blue-positive cells in the villi[59].

Intussusception of the small intestine (Figures 4.29 and 4.30) of rats treated with centrally acting α-adrenergic agonists was observed in our laboratories and may have been due to increased peristalsis. No apparent evidence of blockage, adhesions, necrosis or fibrosis was associated with the lesion.

Lymphangiectasia occurs in protein-losing enteropathies and is generally believed to be the result of obstruction of lymph flow rather than of changes in the mucosal lacteals. Obstruction of the mesenteric lymphatics produces hypoproteinaemia and lymphangiectasia. We have also observed lacteal dilatation as an induced change. This lesion developed in monkeys treated with an immunomodulator and in rats with a novel antihypertensive agent (Figure 4.31). In both cases no lymphatic obstruction was obvious and the mesenteric lymph nodes were histologically normal.

Exocrine Pancreas

Toxic changes are only rarely produced in the exocrine pancreas and are listed in Table 4.4.

Table 4.4 Induced lesions of the exocrine pancreas

Degranulation
Acinar atrophy
Acinar degeneration
Necrosis
Pancreatitis
Acinar hyperplasia/hypertrophy
Fatty change
Interstitial cell vacuolation
Hepatocyte-like cells

Degranulation (loss of zymogen granules) is seen in moribund and fasted animals. This change represents a physiological feature rather than a pathological process. Changes in pancreatic acinar tissue are detected in rats treated with high doses of the diuretic furosemide. The cells are degranulated and atrophic and the lesion probably reflects dehydration due to a severe effect on pancreatic secretion. The number of zymogen granules is shown to decrease with food deprivation[60]. Ultrastructural investigations show that the zymogen granules undergo crinophagy by fusing with lysosomes.

Atrophy of the acinar pancreatic tissue may be induced by a variety of procedures: hypophysectomy[61]; starvation; protein deprivation; protein inhibitors; ethionine (a non-metabolizable amino acid analogue); duct ligation; and copper deficiency[62]. Degranulation is a common early feature of acinar cell atrophy (Figure 4.32) and loss of these eosinophilic zymogen granules contributes to the overall basophilia. The change may be associated with degrees of ectasia characterized by dilatation of the acinar and/or ductular lumina. The cells appear shrunken with pyknotic and karyorrhexic nuclei. Individual cell deletion by apoptosis may be a prominent feature. Apoptosis is a type of single cell death[63] which occurs in normal tissue cell turnover but is enhanced in some pathological conditions. It may be associated with several types of degenerative pancreatic lesions but in our experience can occur as a primary lesion in its own right. It is characterized, by light microscopy (Figure 4.33), by the presence of large, ovoid eosinophilic cytoplasmic bodies which may contain basophilic nuclear fragments. The acinar cells are usually degranulated and focally single cells appear shrunken with nuclear pyknosis and karyorrhexis. No inflammatory reaction is present. The affected cells subsequently become fragmented into membrane-bound bodies (or remain as a single body) which are rapidly phagocytosed by adjacent cells[63]. At this stage the apoptotic bodies appear as membrane-bound inclusions within otherwise normal pancreatic acinar cells (Figure 4.34). They are distinguishable from autophagic vacuoles by the presence of identifiable nuclear fragments[63]. The cause of the death of individual acinar cells is unknown in many cases but in one study, in cynomolgus monkeys, apoptosis was associated with dilatation of the rough endoplasmic reticulum and inclusions containing groups of small electron-dense bodies, often multilamellar in appearance. These inclusions

may have represented a degree of cell damage sufficient to induce subsequent death by apoptosis.

In our laboratories, following a recovery period in a study in which apoptosis was induced in rat pancreas, enhanced mitotic activity was observed in acinar cells (Figure 4.35). This probably indicates the re-establishment of homeostatic control of cell numbers.

The interpretation of apoptosis as a treatment-related change requires a note of caution, particularly in studies with beagle dogs. In this species we, and others[64], have noted the presence of these cytoplasmic inclusions in a relative high percentage of untreated, healthy animals. Apoptosis of acinar cells is described in rats in which exocrine hyperplasia and hypertrophy are induced by a raw soya flour diet, and then involution induced by the return to a normal laboratory diet[65]. Severe acinar atrophy may progress until all acinar cells are lost and replaced by adipose tissue with only the ducts, vasculature and islets remaining. Rats and mice appear more tolerant of this condition than dogs which show severe clinical signs of pancreatic insufficiency.

Degenerative changes in acinar cells of zinc-deficient rats[66] involve reduced numbers of zymogen granules, accumulation of lipid, and prominent lysosomes. It is suggested that zinc deficiency may have an inhibitory effect in protein synthesis.

Multilamellar bodies may be induced in rat pancreatic acinar cells in association with the development of widespread phospholipidosis by compounds such as triparanol. These bodies are not usually associated with degenerative changes.

Acute necrosis of acinar cells is produced in rats by intraperitoneal and intravenous injections of 4-hydroxyaminoquinoline-1-oxide (4-HAQO) and by puromycin[67,68]. The lesion is likened to human acute haemorrhagic pancreatitis, and extensive fibrosis subsequently develops in some cases. Acute haemorrhagic necrosis is induced in mice fed a choline-deficient diet containing DL-ethionine[69]. The lesion develops within 5 days and is characterized by oedema, haemorrhage, calcium deposition and acinar necrosis.

A form of pancreatitis is induced in rats by chronic manganese exposure[70]. Chronic pancreatitis has been seen as an induced lesion in rats, primates and dogs in our laboratories. The condition was characterized by atrophic and degenerative changes in acinar cells, a variable inflammatory cell infiltrate and often pronounced inter-lobular and periacinar fibrosis (Figures 4.36 and 4.37).

Gastrin is known to exert trophic effects on the pancreas and hypertrophy of acinar cells may be induced by pentagastrin in rats[61].

A relatively high incidence of focal acinar hyperplasia, is recently reported in male rats from groups which received corn oil as a vehicle in gavage studies[71]. Upon review the lesion is about five times more common in corn oil-treated rats than untreated animals. The incidence is found to be related to maximum mean body weights. The lesion comprises circumscribed, oval or spherical groups of prominent acinar cells which have abundant zymogen granules, prominent nucleoli and cause slight compression of the adjacent parenchyma. Histologically similar lesions are also seen during the early stages of azaserine and 4-HAQO-induced pancreatic carcinogenesis.

In addition to hyperplastic foci another distinct focal lesion of cellular alteration is recognized. These foci of hypertrophic acinar cells[72] are characterized by prominent nucleoli, basophilic cytoplasm, variable numbers of zymogen granules, rare mitoses with a low mitotic index

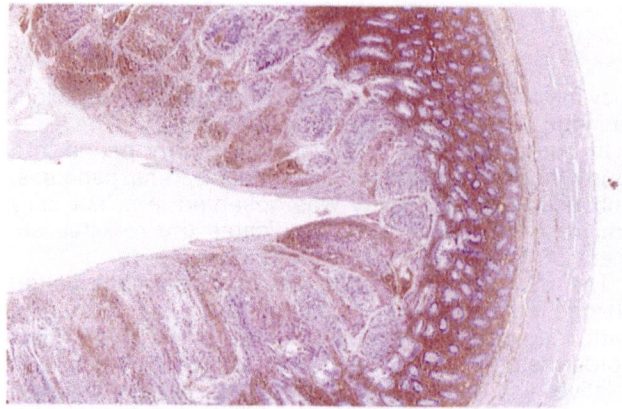

Figure 4.25 Severe haemorrhagic necrosis in the small intestine of a dog. H & E

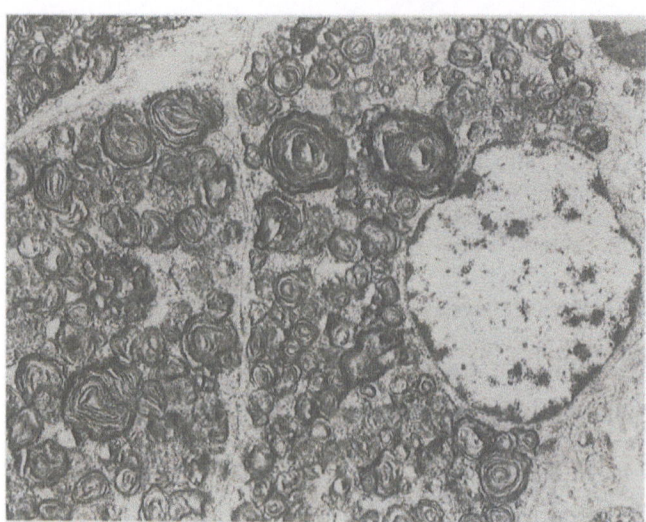

Figure 4.26 Histiocytes from the lamina propria of a rat treated orally with a detergent-like material. Numerous multilamellar bodies in the cytoplasm. Electron micrograph

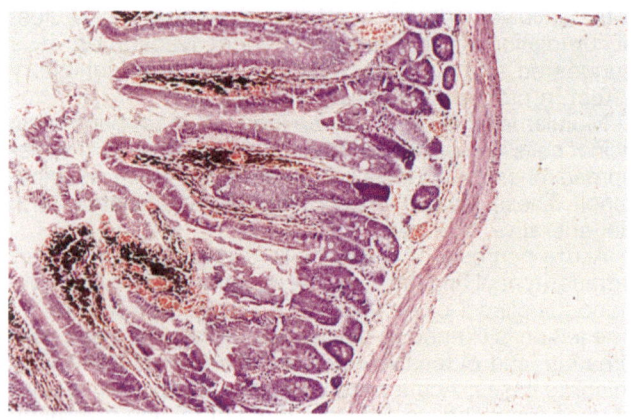

Figure 4.27 Pigment accumulation in histiocytes in the lamina propria at the tips of the villi in a rat following oral administration of a hair dye. H & E

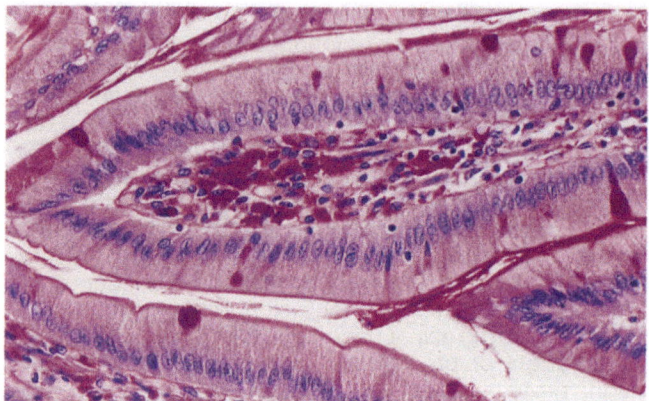

Figure 4.28 Histiocytes in the lamina propria of the duodenum from a rat given a plant extract orally. The material has accumulated in histiocytes and stains positively with PAS. No evidence of degenerative change. PAS

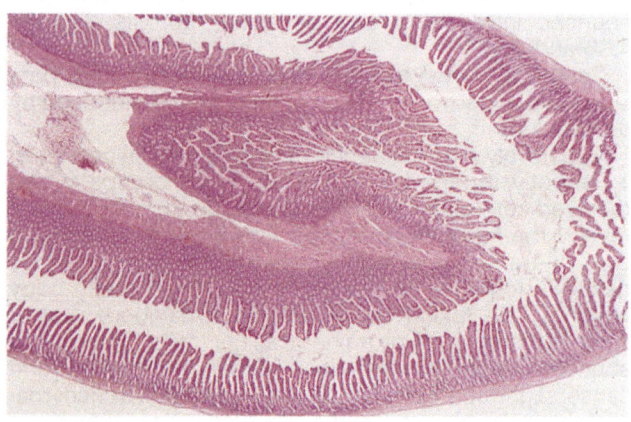

Figure 4.29 Longitudinal section through an intussusception induced in a rat by administration of a centrally acting α-adrenergic agonist. The 'telescope effect' is clearly shown. No evidence of inflammatory or degenerative changes. H & E

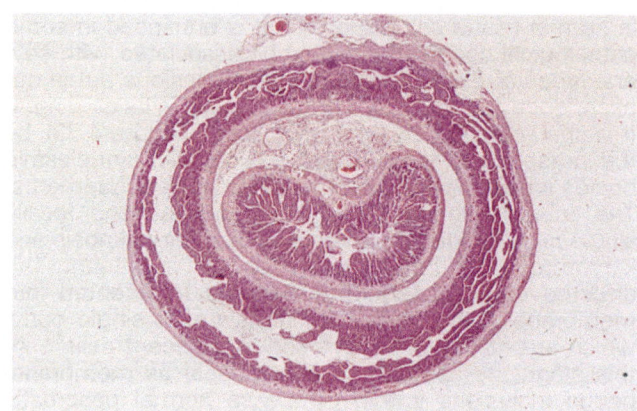

Figure 4.30 Transverse section through an induced intussusception in a rat. Treatment regime as in Figure 4.29, and again there is no evidence of inflammatory or degenerative changes. H & E

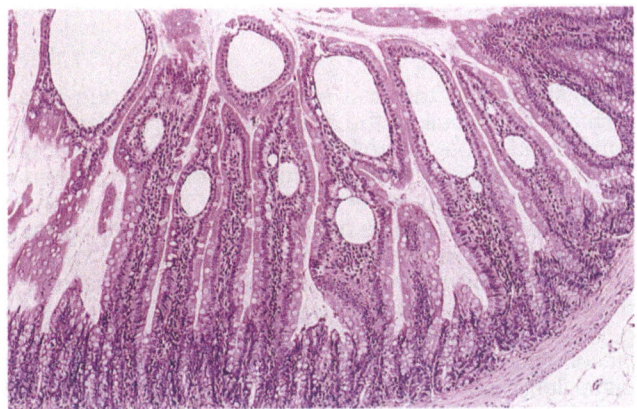

Figure 4.31 Dilated lacteals at the tips of the villi from a rat treated with a novel antihypertensive drug. The lesion is not associated with a significant inflammatory reaction and no lesions were detected in lymphatics elsewhere or in the mesenteric lymph nodes. This change was rapidly reversible on cessation of treatment. H & E

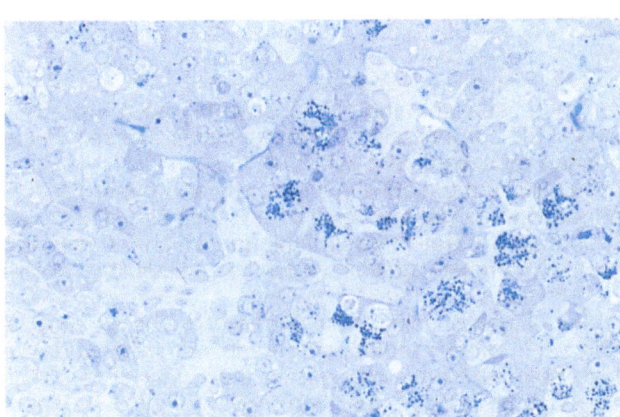

Figure 4.32 Pancreas from a rat showing acinar degranulation and occasional apoptotic cells. Blue-stained zymogen granules are present in only a few acinar cells. 1 µm section. Toluidine Blue

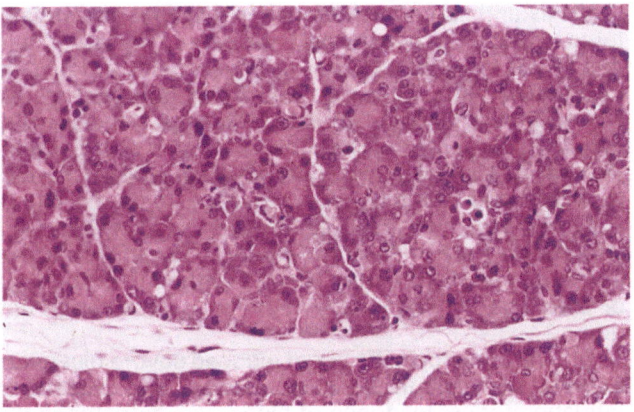

Figure 4.33 Pancreas showing apoptosis of acinar cells induced in a rat following inhalation of an industrial chemical. The apoptotic cells appear as rounded, eosinophilic bodies with basophilic nuclear fragments. H & E

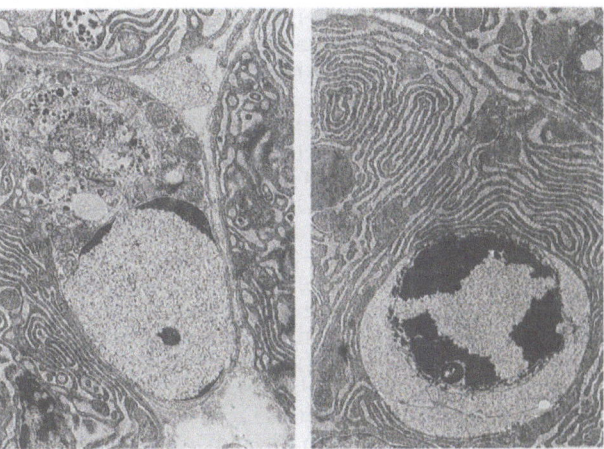

Figure 4.34 Apoptosis in the pancreas of a monkey. In one case an acinar cell appears shrunken with karyorrhexis. This represents an early stage of apoptosis. The other case shows an apoptotic inclusion within the cytoplasm of another acinar cell. Electron micrograph

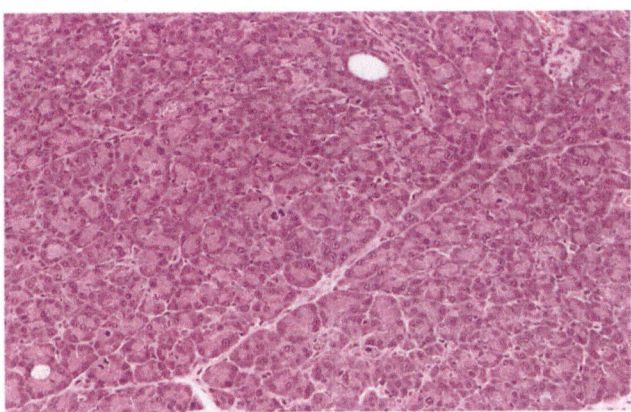

Figure 4.35 Mitosis of rat pancreatic acinar cells. In this study apoptosis was detected at an earlier stage (see Figure 4.33), but following a recovery period without treatment increased mitotic activity is observed. H & E

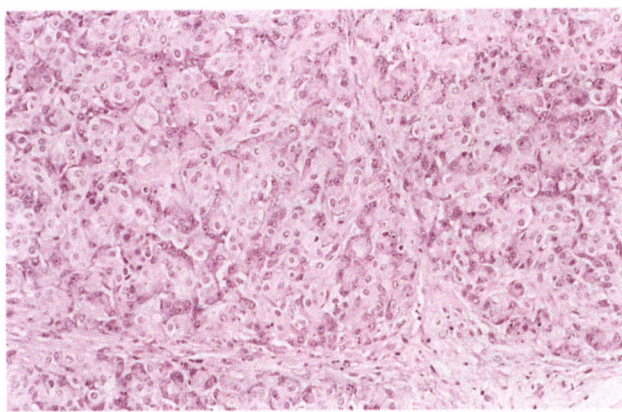

Figure 4.36 Chronic pancreatitis in a monkey induced by a novel anticancer drug. Acinar cells appear degranulated and disorganized with focal single cell degeneration. Interlobular fibrosis is also present. H & E

and increased cell and acinar size (Figure 4.38). They cause little compression of adjacent acini. These foci are induced by azaserine 4-HAQO[72].

A combined exocrine hypertrophy and hyperplasia is induced in rats fed raw soya flour[65]. This diet is believed to contain a potent trypsin inhibitor which induces the release of cholecystokinin which has a trophic effect on the pancreas.

Vacuolation of acinar cells due to fatty change may be induced in rats by prolonged ethanol adminstration. We have observed fatty changes in the acinar cells of the rat pancreas from studies with novel fungicides (Figure 4.39). Extensive hepatic fat deposition was also detected in these studies. The pancreatic acinar cells initially became degranulated and atrophic with the subsequent accumulation of fine fat droplets (Figures 4.40 and 4.41).

Prominent vacuolated cells in the exocrine interstitium (Figure 4.42) have been seen in cynomolgus monkeys treated with high doses of a novel antibiotic. This lesion was associated with the detection of similar cells in a wide variety of organs. The origin of these cells was difficult to assess since ultrastructurally they contained few recognizable organelles, but they most likely represented histiocytes. The vacuoles contained traces of moderately electron-dense material, but no other recognizable structures.

One of the most spectacular and interesting induced changes in pancreatic tissue has been the reported transformation or transdifferentiation of acinar cells into hepatocyte-like cells (Figures 4.43 and 4.44). These cells are described following administration of the pancreatic carcinogen N-nitroso-bis-(2-oxopropyl)amine, to hamsters, previously fed a methionine-deficient diet, in which pancreatic regeneration is initiated by a single intraperitoneal methionine injection[73.] The cells respond in a manner similar to that of hepatocytes to a variety of experimental conditions including: peroxisome proliferation with hypolipidaemic drugs; proliferation of smooth endoplasmic reticulum with phenobarbital; and mitotic activity following subtotal hepatectomy. In rats, hepatocyte-like cells are induced more directly with the peroxisome proliferator ciprofibrate[74] and, more recently, after dietary copper depletion and repletion. The cells are morphologically indistinguishable from hepatocytes and are usually located around islets. The ability of acinar cells to transform into hepatocytes is perhaps less surprising when viewed in the context of their common origin from gut entoderm.

Large Intestine

Lesions of the large intestine are rarely encountered in routine toxicity studies. Induced lesions of the large intestine are listed in Table 4.5.

Table 4.5 Induced lesions of the large intestine

Caecal enlargement
Enterocolitis
Ulcerative changes
Submucosal fibrosis
Mucosal hyperplasia

Pronounced caecal enlargement is reported in rats following dietary manipulation involving incorporation of poorly absorbed chemically modified starches and sugars such as sorbitol, mannitol, lactose and polyethylene glycol and magnesium sulphate[75,76]. This enlargement, which is best assessed macroscopically (Figure 4.45), may be accompanied by diarrhoea but is usually not associated with histological changes[75]. It was originally suggested that the enlargement was due to an increase in the bulk of the caecal contents, but later was considered to be controlled by the osmotic value of the caecal contents so that the enlargement represented a process of physiological adaptation. The condition is usually readily reversible on resumption of a normal diet.

Enterocolitis is readily produced in rodents by antibiotics[1]. Penicillin, chlortetracycline, bacitracin and erythromycin all cause lethal acute haemorrhagic colitis in guinea pigs[77]. Clindamycin and lincomycin cause a similar condition in hamsters. Grossly, the caecum, colon and distal ileum are congested, haemorrhagic and distended with fluid. Histologically, there is a mucosal and submucosal congestion, leukocyte infiltration with a mucopurulent exudate, and degeneration and erosion of the surface enterocytes. Other antibiotics including penicillin, cephalosporins, erythromycin, gentamycin, chloramphenicol and tetracyclines and the anti-neoplastic agents methotrexate and 5-fluorouracil all produce enterocolitis in hamsters[77]. In rabbits, lincomycin and clindamycin produce an enterocolitis which mainly involves the caecum and large bowel[77].

NSAIs and some industrial chemicals, when administered orally, may occasionally produce ulcerative changes in the large intestine of rats and mice, and colonic perforation with peritonitis has been detected in our laboratories. Following mucosal damage we observed the development of pronounced fibrous tissue within the wall of the colon (Figure 4.46). This change, in rats, was detected following withdrawal of treatment with a compound which caused episodes of severe abdominal distension. Presumably, the fibrosis developed following a severe inflammatory reaction although at the time of examination little inflammation was detected in any rat.

A novel antineoplastic agent induced severe ulceration and haemorrhage in the colon of dogs (Figure 4.47) in our laboratories. Evidence of blood was detected in the faeces. No lesions were present at other levels of the gastrointestinal tract. This, in our experience, represents an unusual predilection site with this type of compond which more frequently affects the small intestine.

In rats and mice, compounds which decrease peristalsis or which cause retention of faecal pellets may rarely cause mucosal mineralization. This lesion is usually characterized by distension of the colon and/or rectum with a diffuse mineralization of the superficial mucosa. No inflammatory reaction is observed.

Colonic mucosal hyperplasia, in our experience, is rarely encountered in toxicity studies but may be seen as a repair process following ulcerative changes (Figure 4.48). Bile and secondary bile acids damage colonic epithelium, and intra-rectal and dietary administration of deoxycholic acid to rats and dietary administration of cholic acid to mice cause damage[78]. Initially inflammation, oedema and necrosis develop, followed by increased mitotic activity and epithelial hyperplasia.

Rectal lesions are rarely encountered during toxicity studies but occasional compounds produce inflammatory and/or ulcerative changes.

References

1. Gralla, E. J. (1975). Adverse drug reactions. *Vet. Clin. N. Am.*, **5**, 699–715
2. Grenby, T. H., and Colley, J. (1983). Dental effects of xylitol compared with other carbohydrates and polyols in the diet of laboratory rats. *Arch. Oral Biol.*, **28**, 745–758
3. Vahlsing, H. L., Feringa, E. R., Britten, A. G. and Kinning, W. K. (1975). Dental abnormalities in rats after a single large dose of cyclophosphamide. *Cancer Res.*, **35**, 2199–2202

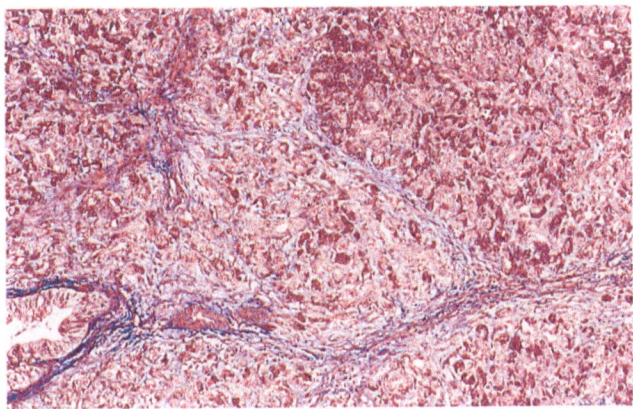

Figure 4.37 From the same case as Figure 4.36. Distinct interstitial fibrosis. Masson's trichrome

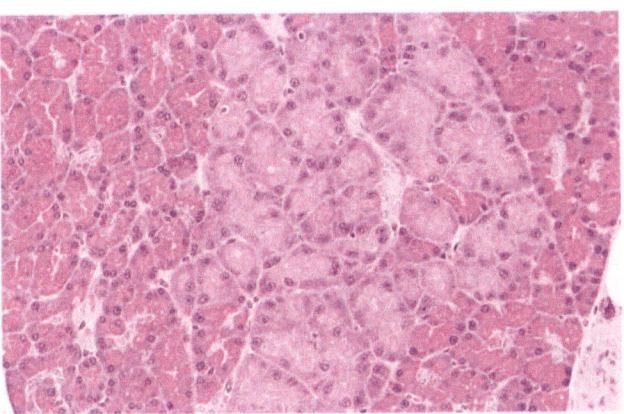

Figure 4.38 Focus of hypertrophic pancreatic acinar cells from a rat treated with an industrial chemical. The cells are enlarged and basophilic. H & E

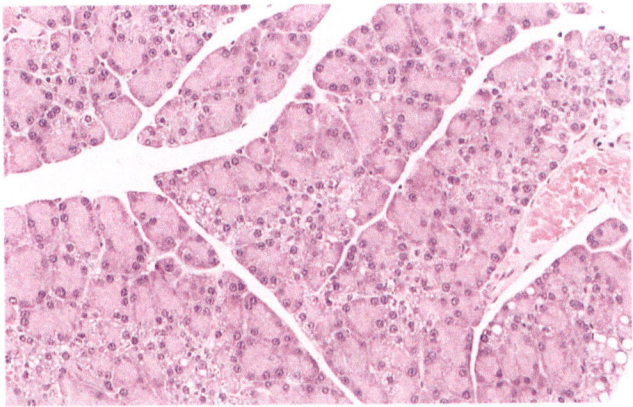

Figure 4.39 Fatty change characterized by fine vacuolation in acinar cells of a rat treated with a novel fungicide. The affected cells contain few zymogen granules. Other acinar cells appear unaffected. H & E

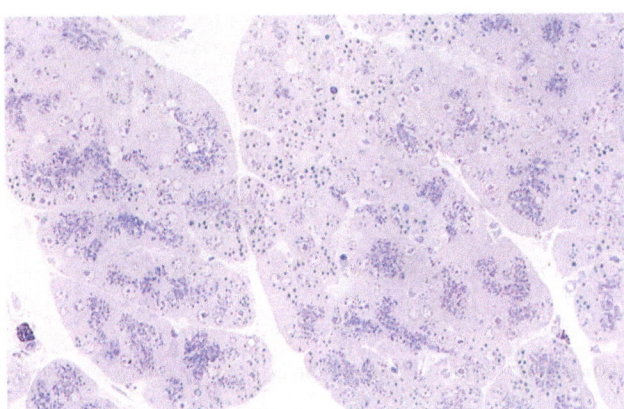

Figure 4.40 Fine fat droplets (stained green) in acinar cells from a rat. From the same study as Figure 4.39. Affected cells contain few zymogen granules (stained blue). 1 μm section. Toluidine Blue

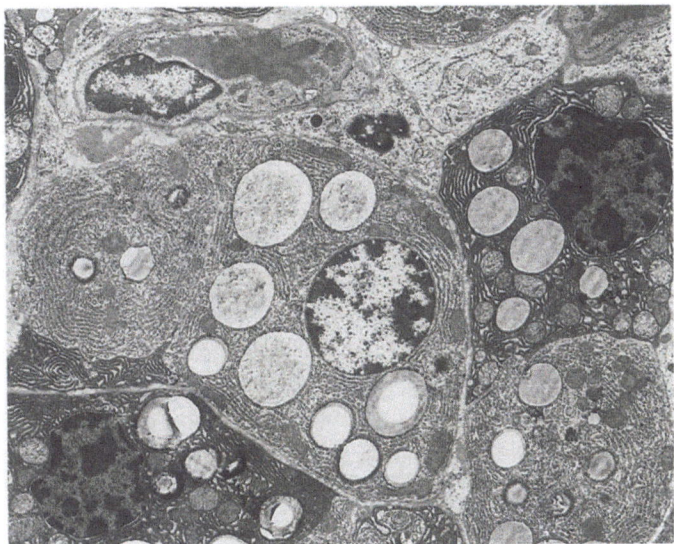

Figure 4.41 Fat droplets in rat pancreatic acinar cells. From the same study as Figures 4.39 and 4.40. Note absence of zymogen granules. Electron micrograph

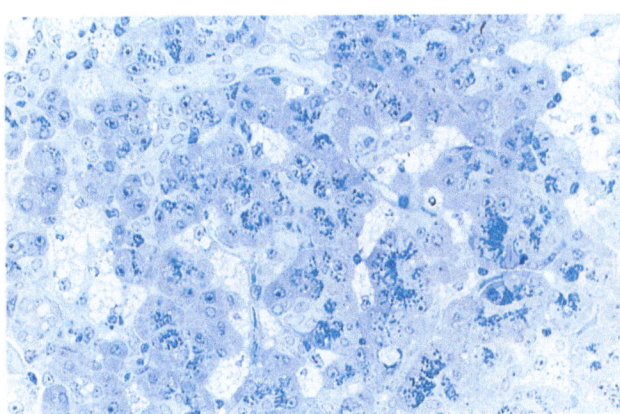

Figure 4.42 Vacuolated cells in the pancreatic interstitium of a monkey treated with a novel antibiotic. These cells are probably macrophages. 1 μm section. Toluidine Blue

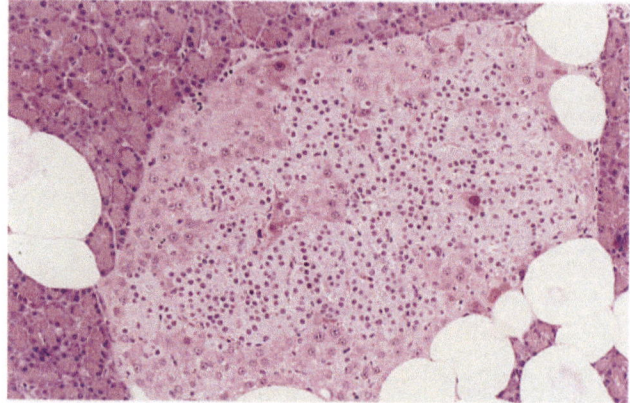

Figure 4.43 Hepatocyte-like cells in and around a rat pancreatic islet. The adjacent acinar and islet cells appear unaffected. These cells are believed to arise by transdifferentiation of acinar cells and have been induced in rats by the peroxisome proliferator ciprofibrate. H & E

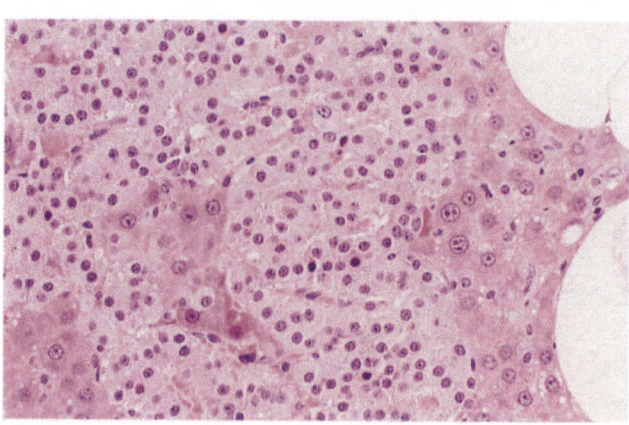

Figure 4.44 Higher power view of Figure 4.43. The hepatocyte-like cells are indistinguishable from hepatocytes and have been shown to respond in a similar way to a variety of exogenous stimuli. H & E

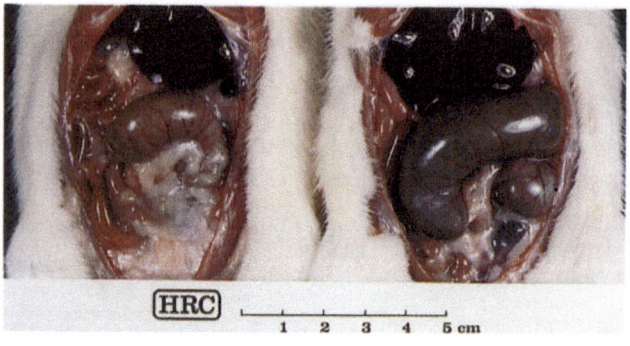

Figure 4.45 Caecal enlargement in a rat treated orally with a sugar alcohol

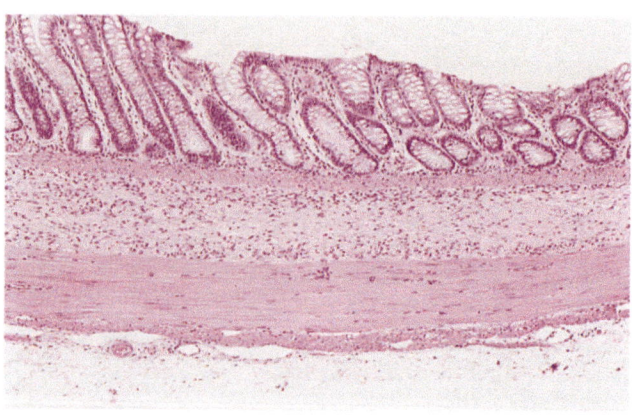

Figure 4.46 Band of fibrous tissue in the submucosa of the colon of a rat, probably a sequel to induced ulcerative changes. H & E

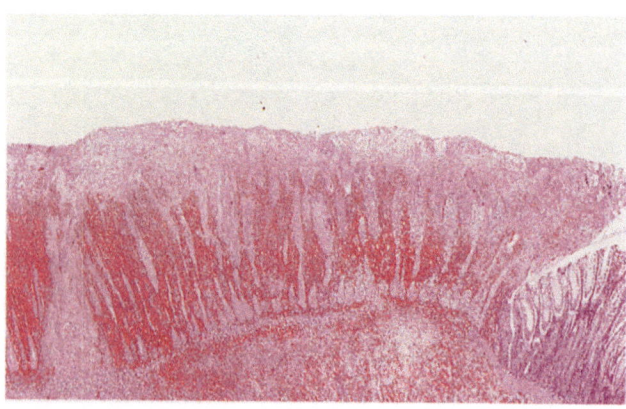

Figure 4.47 Severe mucosal ulceration and haemorrhage in the colon of a dog treated with a novel antineoplastic compound. H & E

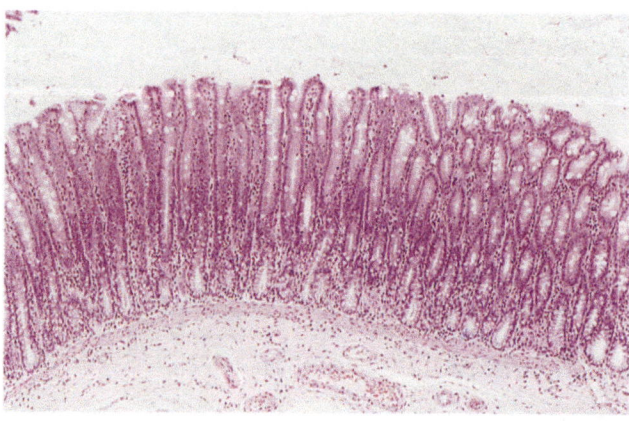

Figure 4.48 Mucosal hyperplasia in the colon of a rat as a sequel to induced ulcerative changes. The epithelium is increased in height and basophilic. H & E

4. Smulow, J. B., Konstantinidis, A. and Sonnenschein, C. (1983). Age-dependent odontogenic lesions in rats after a single i.p. injection of N-nitroso-N-methylurea. *Carcinogenesis*, **4**, 1085–1088

5. Bartelink, A. (1972). Drug-induced diseases of the gastrointestinal tract. In Meyler, L. (ed.) *Drug Induced Diseases*. Vol. 4, pp. 403–421. (Amsterdam: Excerpta Medica)

6. Ryffel, B., Donatsch, P., Madörin, M., Matter, B. E., Rüttimann, G., Schön, H., Stoll, R. and Wilson, J. (1983). Toxicological evaluation of cyclosporin A. *Arch. Toxicol.*, **53**, 107–141

7. van der Wall, E. E., Tuinzing, D. B. and Hes, J. (1985). Gingival hyperplasia induced by nifedipine, and arterial vasodilating drug. *Oral Surg.*, **60**, 38–40

8. Staple, P. H., Reed, M. J., Mashimo, P. A., Sedransk, N. and Umenoto T. (1978). Diphenylhydantoin gingival hyperplasia in *Macaca arctoides*: prevention by inhibition of dental plaque deposition. *J. Periodontol.*, **49**, 310–325

9. Tryphonas, L., Arnold, D. L., Zawidzka, Z., Mes. J., Charbonneau, S. and Wong J. (1986). A pilot study in adult rhesus monkeys treated with Aroclar 1254 for two years. *Toxicol. Pathol.*, **14**, 1–10

10. Eveson, J. W, (1981). Animal models of intra-oral chemical carcinogenesis: a review. *J. Oral Pathol.*, **10**, 129–146

11. Satchell, P. M. and McLeod, J. G. (1981). Megaoesophagus due to acrylamide neuropathy. *J. Neurol. Neurosurg. Psychiatry*, **44**, 906–913

12. Fukuda, M. (1968). The influence of isoprenoline and propranolol on the submaxillary gland of the rat. *Jpn. J. Pharmacol.*, **18**, 185–199

13. Hully, J. R., Benton, H. P. and Alison, M. R. (1984). Isoprenaline-induced cell proliferation in mouse salivary glands: The effect of castration. *Virchows Arch. B: Zellpathol.*, **47**, 95–105

14. Schneyer, C. A. (1962). Salivary gland changes after isoproterenol-induced enlargement. *Am. J. Physiol.*, **203**, 232–236

15. Hall, H. D. and Schneyer, C. A. (1964). Salivary gland atrophy in rat induced by liquid diet. *Proc. Soc. Exp. Biol. Med.*, **117**, 789–793

16. Smith, B. and Butler, M. (1978). The effects of long-term propranolol on the salivary glands and intestinal serosa of the mouse. *J. Pathol.*, **124**, 185–187

17. Ulmansky, M., Rubinow, A. and Ungar, H. (1969). Salivary gland regeneration after DL-ethionine poisoning. *Lab. Invest.*, **20**, 230–233

18. Doine, A. I. and Fava-De-Moraes, F. (1979). Histochemistry of the submandibular salivary gland of castrated male mice treated with androgens and anabolic steroids. *Arch. Oral Biol.*, **24**, 569–574

19. Harvey, H. (1952). Sexual dimorphism of submaxillary glands in mice in relation to reproductive maturity and sex hormones. *Physiol. Zool.*, **25**, 205–222

20. Gresnik, E. W. and Barka, T. (1980). Precocious development of granular convoluted tubules in the mouse submandibular gland induced by thyroxine or by thyroxine and testosterone. *Am. J. Anat.*, **159**, 177–185

21. Steidler, N. E. and Reade, P. C. (1982). An Immunohistochemical and histological study of the influence of the testes and adrenal glands on epidermal growth factor-containing cells in the submandibular salivary glands of male mice. *J. Anat.*, **135**, 413–421

22. Feron, V. J. and Wensvoort, P. (1972). Gastric lesions in rats after the feeding of sulphite. *Path. Eur.*, **7**, 103–111

23. Rodrigues, C., Lok, E., Nera, E., Iverson, F., Page, D., Karpinski, K. and Clayson, D. B. (1986). Short-term effects of various phenols and acids on the Fischer 344 male rat forestomach epithelium. *Toxicology*, **38**, 103–117

24. St. John, D. J. B. (1975). Gastric mucosal damage by aspirin. *CRC Crit. Rev. Toxicol.*, **3**, 317–344

25. Shriver, D. A., White, C. B., Sandor, A. and Rosenthale, M. E. (1975). A profile of the rat gastrointestinal toxicity of drugs used to treat inflammatory diseases. *Toxicol. Appl. Pharmacol.*, **32**, 73–83

26. Wilhelmi, G. (1974). Species differences in susceptibility to the gastro-ulcerogenic action of anti-inflammatory agents. *Pharmacology*, **11**, 220–230

27. Rainsford, K. D., Fox. S. A. and Osborne, D. J. (1984). Comparative effects of some non-steroidal anti-inflammatory drugs on the ultrastructural integrity and prostaglandin levels in the rat gastric mucosa: relationship to drug uptake. *Scand. J. Gastroenterol.*, **19**, (Suppl. 101), 55–68

28. Robert, A., Lancaster, C., Davis, J. P., Field, S. O. and Nezamis, J. E. (1984). Distinction between antiulcer effect and cytoprotection. *Scand. J. Gastroenterol.*, **19**, (Suppl. 101), 69–72

29. Badylack, S. F. and van Vleet, J. F. (1982). Tissue γ-glutamyl transpeptidase activity and hepatic ultrastructural alterations in dogs with experimentally induced glucocorticoid hepatopathy. *Am. J. Vet. Res.*, **43**, 649–655

30. Hollander, D., Tarnawski, A., Gergely, H. and Zipser, R. D. (1984). Sucralfate protection of the gastric mucosa against ethanol-induced injury: a prostaglandin-mediated process? *Scand. J. Gastroenterol.*, **19**, (Suppl. 101), 97–102

31. Puurenen, J., Huttunen, P. and Hirvonen, J. (1980). Is ethanol-induced damage of the gastric mucosa a hyperosmotic effect? Comparative studies on the effects of ethanol, some other hyperosmotic solutions and acetylsalicylic acid on rat gastric mucosa. *Acta Pharmacol. Toxicol.*, **47**, 321–327

32. Money, S. R., Cheron, R. G., Jaffe, B. M. and Zinner, M. J. (1986). The effects of thyroid hormones on the formation of stress ulcers in the rat. *J. Surg. Res.*, **40**, 176–180

33. Ainge, G. and Poynter, D. (1981). H$_2$-Receptor antagonists: ultrastructure of canine parietal cells after long term treatment with ranitidine. *Scand. J. Gastroenterol.*, **16** (Suppl. 70), 143–154

34. Betton, G. R. and Salmon, G. K. (1984). Pathology of the forestomach in rats treated for 1 year with a new histamine H$_2$-receptor antagonist, SK&F 93479 trihydrochloride. *Scand. J. Gastroenterol.*, **19**, (Suppl. 101), 103–108

35. Streett, C. S., Cimprich, R. E. and Robertson, J. L. (1984). Pathologic findings in the stomachs of rats treated with the H$_2$-receptor antagonist tiotidine. *Scand. J. Gastroenterol.*, **19**, (Suppl. 101), 109–117

36. Poynter, D., Pick, C. R., Harcourt, R. A., Selway, S. A. M., Ainge, G., Harman, I. W., Sparling, N. W., Fluck, P. A. and Cook, J. L. (1985). Association of long lasting unsurmountable histamine H$_2$ blockade and gastric carcinoid tumours in the rat. *Gut*, **26**, 1284–1295

37. Ekman, L., Hansson, E., Havu, N., Carlsson, E. and Lundberg, C. (1985). Toxicological studies on omeprazole. *Scand. J. Gastroenterol.*, **20** (Suppl. 108), 53–69

38. Beems, R. B., Spit, B. J., Koëter, H. B. W. M. and Feron, V. J. (1982). Nature and histogenesis of sulfite-induced gastric lesions in rats. *Exp. Mol. Pathol.*, **36**, 316–325

39. Crean, G. P., Marshall, M. W. and Rumsey, R. D. E. (1969). Parietal cell hyperplasia induced by the administration of pentagastrin to rats. *Gastroenterology*, **57**, 147–155

40. Halter, F., Meyrat, P., Fritsche, R., Müller, O., Lentze, M. J. and Koelz, H. R. (1984). Both topical and systemic treatments with 16, 16–dimethyl prostaglandin E$_2$ are atrophic to rat gastric mucosa. *Scand. J. Gastroenterol.*, **19**, (Suppl. 101), 47–53

41. Kramer, A. W., Dougherty, W. J., Belson, A. R. and Iatropoulos, M. J. (1985). Morphologic changes in the gastric mucosa of rats and dogs treated with an analog of prostaglandin E$_1$. *Toxicol. Pathol.*, **13**, 26–35

42. Altmann, G. G. (1972). Influence of starvation and refeeding on mucosal size and epithelial renewal in the rat small intestine. *Am. J. Anat.*, **133**, 391–400

43. Bastie, M. J., Balas, D., Laval, J., Senegas-Balas, F., Bertrand, C., Frexinos, J. and Ribet, A. (1982). Histological variations of jejunal and ileal mucosal on days 8 and 15 after hypophysectomy in rat; morphometric analysis in light and electron microscopy. *Acta Anat.*, **112**, 321–337

44. Allan, S. G. and Smyth, J. F. (1986). Small intestinal mucosal toxicity of cis-platinum – comparison of toxicity with platinum analogues and dexamethasone. *Br. J. Cancer*, **53**, 355–360

45. Bennett, R. E., Harrison, M. W., Bishop, C. J., Searle, J. and Kerr, J. F. R. (1984). The role of apoptosis in atrophy of the small gut mucosa produced by repeated administration of cytosine arabinose. *J. Pathol.*, **142**, 259–263

46. McPherson, J. R. and Shorter, R. C. (1965). Intestinal lesions associated with triparanol. *Am. J. Dig. Dis.*, **10**, 1024–1030

47. Braide, V. B. C. and Aronson, A. L. (1974). Calcium ethylenediamine tetraacetate toxicity in the rat: sequential light and electron-microscopic studies on chelate-induced enteropathy. *Toxicol. Appl. Pharmacol.*, **30**, 52–62

48. Murgatroyd, L. B. (1980). A morphological and histochemical study of a drug-induced enteropathy in the Alderley Park rat. *Br. J. Exp. Pathol.*, **61**, 567–578

49. Fell, B. F., Smith, K. A. and Campbell, R. M. (1963). Hyper-

trophic and hyperplastic changes in the alimentary canal of the lactating rat. *J. Pathol. Bacteriol.*, **85**, 179–188

50. Wall, A. J., Middleton, W. R. J., Pearse, A. G. E. and Booth, C. C. (1970). Intestinal mucosal hyperplasia following induced hyperthyroidism in the rat. *Virchows Arch. B: Zellpathol.*, **6**, 79–87

51. Szabo, S. (1978). Duodenal ulcer disease. *Am. J. Pathol.*, **93**, 273–276

52. Stewart, T. H. M., Hetenyi, C., Rowsell, H. and Orizaga, M. (1980). Ulcerative enterocolitis in dogs induced by drugs. *J. Pathol.*, **131**, 363–378

53. Fleischman, R. W., Schaeppi, U., Heyman, I. A., Phelan, R. S., Rosenkrantz, H. and Ilievski, V. (1974). Preclinical toxicologic evaluation of chromomycin A3 in mice, dogs and monkeys. *Toxicol. Appl. Pharmacol.*, **27**, 259–270

54. Szczech, G. M., Carlton, W. W. and Tuite, J. (1973). Ochratoxicosis in beagle dogs. *Vet. Pathol.*, **10**, 219–231

55. Diener, R. M., Shoffstall, D. H. and Earl, A. E. (1965). Production of potassium-induced gastrointestinal lesions in monkeys. *Toxicol. Appl. Pharmacol.*, **7**, 746–755

56. Visscher, G. E., Robison, R. L. and Hartman, H. A. (1980). Chemically induced lipidosis of the small intestinal villi in the rat. *Toxicol. Appl. Pharmacol.*, **55**, 535–544

57. Gray, J. E., Weaver, R. N., Sinkula, A. A., Schurr, P. E. and Moran, J. (1974). Drug-induced enteropathy characterised by lipid in macrophages. *Toxicol. Appl. Pharmacol.*, **27**, 145–157

58. Driezen, S., Levy, B. M. and Bernick, S. (1971). Diet induced jejunal lipodystrophy in the Cotton top marmoset. *Proc. Soc. Exp. Biol. Med.*, **138**, 7–11

59. Gona, O. (1981). Prolactin and ergocryptine effects on mucus glycoproteins of the rat ileum. *Histochem. J.*, **13**, 101–107

60. Kitagawa, T. and Ono, K. (1986). Ultrastructure of pancreatic exocrine cells of the rat during starvation. *Histol. Histopathol.*, **1**, 49–57

61. Maysten, P. D. and Barrowman, J. A. (1973). Influence of chronic administration of pentagastrin on the pancreas in hypophysectomised rats. *Gastroenterology*, **64**, 391–399

62. Fell, B. F., King, T. P. and Davies, N. T. (1982). Pancreatic atrophy in copper-deficient rats; histochemical and ultrastructural evidence of a selective effect on acinar cells. *Histochem. J.*, **14**, 665–680

63. Wyllie, A. H. (1981). Cell death: a new classification separating apoptosis from necrosis. In Bowen, I. D. and Luckshin, R. A. (eds.) *Cell Death in Biology of Pathology*. pp. 9–33. (London: Chapman Hall).

64. Hartman, H. A., Robison, R. L. and Visscher, G. E. (1975). Naturally occurring intracytoplasmic inclusions in the canine exocrine pancreas. *Vet. Pathol.*, **12**, 210–219

65. Oates, P. S. and Morgan, R. G. H. (1986). Random or selective cell death during pancreatic involution following withdrawal of raw soya flour feeding in the rat. *Pathology.*, **18**, 234–236

66. Koo, S. I. and Turk, D. E. (1977). Effect of zinc dificiency on the ultrastructure of the pancreatic acinar cell and intestinal epithelium in the rat. *J. Nutr.*, **107**, 896–908

67. Okamura, K. and Konishi, Y. (1985). Patterns of pancreatic acinar cell necrosis by 4-hydroxyaminoquinoline-1-oxide. *Exp. Pathol.*, **28**, 3

68. Longnecker, D. S. and Farber, E. (1967). Acute pancreatic necrosis induced by puromycin. *Lab. Invest.*, **16**, 321–329

69. Virji, M. A. and Rao, K. N. (1985). Acute haemorrhagic pancreatitis in mice. *Am. J. Pathol.*, **118**, 162–167

70. Scheuhammer, A. M. (1983). Chronic manganese exposure in rats: histological changes in the pancreas. *J. Toxicol. Environ. Health*, **12**, 353–360

71. Eustis, S. L. and Boorman, G. A. (1985). Proliferative lesions of the exocrine pancreas: relationship to corn oil gavage in the national toxicology program. *J. Natl. Cancer Inst.*, **75**, 1067–1073

72. Chiu, T. (1985). Hypertrophic foci of pancreatic acinar cells in rats. *CRC Crit. Rev. Toxicol.*, **14**, 133–157

73. Rao, M. S., Subbarao, V., Luetteke, N. and Scarpelli, D. G. (1983). Further characterisation of carcinogen-induced hepatocyte-like cells in hamster pancreas. *Am. J. Pathol.*, **110**, 89–94

74. Reddy, J. K., Rao, M. S., Qureshi, S. A., Reddy, M. K., Scarpelli, D. G. and Lalwani, N. D. (1984). Induction and origin of hepatocytes in rat pancreas. *J. Cell. Biol.*, **98**, 2082–2090

75. Leegwater, D. C., de Groot, A. P. and van Kalmthout-kuyper, M. (1974). The aetiology of caecal enlargement in the rat. *Food Cosmet. Toxicol.*, **12**, 687–697

76. MacKenzie, K. M., Hauck, W. N., Wheeler, A. G. and Roe, F. J. C. (1986). Three-generation reproduction study of rats ingesting up to 10% sorbitol in the diet – and a brief review of the toxicological status of sorbitol. *Food Cosmet. Toxicol.*, **24**, 191–200

77. Rifkin, G. D. and Fekerty, F. R. (1985). Antibiotic-induced entercolitis in animals. In Pfeiffer, C. J. (ed.) *Animal Models for Intestinal Disease*. CRC Series on Gastrointestinal Disease. pp. 124–133

78. Bird, R. P., Schneider, R., Stamp. D. and Bruce, W. R. (1986). Effect of dietary calcium and cholic acid on the proliferative indices of murine colonic epithelium. *Carcinogenesis*, **7**, 1657–1661

The Urinary System

5

The kidney is frequently a target organ in routine toxicity testing. This is perhaps not surprising as, like the liver, it is a major route of xenobiotic excretion. Also like the liver, the kidney can metabolize and even accumulate certain chemicals[1]. The various renal functions, principally glomerular filtration and tubular transport, require a relatively high blood flow (approx. 25% of cardiac output). Therefore, the kidney may be exposed to compounds which achieve measurable plasma concentrations but are not excreted through the organ to any great extent. Many factors, such as molecular size, lipid solubility and protein binding, interact to determine the route and speed of elimination of compounds. Ultimately, for a noxious chemical, the nephrotoxic potential is determined by the amount of compound present and the duration of exposure.

Other portions of the urinary tract, i.e. ureters, urinary bladder and urethra, are rarely involved in toxicological processes. The ureters, bladder, most of the urethra and also the pelvis of the kidney are lined by transitional epithelium. Chemicals carried in the urine may injure this urothelium, the sequelae of which include necrosis, ulceration, repair and reactive hyperplasia. Systemic toxins generally do not affect the lower urinary tract.

Kidney

Induced morphological lesions occur in particular cells or parts of the kidney. However, with prolonged treatment, many chemicals damage more than one cell type or area, and the end results can appear morphologically similar, i.e. misshapen kidneys with loss of nephrons and varying degrees of interstitial reaction. Conventionally, the kidney is divided into four anatomical zones, each containing different parts of the nephrons:

  (i) the cortex contains glomeruli, proximal convoluted tubules (S_1, S_2) and distal tubules;

  (ii) the outer stripe of the outer medulla contains the proximal straight tubule (S_3) and distal tubules;

  (iii) the inner stripe of the outer medulla contains the thin limb of Henle and distal tubules; and

  (iv) the inner medulla contains the thin limb of Henle and collecting ducts.

Where possible in this chapter, lesions are described according to these anatomical zones. However, in routine toxicological studies, nephrotoxic change often affects more than one portion of the nephron and hence morphological changes appear in several zones (Table 5.1)

Table 5.1 Induced lesions of the kidney

Glomerulus
  Direct injury and glomerulosclerosis
  Mesangial changes
  Immunologically-mediated injury
  Progressive glomerulonephrosis

Vasculature
  Atherosclerosis
  Mineralization
  Thrombosis
  Juxtaglomerular cell hypertrophy/hyperplasia

Tubules
  Degeneration and necrosis
  Vacuolation
  Inclusions
  Hypertrophy
  Hyperplasia
  Crystals
  Mineralization
  Dilatation and cysts

Papilla
  Necrosis
  Urothelial hyperplasia

Glomerulus

In out experience, glomerular changes are rarely found in routine toxicity testing. The histological appearance of the normal glomerulus in haematoxylin and eosin stained sections in laboratory animals is frequently indefinite. Fine or subtle changes may consequently be obscured in routine preparations. Examination of perfusion-fixed, 1 µm resin sections and electron microscopy are more useful in these cases. However, as proteinuria is a reasonably good indicator of glomerular dysfunction in toxicity studies, such a finding can be a trigger for fuller investigations.

Conventionally, induced glomerular changes are described as direct or immunologically-mediated (indirect). A well-known example of direct injury is with the aminonucleoside of puromycin where, ultrastructurally, epithelial cells lose their foot processes and become detached from the basement membrane[2]. A progressive glomerulosclerosis subsequently develops characterized by thickened basement membranes, mesangial cell proliferation and segmental hyalinization[3]. Such changes are similar to those encountered in the aging laboratory rat with spontaneous progressive glomerulonephrosis[4].

Other examples of direct glomerular injury include: phorbial myristate acetate which, ultrastructurally, shows accumulation of neutrophils in glomerular capillaries and endothelial blebs with separation from basement membrane[4,5]; and adriamycin which induces glomerulosclerosis in rats[6].

In dogs which have become diabetic with prolonged administration of progestational drugs[7], a form of glomerulosclerosis may be encountered which is similar to the Kimmelstiel-Wilson lesion in man (Figure 5.1). Glomerulosclerosis is also reported in dogs and monkeys with alloxan-induced diabetes[8,9]. Rats with streptozotocin-induced diabetes show basement membrane thickening and increased mesangial volume[10].

In phospholipidosis induced by compounds such as tilorone, chlorphentermine and chloroquine, multilamellar bodies may be detected in the glomerular podocytes (Figure 5.2). This condition does not appear to provoke degenerative changes.

In addition to glomerular endothelial and epithelial cell damage, mesangial cells may sometimes show morphological changes, usually in the form of cytoplasmic alterations or inclusions. The macrophagic mesangial cells can ingest circulating particulate or lipoid material (Figures 5.3 and 5.4). Parenteral administrations of macromolecular substances such as polyvinyl alcohol, gum acacia, pectins, methyl cellulose and perfluorochemicals produce such changes[11-13].

Immunologically-mediated glomerular injury is extremely rare in laboratory animals from routine toxicity tests. Administration of D-penicillamine[14], gold[15] or mercury[16] is associated with deposition of immune complexes. These and other animal models, such as acute and chronic serum sickness, are used in screening therapeutic compounds which might prevent the deposition of, or remove glomerular immune complexes[17-20] (Figures 5.5, 5.6 and 5.7). In man, immune-mediated glomerular disease is associated with many compounds including pharmaceutical preparations (for review see Ref. 4).

Progressive glomerulonephrosis in rats is spontaneous, progressive, age-related and it exhibits both glomerular and tubular lesions[21]. The development of the condition can be enhanced or inhibited by numerous factors such as diet and stress, and also the administration of pharmaceutical and chemical substances[22,23]. Prolactin appears to have a role in the aetiology of this disease[24] and it is possible that many of the factors or compounds influencing the disease are in fact altering circulating prolactin levels.

Vasculature

Toxic damage to the renal vasculature in routine toxicity studies is uncommon. Systemic effects on blood vessels may also be found in the kidney, e.g. atherosclerotic lesions in non-human primates on atherogenic diets (Figure 1.36), and metastatic mineralization as a sequel to renal damage and hyperparathyroidism. In the spontaneous hypertensive (SH) rat, renal arteriolar changes occur relatively early in life in association with elevated blood pressure. These changes consist of either fibrinoid necrosis of the media or a proliferative form with obliteration of the lumen (Figure 5.8). This feature allows the use of the SH rat as a suitable animal model for the renal vascular changes found in some patients treated with the immunosuppressant, cyclosporine[25]. We have noted tubular degeneration and thrombus formation in monkeys treated with high doses of a novel hypolipidaemic agent (Figure 5.9).

Antihypertensive agents which act by inhibiting the action of angiotensin I converting enzyme (ACE), cause hypertrophy and hyperplasia of renin secreting cells in the juxtaglomerular apparatus. Morphologically, the change is most obvious as hyperplasia of the juxtaglomerular cells surrounding afferent arterioles (Figures 5.10 and

5.11). Juxtaglomerular hyperplasia is found in rats, mice, dogs and monkeys and it is reversible on cessation of dosing[26,27]. The hyperplasia most probably results from continual stimulation of renin secreting cells due to lack of feedback inhibition by angiotensin II[26].

Tubules

In our experience, the proximal tubule is a frequent site for induced renal damage. Not uncommonly, when the proximal tubule displays toxic damage, other tubular portions of the nephron are spared. Differences in the site of tubular toxic change are in most instances inexplicable. In the rat, ischaemia and heavy metals cause preferential necrosis in the S_3 segment of the proximal tubule, while certain antibiotics are toxic to the S_2 region. Many factors, including blood flow, transport of compound, binding sites and metabolic activity, may be responsible for the predilection sites of induced lesions.

Numerous, structurally unrelated compounds cause tubular necrosis but the morphological picture of necrosis and its sequelae remain essentially the same. Following the initial acute nephrotoxic insult, varying degrees of regeneration and interstitial inflammation ensue. In fact, in toxicity studies where daily dosing is mandatory, the processes of necrosis, repair, inflammation and fibrosis can be observed simultaneously (Figure 5.12). The stages of renal tubular degeneration and necrosis have been extensively studied and seven are described[28,29]. The first three stages show reversible change and include loss of glycogen and microvilli, vesiculation, nuclear clumping, and swelling of endoplasmic reticulum. Beyond stage 3, irreversible changes include loss of nuclear staining and digestion of cell contents. Most nephrotoxic compounds can cause this sequence of changes leading to cell death, but different patterns may emerge depending on speed of onset, severity of insult, and extent of regeneration. Tubular basophilia (Figure 5.13) is probably the most frequently encountered characteristic of induced nephropathies, particularly in repeat-dose studies. It may be a sequel to degenerative conditions or represent excessive cell turnover. The pathogenesis of this tinctorial change may sometimes be uncertain, as both atrophic and regenerative tubules appear basophilic.

Tubular necrosis (Figures 5.14 and 5.15) is encountered in laboratory animals with many compounds including aminoglycoside and cephalosporin antibiotics[30,31], heavy metals[32] and halogenated hydrocarbons[33].

Tubular vacuolation may precede degeneration and necrosis, but may also indicate a reversible change, e.g. scattered vacuolization with cyclosporin treatment (Figure 5.16) or extensive uniform vacuolization found after intravascular infusions of hypertonic sugar solutions ('osmotic nephrosis') or some radio-contrast agents (Figure 5.17). Vacuolation may also indicate fat deposition as a toxic response in proximal convoluted tubules. In our experience this is a rare induced lesion.

Nuclear and cytoplasmic inclusions are relatively common findings in toxicity testing. Cytoplasmic inclusions are more common than nuclear. Intranuclear inclusions, similar to those seen in lead poisoning of domestic animals, are occasionally encountered. We have observed rounded, eosinophilic, intranuclear inclusions in rats treated with a novel pharmaceutical (Figure 5.18). The range of cytoplasmic tubular inclusion bodies is extensive. With some agents such as cyclosporine[34], the inclusions are red (Figures 5.16 and 5.19), whereas with others (oestrogens, neuroleptic drugs) the inclusions

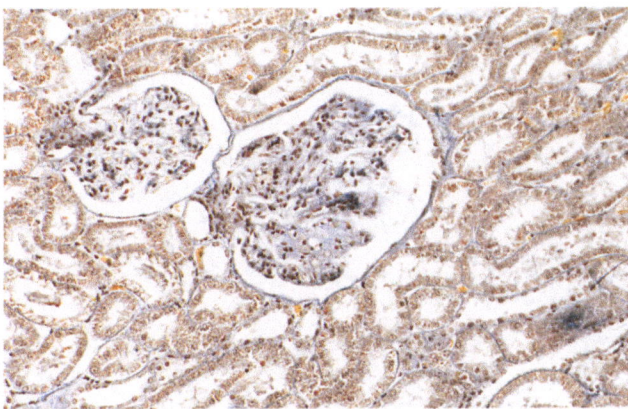

Figure 5.1 Glomerulosclerosis, in a diabetic beagle dog. Diabetes was induced by chronic administration of a progestational agent. The section shows partial hyalinization of the glomerular tuft and resembles the Kimmelstiel-Wilson lesion in man. Masson's trichrome

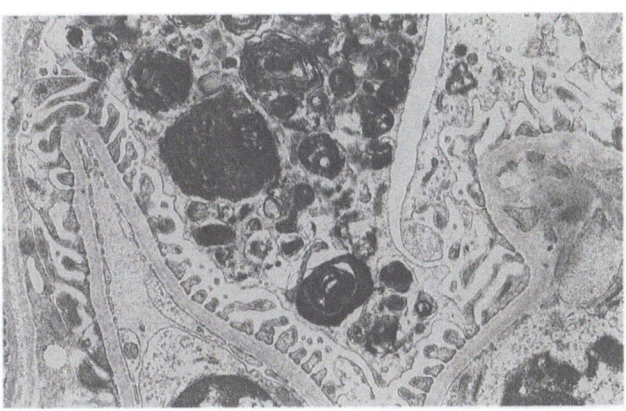

Figure 5.2 Numerous multilamellar bodies in a podocyte from the glomerulus of a dog treated with an amphiphilic cationic drug. These inclusions are characteristic of phospholipidosis. Electron micrograph

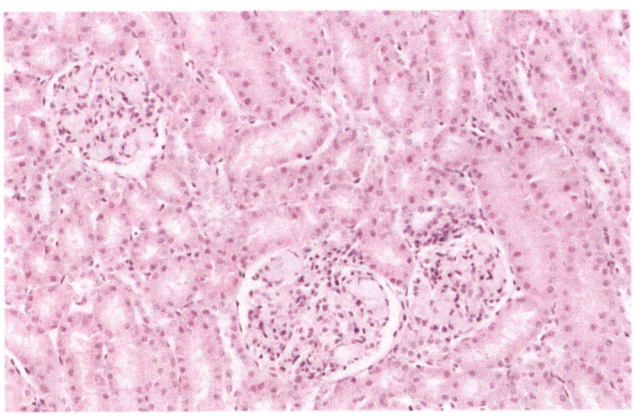

Figure 5.3 Mesangial accumulation of amorphous material in the glomeruli of a dog, following intravascular administration of a potential anticancer compound. The globular appearance of the glomeruli was also present in macrophages in other locations throughout the body. H & E

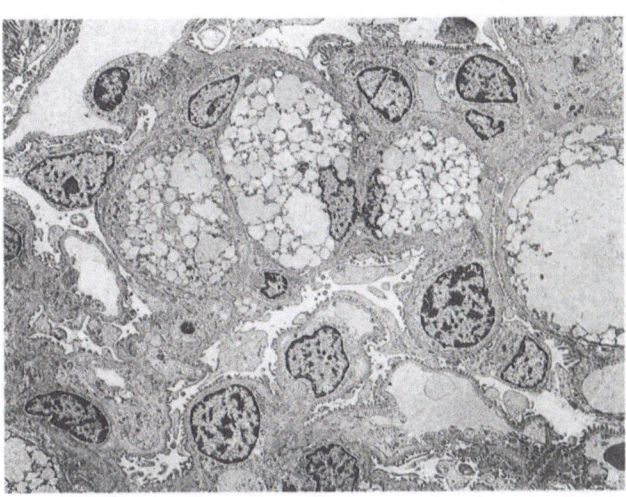

Figure 5.4 Ultrastructural details of a dog glomerulus from the same study as Figure 5.3. Irregular electron-lucent inclusions in mesangial cells. No evidence of degenerative change. Electron micrograph

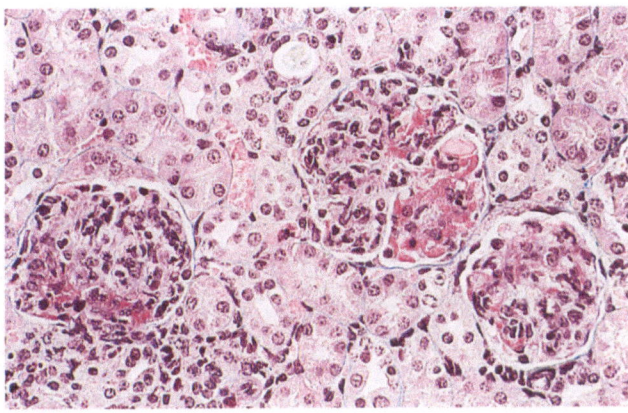

Figure 5.5 Glomerulonephritis in a New Zealand black and white hybrid mouse. These mice develop autoimmune glomerulonephritis at 3–6 months of age. This section shows early changes which consist of thickened capillary basement membranes by deposition of immunoglobulin and complement, and a tubular cast. The mouse disease is regarded as a suitable animal model of human systemic lupus erythematosus. Chromotrope–Aniline Blue

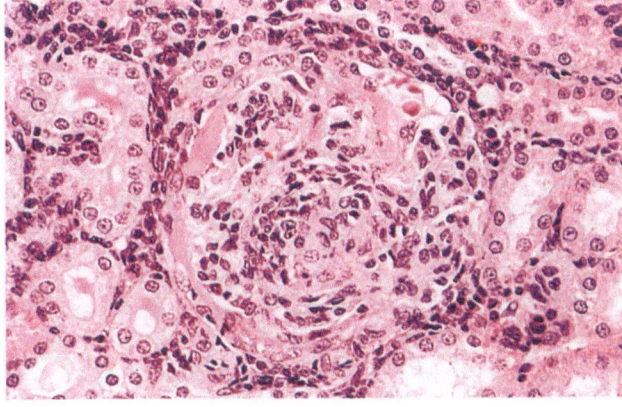

Figure 5.6 Acute serum sickness in a New Zealand white rabbit. This section shows a highly cellular glomerular tuft with fibrin deposition in Bowman's space and in the mesangium. This model is frequently used to assess the therapeutic or preventative effect of drugs on glomerulonephritis. H & E

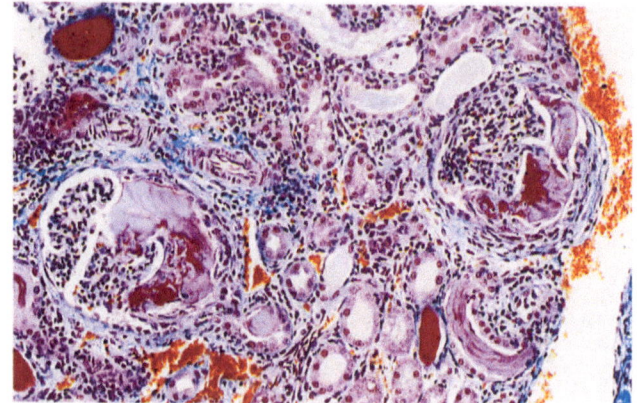

Figure 5.7 Acute serum sickness in a New Zealand white rabbit. Similar to Figure 5.6, but shows more severe change together with some interstitial reaction. Martius Scarlet Blue

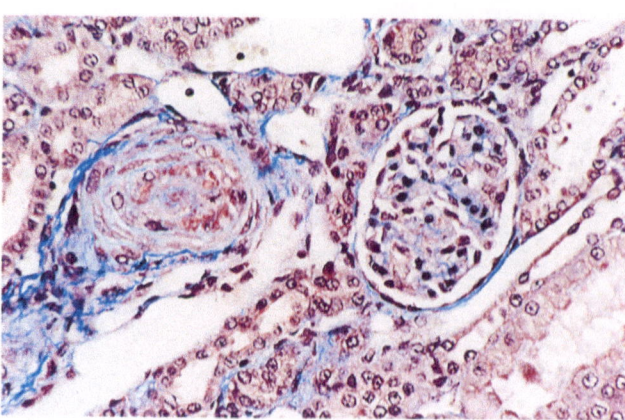

Figure 5.8 Arteriolar lesion in a spontaneously hypertensive rat treated with high doses of cyclosporin. The photomicrograph shows a proliferative lesion with obliteration of the lumen. Chromotrope–Aniline Blue

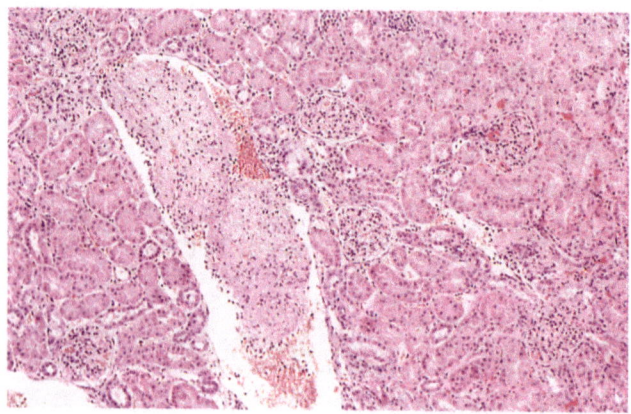

Figure 5.9 Thrombus formation in an arcuate vein of a monkey treated with high doses of a novel hypolipidaemic agent. Widespread renal thrombi were associated with tubular degenerative changes.   H & E

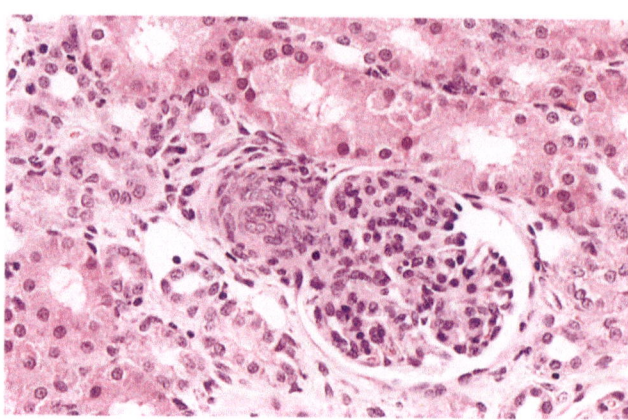

Figure 5.10 Hyperplasia of juxtaglomerular cells surrounding an afferent arteriole in a dog, following long term administration of an angiotensin I converting enzyme inhibitor.   H & E

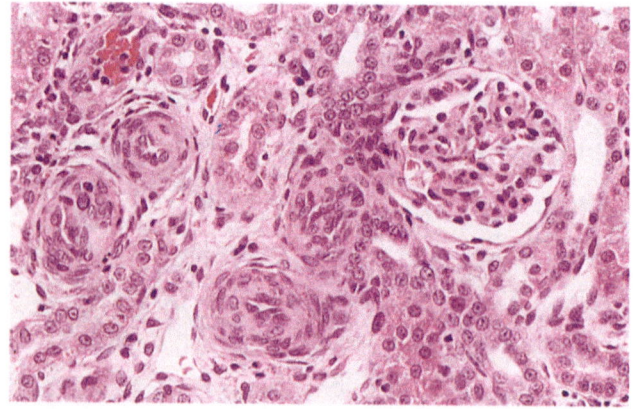

Figure 5.11 Similar lesion to Figure 5.10, but in this dog the hyperplasia of juxtaglomerular cells is more pronounced and appears to involve the efferent as well as the afferent arterioles. Blood vessels appear to have markedly reduced lumina.   H & E

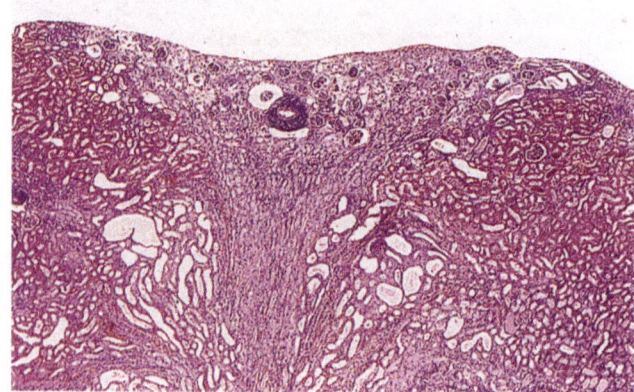

Figure 5.12 Wedge-shaped cortical scarring with capsular depression in a mouse. There is focal tubular atrophy and loss within the lesion. Adjacent areas show inflammation and tubular dilatation.   H & E

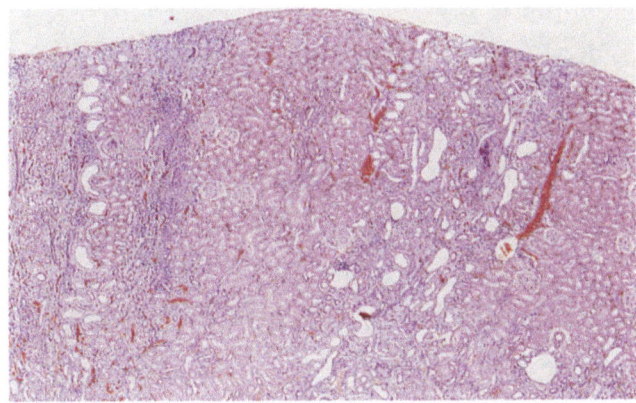

Figure 5.13 Areas of tubular basophilia and dilatation in a mouse kidney. From a toxicity study with a novel herbicide. H & E

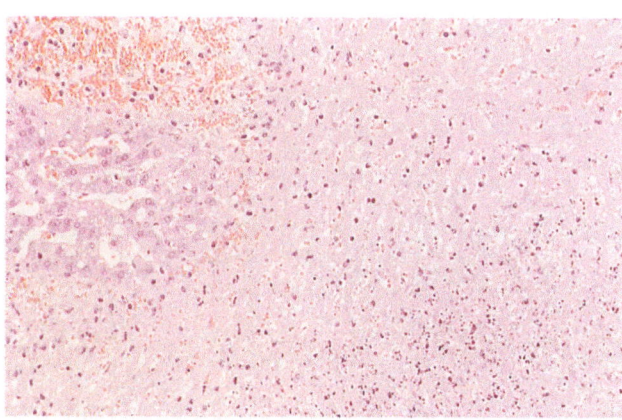

Figure 5.14 Kidney of a rat treated with gentamicin. The photomicrograph shows widespread acute necrosis of proximal tubules with a mild interstitial inflammatory infiltrate. Chromotrope–Aniline Blue

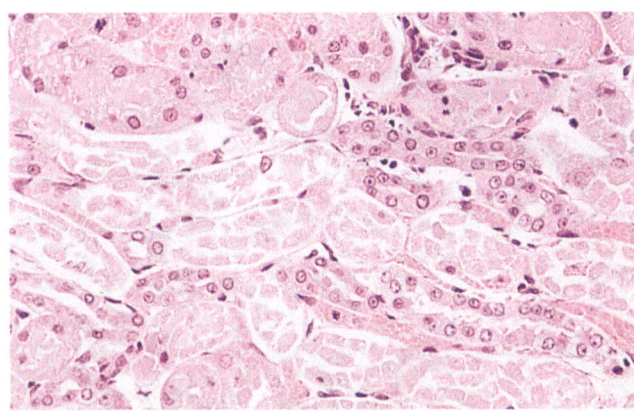

Figure 5.15 Kidney of a rat treated with an industrial chemical, showing necrosis of proximal convoluted tubules. H & E

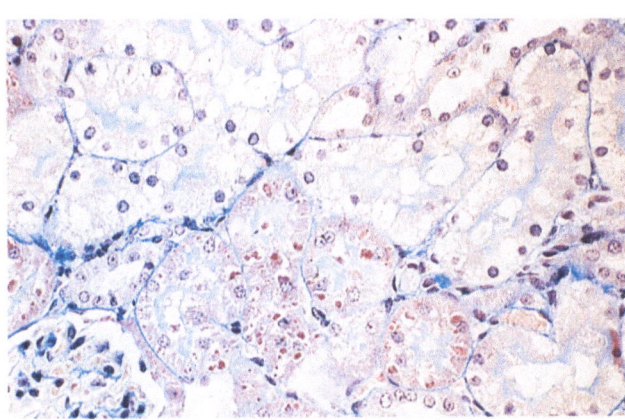

Figure 5.16 Vacuolization in the proximal tubules of a rat kidney following treatment with cyclosporine. There is variability in the degree of vacuolization between adjacent cells. Ultrastructurally, the vacuoles are due to dilatation of endoplasmic reticulum. Nearby proximal tubular cells contain red inclusion bodies of varying size which stain positively with PAS but negatively with Oil Red O. Ultrastructurally, the inclusions are enlarged lysosomes and occasionally giant mitochondria. Chromotrope–Aniline Blue

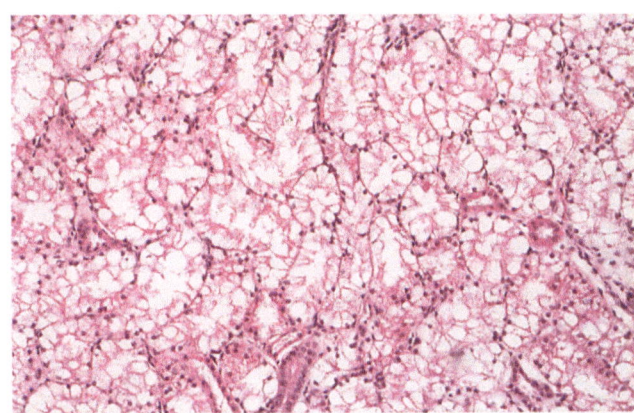

Figure 5.17 Vacuolization in the proximal tubules of a monkey kidney following infusion of a radio-contrast material. A similar histological picture is found in laboratory animals following rapid infusion of hypertonic sugar solutions. The histological appearance is often termed 'osmotic nephrosis'. H & E

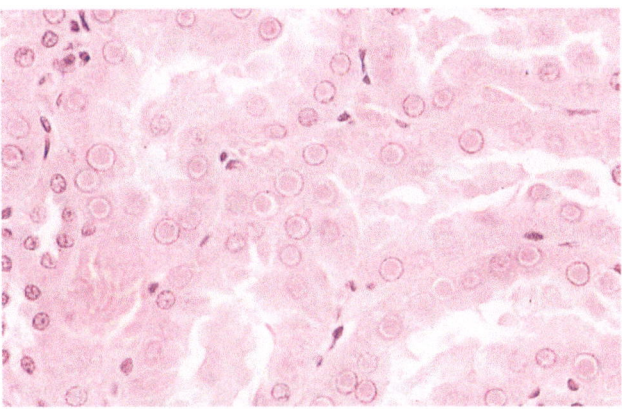

Figure 5.18 Intranuclear inclusions in tubular cells in a rat kidney. These eosinophilic inclusions are found in the majority of proximal tubular cells following the administration of a compound designed to promote peripheral nerve regeneration. The inclusions stained negatively with Oil Red O, PAS and MethylGreen–pyronine. They are not associated with degenerative or functional changes. H & E

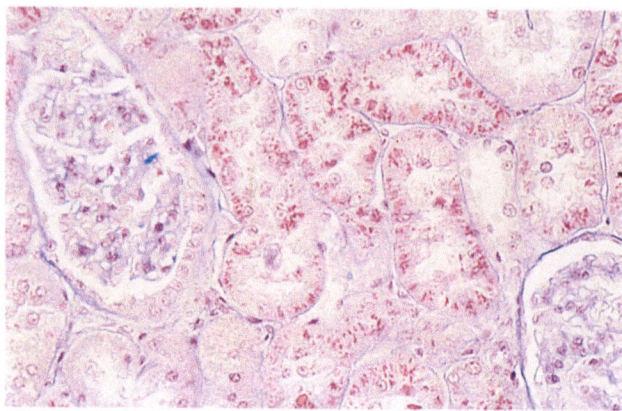

Figure 5.19 Multiple small intracytoplasmic hyaline droplets in proximal tubular epithelial cells of a male rat. This change was present only in males and although produced by a novel pharmaceutical compound it is indistinguishable from 'hydrocarbon nephropathy'. In this case, there is no evidence of epithelial degeneration. Martius Scarlet Blue

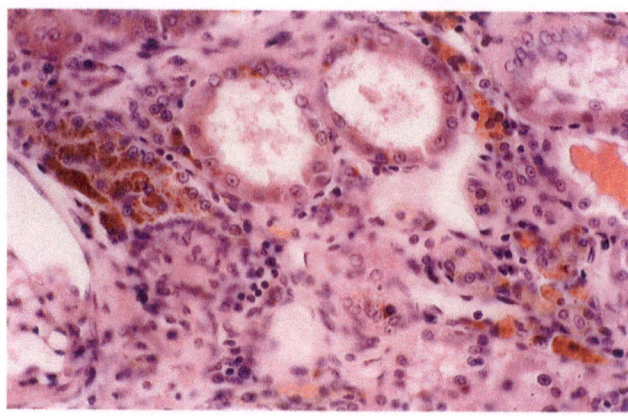

Figure 5.20 Brown pigmentation (lipofuscin) due to neuroleptic drug treatment in an aged rat. In the treated young rat this lipopigment is found in tubular epithelial cells. However, in the aged rat with loss of nephrons due to spontaneous progressive glomerulonephrosis, the pigment is found in macrophages within nonfunctional atrophic tubules and in the interstitium. This pigment was also present in thyroid, brain, liver, heart, spleen and skeletal muscle. H & E

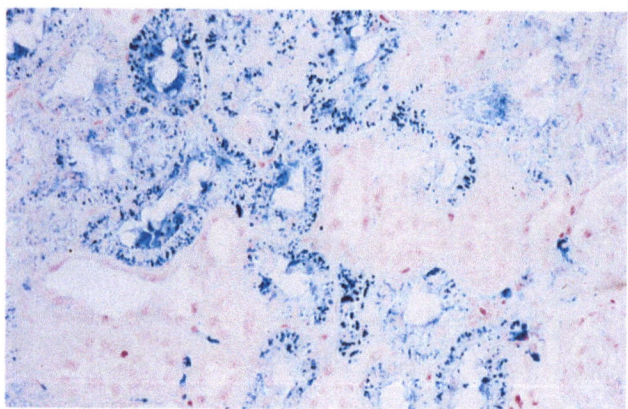

Figure 5.21 Iron pigment deposition in proximal tubule cells of a dog with a drug induced haemolytic anaemia. Perl's stain

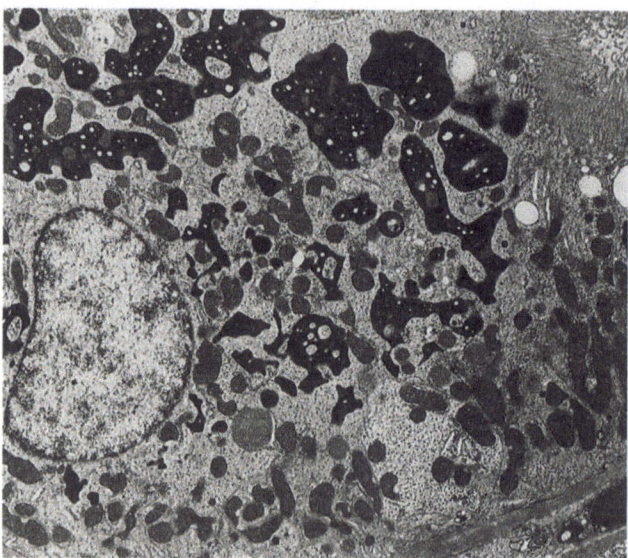

Figure 5.22 Irregular electron-dense inclusions in proximal convoluted tubule of a male rat with 'hydrocarbon nephropathy'. Electron micrograph

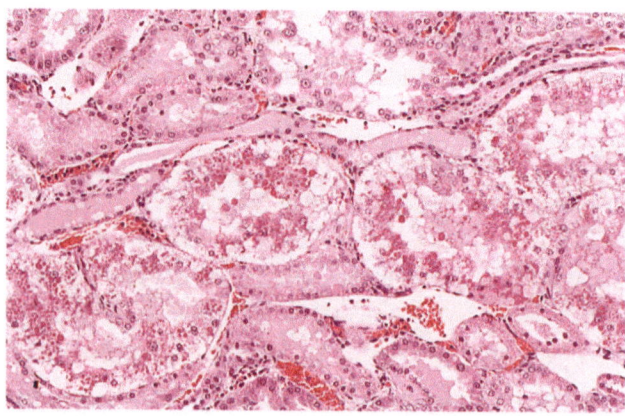

Figure 5.23 Pronounced vacuolar degeneration and hyaline droplet formation in proximal tubular epithelial cells. Tubules are considerably dilated. In comparison with Figure 5.19, this photomicrograph is from a severe case of 'hydrocarbon nephropathy' in a male rat. Female rats did not develop such histological changes. H & E

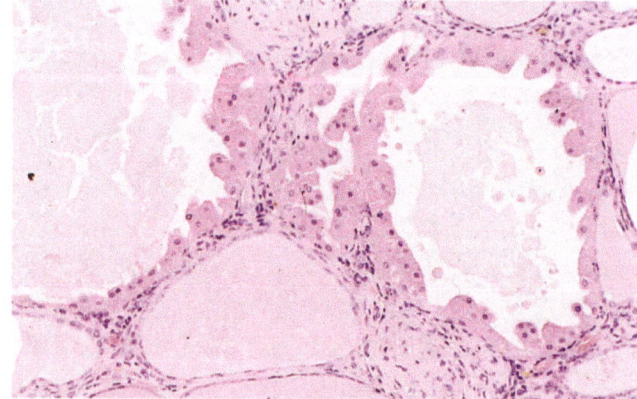

Figure 5.24 Renal tubular hypertrophy in a rat. This photomicrograph shows enlarged tubules lined by a single layer of large eosinophilic epithelial cells, which tend to have distally located nuclei. This form of hypertrophy occurs spontaneously in aging rats but the incidence can increase following administration of drugs and chemicals. H & E

appear as brown pigments (Figure 5.20). Some of these inclusions contain lipofuscin and others may represent the test compound or its metabolites. In haemolytic conditions, haemosiderin deposits can be seen in renal tubules (Figure 5.21). In most instances, renal inclusions do not appear to be associated with degenerative or functional alterations. Reversibility of inclusions on cessation of treatment is usually slow or not perceptible.

Hyaline droplet inclusions induced by some hydrocarbons can, however, proceed to necrosis. Such hydrocarbon-induced droplets are peculiar to the male rat[35,36]. The hyaline droplets are strongly eosinophilic and PAS negative. Ultrastructurally, they appear as irregular electron-dense inclusions (Figure 5.22). Female rats and other laboratory animals do not develop 'hydrocarbon nephropathy'. Early alterations consist of hyaline droplet formation which may progress to degenerative change (Figure 5.23). Biochemically, the effect is to exacerbate the accumulation of α_2-microglobulin in proximal tubular cells. This protein is found only in the proximal tubules of adult male rats.

Tubules, particularly proximal convoluted tubules, may show induced ultrastructural changes similar to those found in hepatocytes. These include: SER proliferation with microsomal enzyme inducers; microbody proliferation with hypolipidaemic drugs; and multilamellar bodies with amphiphilic cationic compounds.

Tubular hypertrophy in the rat is characterized by dilated proximal tubules lined by enlarged eosinophilic epithelial cells. These cells usually have distally located nuclei and may appear as finger-like projections into the lumen (Figure 5.24). This age-related lesion occurs spontaneously and the incidence varies between rat strains. Administration of drugs and chemicals may increase the incidence and severity of the hypertrophy[23]. The mechanism of induction is unknown.

Other forms of tubular hypertrophy are also occasionally encountered, i.e. multilayering with enlarged eosinophilic or clear cells (Figure 5.25) or apparent occlusion of the tubular lumen with enlarged clear cells (Figure 5.26). The eosinophilic hypertrophic cells have some resemblance to oncocytes, while the clear cells may represent the 'chromophobic' tubules described by Bannasch[37]. Both these latter forms of tubular hypertrophy can be considered as preneoplastic developments. In our experience, induced tubular hypertrophy is rarely encountered in other laboratory animal species.

Tubular hyperplasia is found spontaneously in rats, particularly with the more severe forms of progressive glomerulonephrosis or as a treatment-related change in most laboratory animal species. The increase in tubular epithelial cells in both instances is most probably compensatory in nature. With many nephrotoxic agents, tubular regenerative hyperplasia may be found within areas of ongoing degeneration[38]. Hyperplastic cells are usually normal in size and tinctorial affinity but may occasionally appear basophilic (Figures 5.27, 5.28 and 5.29). Hyperplasia is seen focally and cells are either heaped, multilayered or form papillary projections into the lumen (Figure 5.30). Mitoses are infrequently encountered. Tubular hyperplasia and nodular hyperplasia are described in rats following cisplatin treatment[38], but the nodular lesion described may well represent neoplasia rather than hyperplasia.

Intratubular crystal deposits are relatively rare in routine toxicity testing. However such deposits are occasionally seen, usually in the outer medulla. They are a consequence of the concentrating properties and/or pH changes in the distal portion of the nephron. Other crystals may be found in the proximal tubules scattered throughout the cortex[39]. The morphological picture and the end result depend mainly on two factors, crystal shape/size and number of nephrons affected. The sequelae include: tubular dilatation and atrophy, pyelonephritis, and interstitial reactions. If many nephrons are blocked or damaged then impairment of urinary flow may lead to a uraemic state. Oxalate[39,40] (Figure 5.31), sulphonamide (Figure 5.32), and several types of unidentified crystals (Figure 5.33) have been encountered in our laboratories. Crystalline deposits may also be encountered in collecting ducts in the renal papilla. Sometimes they provoke hyperplasia of the collecting duct epithelium and inflammation (Figure 5.34). Some crystals are birefringent (Figure 5.35) while others may only be detected as clefts due to their solubility during histological processing.

Intratubular mineralization occurs spontaneously in most laboratory animals but is particularly common in rats and dogs. Deposits can be found in the cortex, medulla and papilla. In the rat, deposits are commonly found at the corticomedullary junction (Figure 5.36) and the incidence tends to be higher in female than in male rats. The chemical composition of deposits is variable[41,42]. Mineralization may be induced by many compounds including parathyroid hormone, calcium gluconate, vitamin D, carbonic anhydrase inhibitors or by dietary means (alteration of calcium/phosphorus ratios). The consequences of induced intratubular mineralization are normally minimal though in severe cases the sequelae listed above for crystal deposits may ensue.

Renal tubular dilatation (Figure 5.37) and cysts may be induced in laboratory animals by a variety of agents. Nephrotoxic agents can cause tubular damage and dilatation with or without an interstitial reaction, and the dilatation is caused at least in part by intratubular stasis. However, certain compounds, notably steroids, when given in high doses cause tubular ectasia in young animals[43]. In these instances the tubular enlargement is not associated with tubular damage. Compounds which interfere with nephron development during the nephrogenic phase may cause severe dilatation and cyst development (Figures 5.38 and 5.39). Administration of long acting adrenal corticosteroids to neonatal animals during the nephrogenic stage causes, within a relatively short period, multiple cysts throughout the cortex[44]. These cysts appear to arise from dilated collecting ducts which have failed to establish continuity with developing nephrons. The cysts are fluid-filled and cause marked enlargement of the organ.

In our experience a number of unrelated substances cause karyomegaly in rodent tubular epithelial cells (Figure 5.40). The alteration may affect all tubular elements or be confined to a particular portion of the tubular system. It may also be preceded by a degenerative episode, but this is not always the case. The karyomegaly may be accompanied by cytomegaly and in a few instances the nuclei are bizarre. Similar changes are also reported with some renal carcinogens[45,46].

Papilla

Many analgesic and most non-steroidal, anti-inflammatory (NSAI) drugs are capable of inducing renal papillary necrosis (RPN) in experimental animals, including monkeys. In addition, several compounds which are structurally unrelated to the analgesic/NSAI group can also induce RPN (for review see Ref. 47). Morphologically, the lesion first appears at the extreme tip of the papilla as foci or areas of interstitial degeneration. As the lesion extends and involves more of the papilla, interstitial

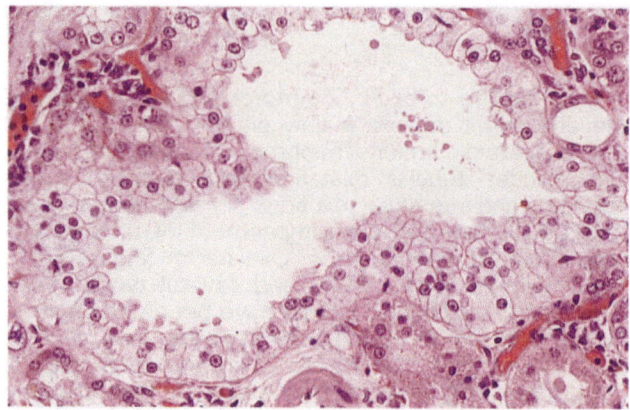

Figure 5.25   Renal tubular hypertrophy in a rat. A dilated tubule lined by enlarged slightly eosinophilic or clear epithelial cells. Focally the epithelial cells show multilayering. As in Figure 5.24, the spontaneous incidence of this lesion may be increased following treatment with drugs and chemicals.   H & E

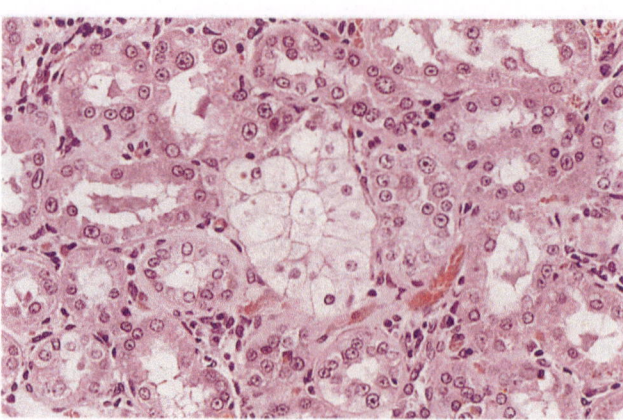

Figure 5.26   Renal tubular hypertrophy in a rat. A slightly dilated tubule containing hypertrophic clear cells. The tubular lumen appears to be occluded.   H & E

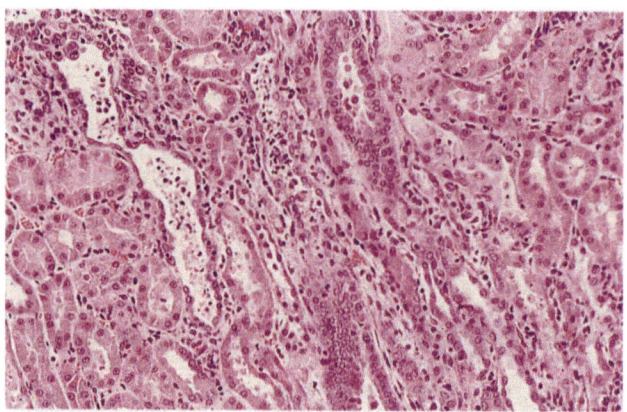

Figure 5.27   Tubular degeneration with ongoing regenerative hyperplasia in a kidney from a rat treated with an industrial chemical. The hyperplastic tubules show epithelial multilayering.   H & E

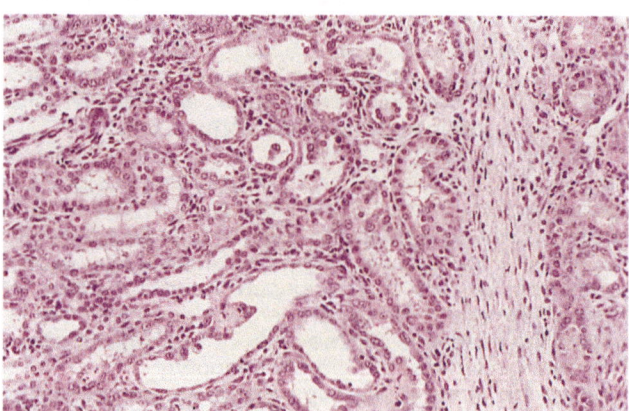

Figure 5.28   Tubular hyperplasia with cortical fibrosis in a rat kidney. This photomicrograph is from the same study as Figure 5.27 and shows, in addition, tubular dilatation and interstitial fibrosis.   H & E

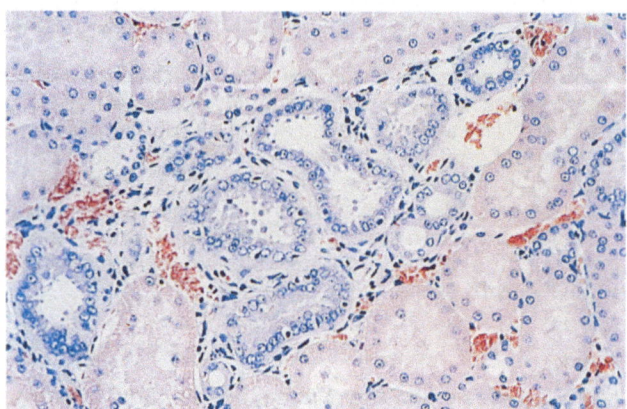

Figure 5.29   Tubular regenerative hyperplasia in the kidney of a rat treated chronically with a novel fungicide. The photomicrograph shows dilated basophilic tubules together with a mild interstitial reaction.   H & E

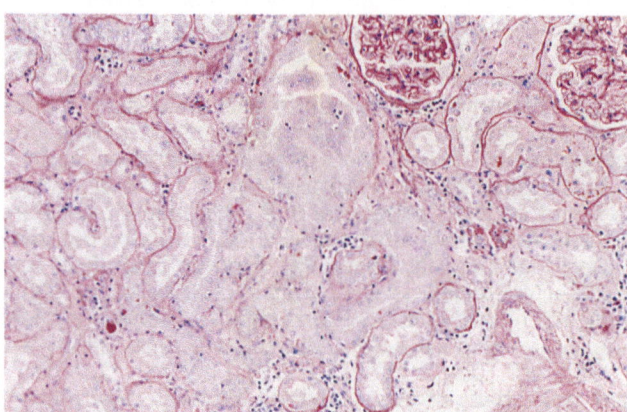

Figure 5.30   Focal tubular hyperplasia in a rat. Slightly dilated tubule partially occluded by hyperplastic epithelial cells forming papillary structures. Mitoses are not detected. The adjacent tubules appear normal.   PAS

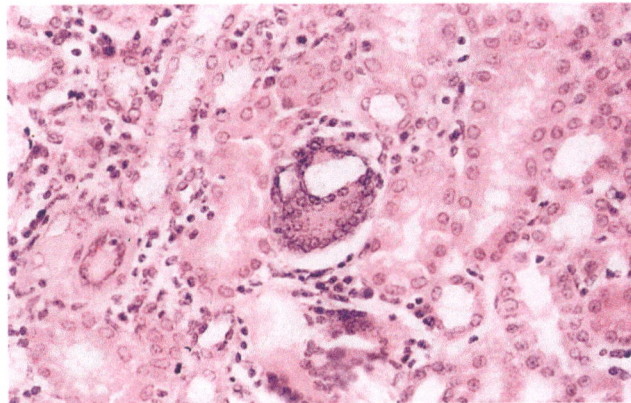

Figure 5.31 Oxalate crystals in a monkey kidney. Proximal tubular cells are heaped around a crystal giving the appearance of multi-nucleate giant cells. Nuclei of these altered cells are small and hyperchromatic. Crystals were present throughout the cortex. H & E

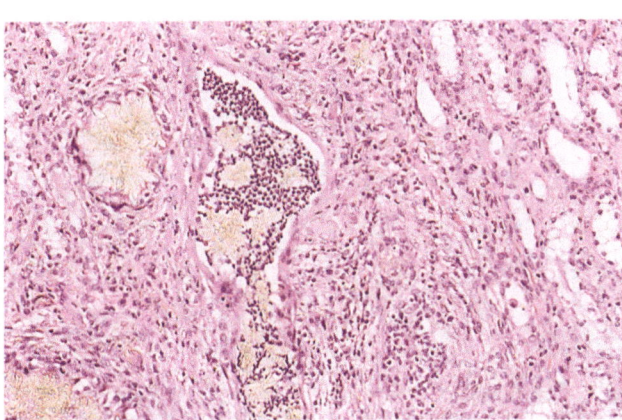

Figure 5.32 Sulphonamide crystals in a dog kidney. Numerous yellow crystals, sometimes radially arranged, are present within tubules and scattered in the interstitium of the outer medulla. An extensive interstitial reaction with tubule loss is present. Centrally, a dilated tubule contains both crystals and neutrophil polymorphs. H & E

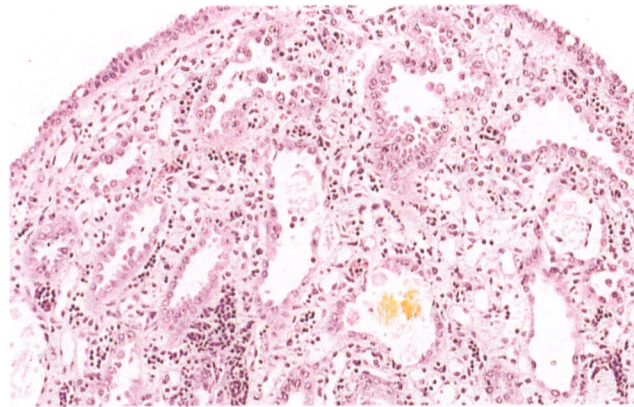

Figure 5.33 Crystals in the papilla of a rat. Bright yellow crystals (probably test compound or metabolites) within collecting ducts causing ductular hyperplasia and interstitial inflammation. H & E

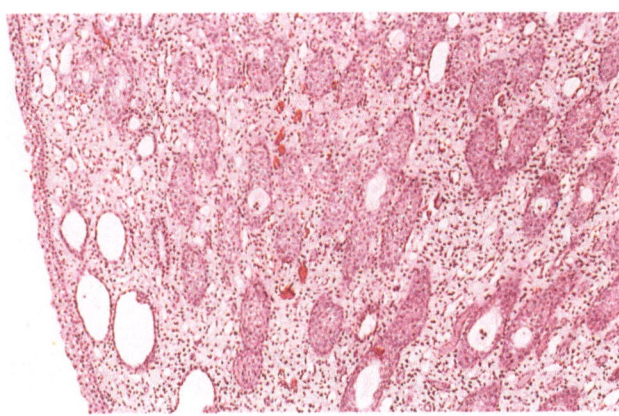

Figure 5.34 Epithelial hyperplasia in the collecting ducts of a dog treated with a novel pharmaceutical. H & E

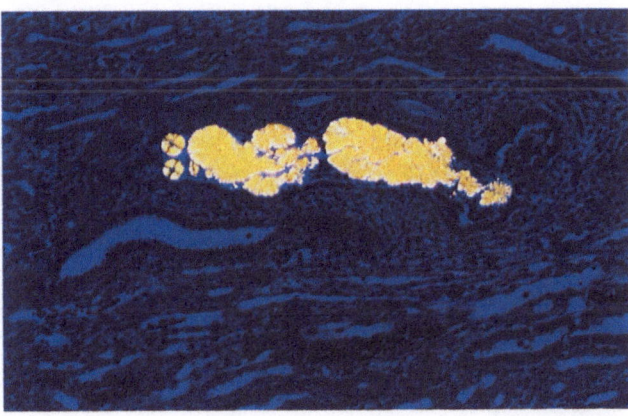

Figure 5.35 Birefringence of crystals in renal medulla of a rat kidney induced by a novel anti-allergic compound. Polarized light.

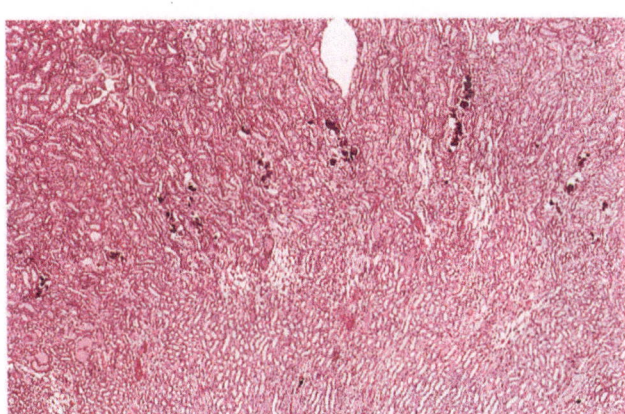

Figure 5.36 Renal mineralization in a rat. Mineral deposits form a 'necklace' at the corticomedullary junction. These deposits can occur spontaneously or following administration of various chemicals, particularly those which alter urinary pH. H & E

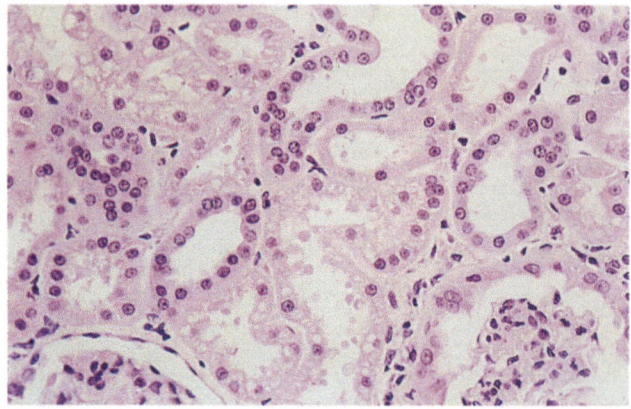

Figure 5.37 Tubular basophilia, dilation and vacuolation in a monkey treated with a novel male antifertility drug. The parietal layer of a Bowman's capsule also shows hypertrophy and basophilia.   H & E

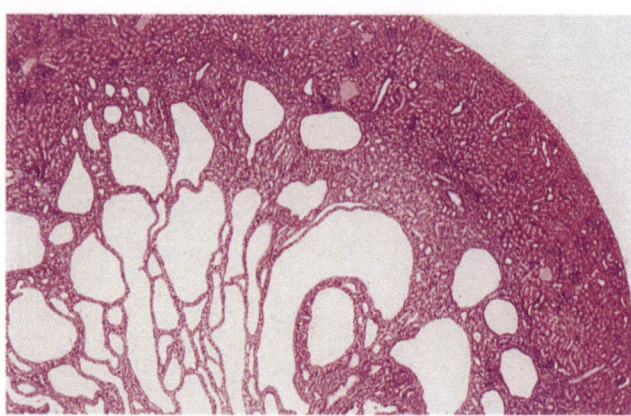

Figure 5.38 Renal tubular dilatation in a young rat. This animal from a reproductive toxicity study, received an insecticide as a neonate via the mother's milk. Extensive tubular dilatation is confined to the medulla.   H & E

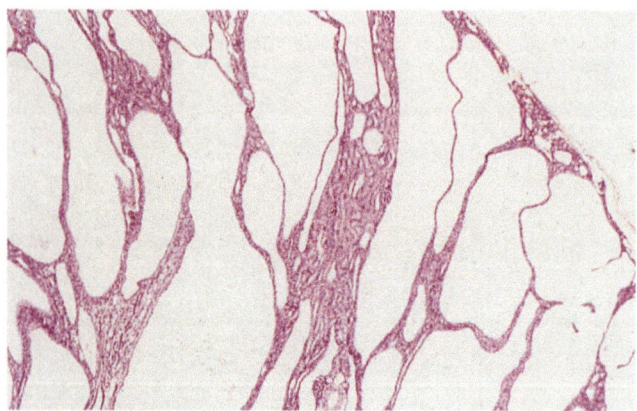

Figure 5.39 Renal tubular cysts in an adult rat. This rat was treated similarly to that in Figure 5.38, but treatment was continued for a longer period. The tubular dilatation and cysts are more pronounced and extend well into the cortex.   H & E

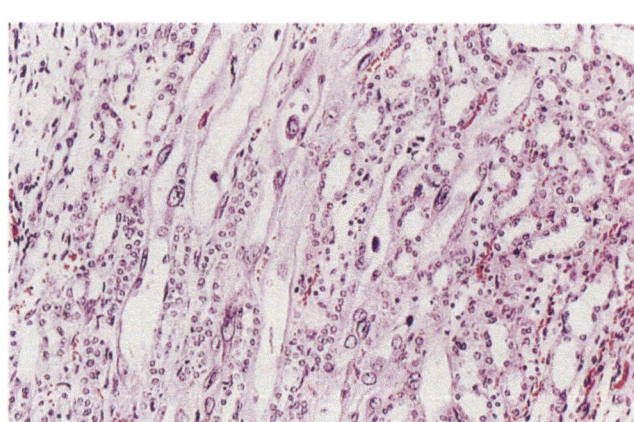

Figure 5.40 Enlarged cells with karyomegaly in the tubular epithelium of a rat treated with an agrochemical compound.   H & E

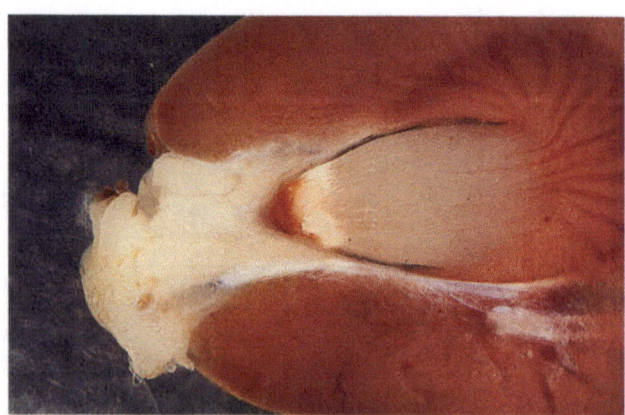

Figure 5.41 Macroscopic appearance of renal papillary necrosis in a rat treated chronically with a non-steroidal anti-inflammatory drug

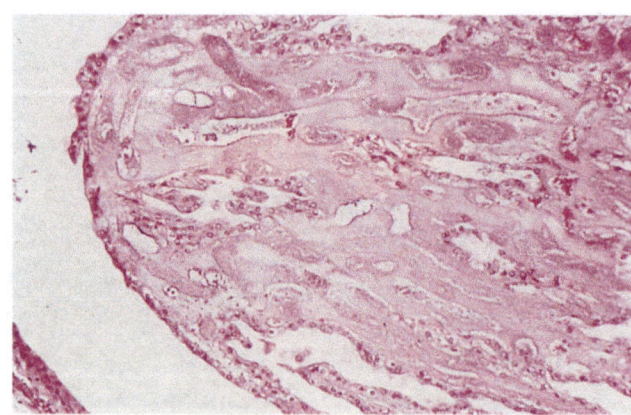

Figure 5.42 Papillary necrosis in a rat treated chronically with a non-steroidal anti-inflammatory drug. In this section, the lesion is extensive and involves tubular, vascular and interstitial elements.   H & E

cells, capillaries and tubules show degenerative change. The whole papilla may eventually become necrotic and may even become detached from the adjacent outer medulla (Figures 5.41–5.45). The lesion usually fails to provoke a cellular reaction. The severity of RPN can be graded histologically[48].

Hyperplasia of the urothelium of the renal papilla and pelvis is noted following the administration of various chemicals (Figure 5.46), including aspirin, phenacetin and sodium saccharin[49,50]. Combined administration of two such compounds appears to exacerbate the hyperplastic response[51]. The urothelium usually shows focal multilayering and the more florid lesions appear endophytic as well as exophytic. Urothelial hyperplasia is also noted as a sequel to RPN.

Ureter

Toxic changes are rarely detected in the ureters. However, compounds which effect the urothelium of the kidney pelvis or bladder may also effect the urothelium of the ureter.

Urinary Bladder

Induced bladder changes are relatively uncommon, and are generally confined to the mucosa (Table 5.2).

Table 5.2 Induced lesions of the urinary bladder

Mucosal necrosis
Mucosal hyperplasia
Calculi

Cystitis is recorded from time to time in most laboratory animals. However, we have not recorded induced cystitis in the absence of mucosal injury. Mucosal damage may be caused by chemical agents, mechanical injury or irradiation. Compounds such as: N-methyl-N-nitrosurea; methyl methane sulphonate; ethyl methane sulphonite; ethyl-sulphonyl naphthalene sulphonamide and cyclophosphamide are cytotoxic to the bladder urothelium and can cause haemorrhage from subepithelial capillaries. In severe cases, large areas of epithelium may slough. Epithelial necrosis is followed rapidly by a reversible hyperplasia (Figures 5.47, 5.48 and 5.49). Erythrophagocytosis by urothelial cells may be observed[52]. Hyperplasias are diffuse or focal and they may be categorized as simple, papillary, nodular or associated with metaplasia[53]. A few substances, however, induce reversible hyperplasia of the urothelium without prior epithelial necrosis (Figure 5.50), e.g. some cytostatic agents, phenacetin, sodium saccharin, and vitamin A deficiency. In addition, foreign bodies including induced bladder calculi can cause hyperplasia which in some cases is severe and extensive (Figures 5.51–5.54).

Bladder calculi may arise spontaneously particularly in rodents. Calculi can also be induced by a variety of means: administration of carbonic anhydrase inhibitors including sulphonamides; administration of chemicals which alter urinary pH; and by dietary manipulation, particularly alteration of the concentrations and ratios of calcium, phosphorus and magnesium. The calculi usually consist of magnesium phosphate, calcium phosphate or calcium oxalate[39,42]. In our experience, induced calculi are usually complex and contain mixtures of mineral salts with a high proportion of oxalates.

It is known that some chemicals, and even chronic inflammatory processes which induce hyperplasia, can also induce neoplasia of the bladder epithelium. Chemicals which are reported to induce irreversible preneoplastic hyperplasias and neoplasias are listed by Kunze[53].

References

1. Pritchard, J. B. (1981). Renal handling of environmental chemicals. In Hook, J. B. (ed.) *Toxicology of the Kidney.* (New York: Raven Press)
2. Ryan, G. B. and Karnovsky, M. S. (1975). An ultrastructural study of the mechanism of proteinuria in aminonucleoside nephrosis. *Kidney Int.*, **8**, 219–232
3. Schöll, A., Hiller, G. W., Gärtner, H. V. and Fischbach, H. (1974). Fokale Glomerulumläsionen im Spätstadium der Aminonucleosidnephrose (ANN) bei Ratten. *Verh. Dtsch. Ges. Pathol.*, **58**, 483
4. Hill, G. S. (1986). Drug-associated glomerulopathies. *Toxicol. Pathol.*, **14**, 37–44
5. Rehan, A., Johnson, K. J., Kunkel, R. G. and Wiggins, R. C. (1985). Role of oxygen radicals in phorbol myristate acetate-induced glomerular injury. *Kidney Int.*, **27**, 503–511
6. Weening, J. J. and Rennke, H. G. (1983). Glomerular permeability and polyanion in adriamycin nephrosis in the rat. *Kidney Int.*, **24**, 157–159
7. Tucker, M. J. (1971). Some effects of prolonged administration of a progestagen to dogs. *Proc. Eur. Soc. Study Drug Toxicity*, **12**, 228–238
8. Bloodsworth, J. M. B. (1965). Experimental diabetic glomerulosclerosis II. The Dog. *Arch. Pathol.*, **79**, 113
9. Gibbs, G. E., Wilson, R. B. and Gifford, H. (1966). Glomerulosclerosis in the long term alloxan diabetic monkey. *Diabetes*, **15**, 258–262
10. Wehner, H. and Petri, M. (1983). Glomerular alterations in experimental diabetes of the rat. *Pathol. Res. Pract.*, **176**, 145–157
11. Teoh, T. B. (1961). The effects of methylcellulose in rats with special reference to splenomegaly, anaemia and the problem of hypersplenism. *J. Pathol. Bacteriol.*, **81**, 33–44
12. Weissmann, S. M., Waldmann, T. A., Levin, E. and Berlin, N. I. (1961). An attempt to produce hypersplenism in the dog, using methylcellulose. *Blood*, **17**, 632–642
13. Nanney, L., Fink, L. M. and Virmani, R. (1980). Perfluorochemicals. Morphologic changes in infused liver, spleen, lung and kidney of rabbits. *Arch. Pathol. Lab. Med.*, **108**, 631–637
14. Batsford, S. R., Rohrbach, R., Riede, U. N., Sandritter, W. and Kluthe, R. (1976). Effects of D-penicillamine administration to rats, induction of renal changes: preliminary communication. *Clin. Nephrol.*, **6**, 394–397
15. Nagi, A. H., Alexander, F. and Barabas, A. Z. (1971). Gold nephropathy in rats – light and electron microscopic studies. *Exp. Mol. Pathol.*, **15**, 354–362
16. Druet, P., Druet, E., Potdevin, F. and Sapin, C. (1978). Immune type of glomerulonephritis induced by $HgCl_2$ in the Brown Norway Rat. *Ann. Immunol.*, **129C**, 777
17. Neild, G. H., Ivory, K., Hiramatsu, M. and Williams, D. G. (1983). Cyclosporine A inhibits acute serum sickness in rabbits. *Clin. Exp. Immunol.*, **52**, 586–594
18. Neild, G. H., Ivory, K. and Williams, D. G. (1986). Effects of cyclosporine on proteinuria in chronic serum sickness in rats. *Clin. Nephrol.*, **25**, 186–188
19. Thaiss, F., Mihatsch, M. J., Batsford, S., Vogt, A. and Schallmeyer, P. (1986). Effect of cyclosporine on *in situ* immune complex glomerulonephritis. *Clin. Nephrol.*, **25**, 181–186
20. Gunn, H. C. and Ryffel, B. (1986). Glomerulonephritis in NZ B/W mice; therapeutic effect of cyclosporine. *Clin. Nephrol.*, **25**, 189–192
21. Gray, J. E. (1986). Chronic progressive nephrosis, rat. In Jones, T. C., Mohr, V. and Hunt, R. D. (eds.) *Urinary System. Monographs of Pathology of Laboratory Animals.* (Heidelberg: Springer Verlag)
22. Saxton, J. A. and Kimball, G. C. (1941). Relation of nephrosis and other disease of albino rats to age and modification of diet. *Arch. Pathol.*, **32**, 951–965
23. Peter, C. P., Burek, J. D. and van Zwieten, M. J. (1986). Spontaneous nephropathies in rats. *Toxicol. Pathol.*, **14**, 91–100
24. Richardson, B. and Luginbühl, H. (1976). The role of prolactin in the development of chronic progressive nephropathy in the rat. *Virchows Arch. A: Pathol. Anat. Histol.*, **370**, 13–19

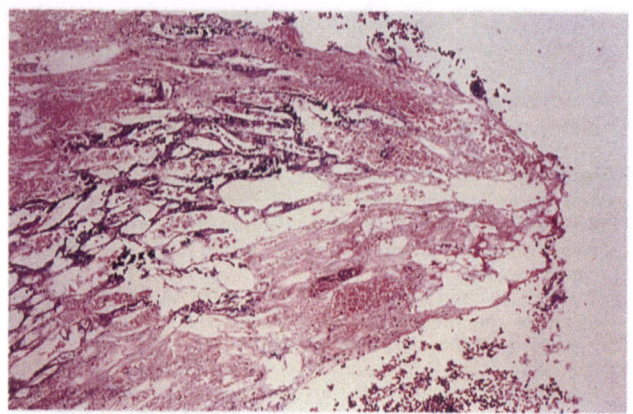

Figure 5.43 Papillary necrosis in a rat treated chronically with a non-steroidal anti-inflammatory drug. Similar to Figure 5.42 but involving whole papilla. Note also mineralization in the necrotic tissue and slight pyelitis.   H & E

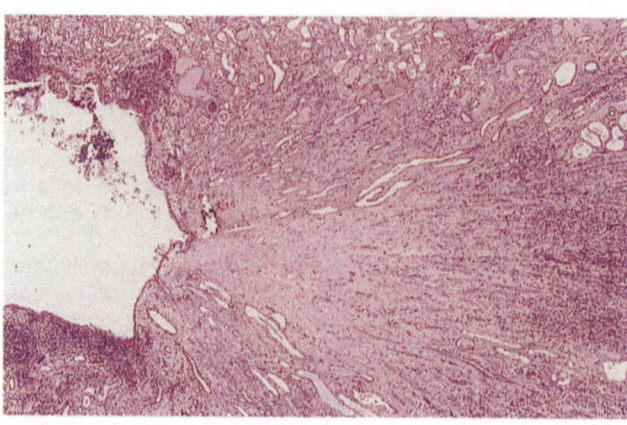

Figure 5.44 Loss of the renal papilla in a rat treated with a non-steroidal anti-inflammatory drug. The papilla has become detached resulting in minor pyelitis and some scarring in the outer medulla.   H & E

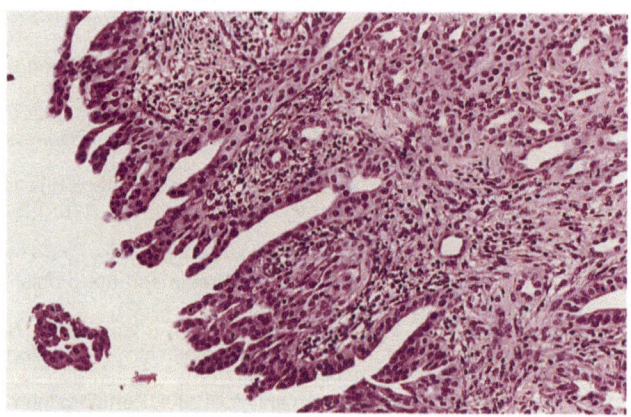

Figure 5.45 Papillitis with extensive proliferation of the urothelium following degeneration and necrosis of the tip of the papilla. This case is from a monkey treated with a non-steroidal anti-inflammatory drug.   H & E

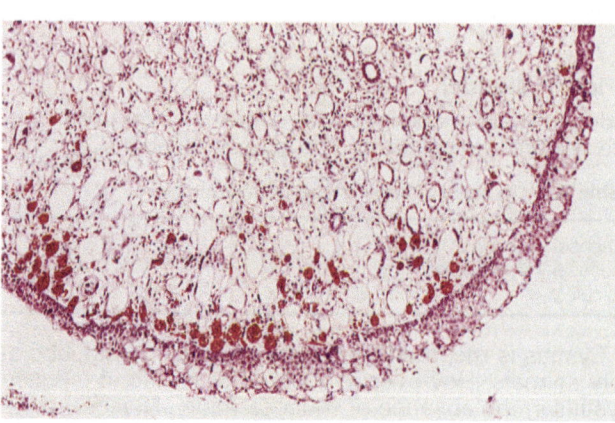

Figure 5.46 Papilla from a rat treated with a novel H$_2$-antagonist drug, showing congestion with vacuolation and hyperplasia of the overlying urothelium.   H & E

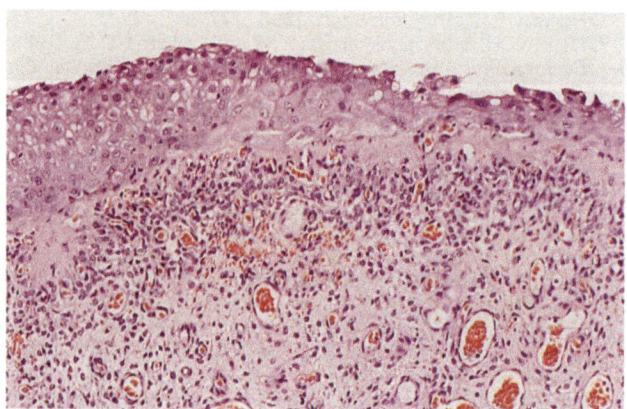

Figure 5.47 Erosion and hyperplasia of the bladder mucosa with submucosal inflammation in a dog treated with a novel pharmaceutical compound.   H & E

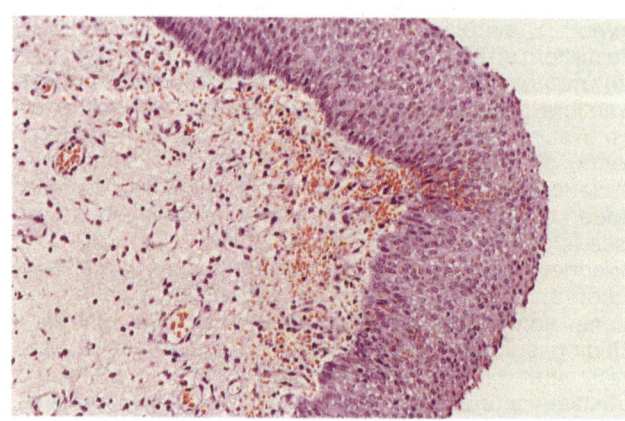

Figure 5.48 Pronounced mucosal hyperplasia in the bladder of a dog, together with submucosal haemorrhage, oedema and inflammation. From the same study as Figure 5.47.   H & E

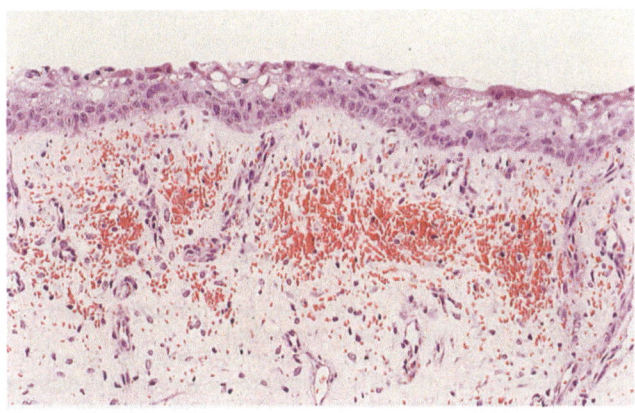

Figure 5.49 Mucosal vacuolation with submucosal haemorrhage in a dog bladder. This case is from the same study as Figure 5.47. H & E

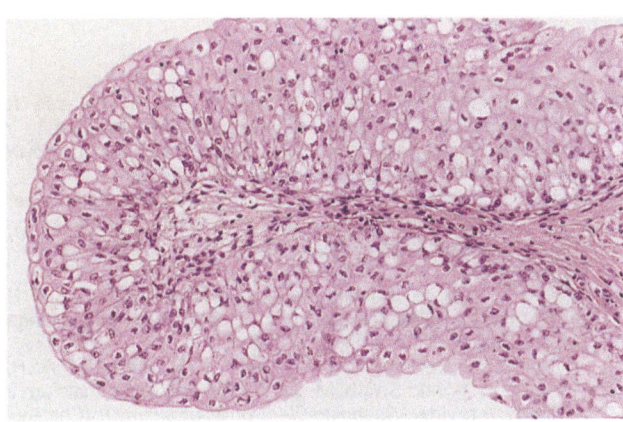

Figure 5.50 Mucosal hyperplasia and marked vacuolation of the epithelium from the urinary bladder of a monkey treated with an antineoplastic compound. H & E

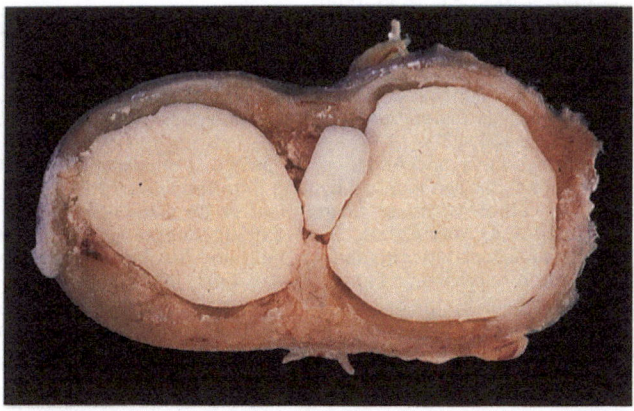

Figure 5.51 Urinary bladder calculi. Macroscopic photograph showing a rat bladder greatly distended by a few large calculi. Note the thickened appearance of the bladder wall. Calculi can occur spontaneously or can be induced by a variety of treatments including dietary manipulation

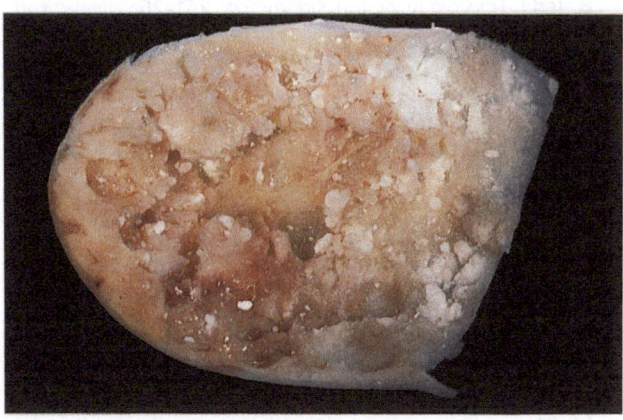

Figure 5.52 Urinary bladder calculi. Macroscopic photograph of an enlarged bladder containing numerous calculi. The mucosa appears rough with papillary projections

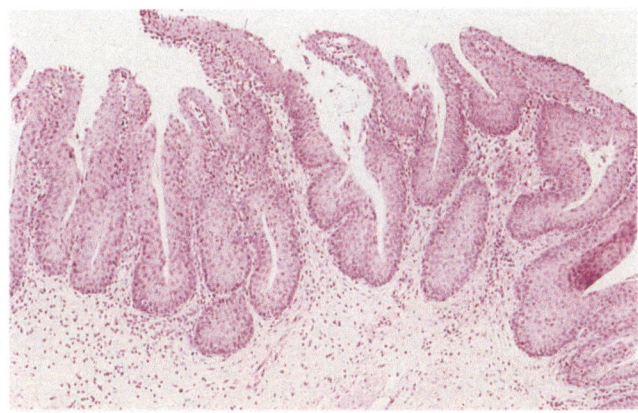

Figure 5.53 Marked mucosal hyperplasia of the bladder associated with treatment-induced calculi (not shown) in a rat. H & E

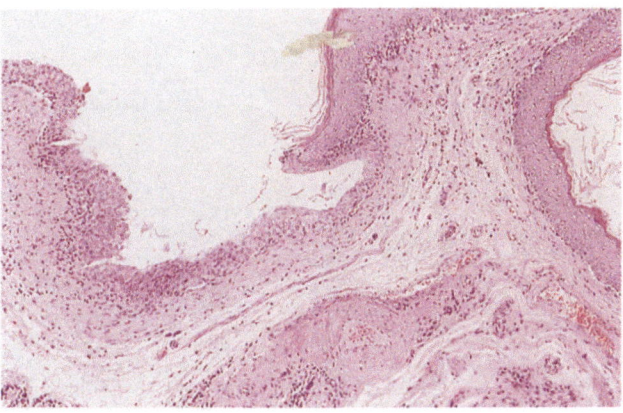

Figure 5.54 Mucosal hyperplasia and squamous metaplasia associated with induction of bladder calculi (not shown) in a rat. H & E

25. Ryffel, B., Siegl, H., Petric, R., Müller, A. M., Hauser, R. and Mihatsch, M. J. (1986). Nephrotoxicity of cyclosporine in spontaneously hypertensive rats: effects on blood pressure and vascular lesions. *Clin. Nephrol.*, **25**, 193–198

26. Zaki, F. G., Keim, G. R., Takii, Y. and Inagami, T. (1982). Hyperplasia of juxtaglomerular cells and renin localization in kidneys of normotensive animals given Captopril. *Ann. Clin. Lab. Sci.*, **12**, 200–215

27. Ohtaki, T., Imai, K., Yoshimuna, S. and Hashimoto, K. (1981). Three months subacute toxicity of Captopril in beagle dogs. *Toxicol. Sci.*, **6**, (Suppl. II), 247–279

28. Trump, B. F., Berezesky, I. K., Laiho, K. V., Osornio, A. R., Mergner, W. S. and Smith, M. W. (1980). The role of calcium in cell injury. A review. *Scanning Electron Microscopy II.* (Chicago: SEM Inc., AMF O'Hare)

29. Bulger, R. E. (1985). Relating morphological and functional changes following toxic injury. In Bach, P. H. and Lock, E. A. (eds) *Renal Heterogeneity and Target Cell Toxicity.* Proceedings of the Second International Symposium on Nephrotoxicity, University of Surrey, pp. 71–82. (Chichester: John Wiley and Sons)

30. Hottendorf, G. H. and Williams, P. D. (1986). Aminoglycoside nephrotoxicity. *Toxicol. Pathol.*, **14**, 66–72

31. Wold, J. S. (1981). Cephalosporin nephrotoxicity. In Hook, J. B. (ed.) *Toxicology of the Kidney*, pp. 251–266. (New York: Raven Press)

32. Bulger, R. E. (1986). Renal damage caused by heavy metals. *Toxicol. Pathol.*, **14**, 58–65

33. Kluwe, W. M. (1981). The nephrotoxicity of low molecular weight halogenated alkane solvents, pesticides and chemical intermediates. In Hook, J. B. (ed.) *Toxicology of the Kidney.* pp. 179–226. (New York: Raven Press)

34. Mihatsch, M. J., Ryffel, B., Hermle, M., Brunner, F. P. and Thiel, G. (1986). Morphology of cyclosporine nephrotoxicity in the rat. *Clin. Nephrol.*, **25**, 2–8

35. Phillips, D. R. and Cockrell, B. Y. (1984). Kidney structural changes in rats following inhalation exposure to C_{10}–C_{11} isoparaffinic solvent. *Toxicology*, **33**, 261–273

36. Alden, C. L. (1986). A review of unique male rat hydrocarbon nephropathy. *Toxicol. Pathol.*, **14**, 109–111

37. Bannasch, P. (1976). Chemical carcinogenesis; early morphological and cytochemical changes. *Proc. Eur. Soc. Toxicol.*, **17**, 21–31

38. Bulger, R. E. and Dobyan, D. C. (1984). Proliferative lesions found in rat kidneys after a single dose of cisplatin. *J. Natl. Cancer Inst.*, **73**, 1235–1242

39. Khan, S. R. and Woodward, J. C. (1986). Calcium oxalate urolithiasis, rat. In Jones, T. C., Mohr, U. and Hunt, R. D. (eds.) *Urinary System. Monographs on Pathology of Laboratory Animals* pp. 355–360. (Heidelberg: Springer-Verlag)

40. Prentice, D. E. and Majeed, S. K. (1978). Oral toxicity of polyethylene glycol (PEG 200) in monkeys and rats. *Toxicol. Lett.*, **2**, 119–122

41. Greaves, P. and Faccini, J. M. (1984). *Rat Histopathology.* (Amsterdam: Elsevier)

42. Woodward, J. C. and Khan, S. R. (1986). Phosphate urolithiasis, rat. In Jones, T. C., Mohr, U. and Hunt, R. D. (eds.) *Urinary System. Monographs on Pathology of Laboratory Animals*, pp. 364–368. (Heidelberg: Springer-Verlag)

43. Kime, S. W., McNamara, J. J., Luse, S., Farmer, S., Silbert, C. and Bricker, N. S. (1962). Experimental polycystic renal disease in rats: electron microscopy, function, and susceptibility to pyelonephritis. *J. Lab. Clin. Med.*, **60**, 64–78

44. Perey, D. Y. E., Herdman, R. C. and Good, R. A. (1967). Polycystic renal disease; a new experimental model. *Science*, **158**, 494–496

45. Dees, J. H., Heatfield, B. M., Reuber, M. D. and Trump, B. F. (1980). Adenocarcinoma of the kidney. III. Histogenesis of renal adenocarcinomas induced in rats by *N*-(4-fluoro-4-biphenyl)acetamide. *J. Natl. Cancer Inst.*, **64**, 1537–1545

46. Hard, G. C. and Butler, W. (1971). Morphogenesis of epithelial neoplasms in the rat kidney by dimethylnitrosamine. *Cancer Res.*, **31**, 1496–1505

47. Bach, P. M. and Bridges, J. W. (1985). Chemically-induced renal papillary necrosis and upper urothelial carcinoma. *Crit. Rev. Toxicol.*, **15**, Issues 3 and 4

48. Henry, M. A., Sweet, R. S. and Tange, T. D. (1983). A new reproducible experimental model of analgesic nephropathy. *J. Pathol.*, **139**, 23

49. Johansson, S. and Angervall, L. (1976). Urothelial changes of the renal papillae induced by long term feeding of phenacetin. *Acta Pathol. Microbiol. Scand. Sect. A*, **84**, 375–383

50. Miller, T. D. and Cohen, S. M. (1983). Alterations in the rat kidney associated with sodium saccharin feeding: A scanning electron microscopic study. *Toxicol. Lett.*, **20**, 177–181

51. Johansson, S. L., Sakata, T., Hasegawa, R., Zenser, T. V., Davis, B. B. and Cohen, S. M. (1986). The effect of long term administration of aspirin and sodium saccharin on the rat kidney. *Toxicol. Appl. Pharmacol.*, **86**, 80–92

52. Wakefield, J. St. J. and Hicks, R. M. (1974). Erythrophagocytosis by the epithelial cells of the bladder. *J. Cell Sci.*, **15**, 555–573

53. Kunze, E. (1986). Hyperplasia, urinary bladder, rat. In Jones, T. C., Mohr, V. and Hunt, R. D. (eds.) *Urinary System. Monographs of Pathology of Laboratory Animals.* (Heidelberg: Springer-Verlag)

The Reproductive System

6

Toxic injury to the gonads may be due to either direct or indirect toxicity. Certain agents exert their toxic influence directly on the gonads without any mediation through other endocrine organs. Some of these compounds are locally metabolized and biotransformed into toxic radicals. Others cause gonadal toxicity indirectly by mediation through hormonal control, either at the gondal or at the pituitary–hypothalamic level. It is important to use sexually mature animals for toxicity studies in which lesions are likely to be encountered in the reproductive system since many induced changes can mimic the morphological features of immaturity. The vast majority of the induced lesions recorded in the reproductive tract during toxicity studies are produced by sex hormones and allied compounds.

Female Reproductive System

Ovaries

The inducible ovarian changes include those affecting follicles, corpora lutea, stroma and the surface mesothelium (Table 6.1). Although beyond the scope of this text, a thorough understanding of the morphology of the ovaries and other reproductive organs at various phases of the oestrous cycle of the different species is essential for the interpretation of possible induced changes. Treatment-related effects on ovarian morphology often resemble changes occurring during different phases of the oestrous cycle, albeit in an exaggerated and persistent manner.

Table 6.1 Induced ovarian lesions

Oocyte destruction
Atrophy
Atretic follicles
Absence of corpora lutea
Persistence of corpora lutea
Tubular hyperplasia
Follicular cysts
Mesothelial hyperplasia
Mesovarial smooth muscle hyperplasia

A few polycyclic aromatic hydrocarbons, chemotherapeutic agents and ionizing radiation cause oocyte destruction with evidence of pyknosis and cytolysis[1,2]. Primordial follicles of rats and mice are especially radiosensitive. In the early stages of radiation injury, there is necrosis of the ovarian germ cells, which initially affects small oocytes of the primordial follicles[1]. Polycyclic aromatic hydrocarbon-induced injury is confined to germ cells; the surrounding granulosa cells and ovarian stroma are unaffected[2]. As oocyte destruction is irreversible, oocyte or follicle counts are useful for detecting and measuring follicular atresia. Those agents which impede cell growth ultimately interfere with the development of follicles leading to follicular atresia, decline in the number of follicles and even ovarian atrophy. Atrophic ovaries are small and shrunken with reduction of cortical structures, no corpora lutea and large areas devoid of follicles.

Hormonal compounds which inhibit the oestrous cycle produce an ovarian morphology similar to that in resting or anoestrous phase. Prolonged treatment of primates, dogs or rodents with contraceptive steroids produces ovaries without corpora lutea, arrest of follicular development, increased numbers of atretic follicles and even partial atrophy of the ovarian cortex (Figures 6.1 and 6.2). Gonadotrophin-mediated inhibition of follicular development results in excessive numbers of immature secondary follicles (Figure 6.3) in dogs[3]. Absence of corpora lutea (Figures 6.4 and 6.5), a common expression of inhibition of ovarian function, is seen in rats after prolonged treatment with oestrogens[4]. Conversely, transient deviations in gonadotrophins result in delayed luteolysis causing persistent corpora lutea and a consequent increase in their numbers. Prolactogenic compounds, such as butyrophenones, disturb the oestrous cycle and increase the size and number of corpora lutea in rats[5]. Bromocriptine and lergotril, which lower circulating prolactin concentrations, also cause persistence of corpora lutea in rats[6]. In our experience the occurrence of increased numbers of corpora lutea is not uncommon in rodent toxicity studies with many other unrelated compounds. Ovarian weights and corpora lutea counts are frequently useful in such cases. Standardization of the plane of histological sectioning is essential for proper evaluation. The mechanism responsible for the occurrence of increased numbers of corpora lutea is poorly understood.

In the ovaries of some strains of aged rats tubular structures, lined by cells like Sertoli's cells, are seen in the ovarian medulla. These structures can be induced by hypophysectomy and by growth hormone administration[7,8]. Hyperplasia of these tubules has been observed (Figure 6.6) in our laboratories in rats treated with a novel agrochemical, subsequently shown to have antiandrogenic properties.

Ovarian cysts are occasionally recorded in rats treated with oestrogenic compounds[9]. An increased incidence of ovarian cysts (Figure 6.7) is observed in rats treated with high levels of β-stimulants[10]. These follicular cysts vary markedly in size and usually have a thin wall lined by cuboidal or flattened granulosa cells. Prolonged treatment with bromocriptine also produces increased numbers of follicular cysts in rats[11].

Certain synthetic oestrogens affect the ovarian mesothelium of dogs (Figure 6.8) and induce marked papillary mesothelial hyperplasia[12].

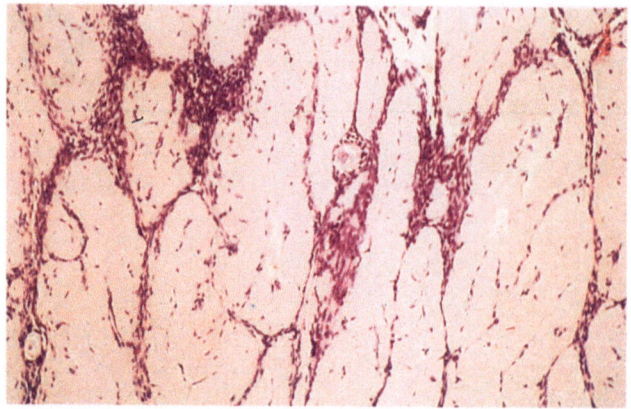

Figure 6.1 Atretic follicles in the ovary of a monkey following prolonged treatment with a progestational compound. Note the acellular hyalinized areas within the affected follicles. H & E

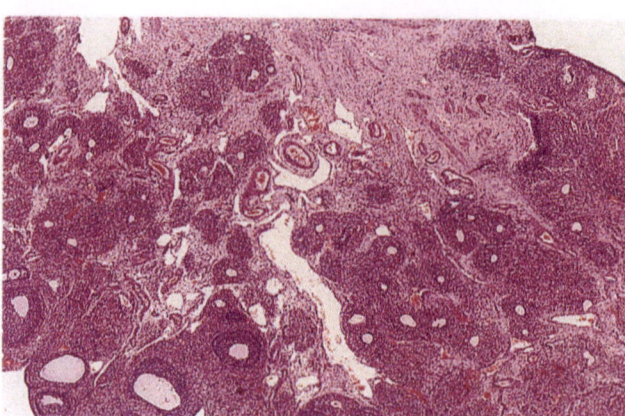

Figure 6.2 Absence of corpora lutea and secondary follicles in the ovary of a rat treated with an industrial chemical. The primordial follicles show oocyte destruction associated with interstitial gland hyperplasia. H & E

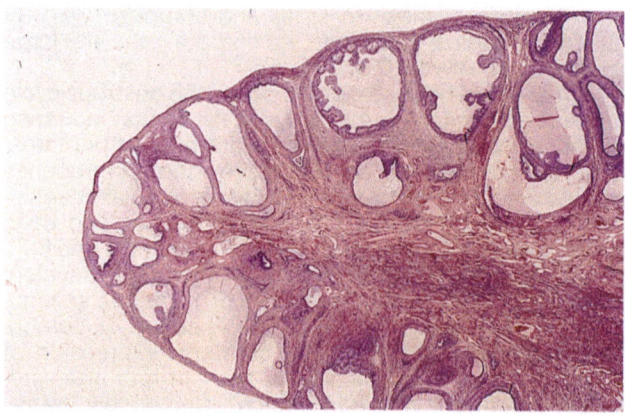

Figure 6.3 Several secondary follicles at a similar stage of development in a dog ovary. The lesion is presumed to have developed as a result of continued gonadotrophic inhibition. H & E

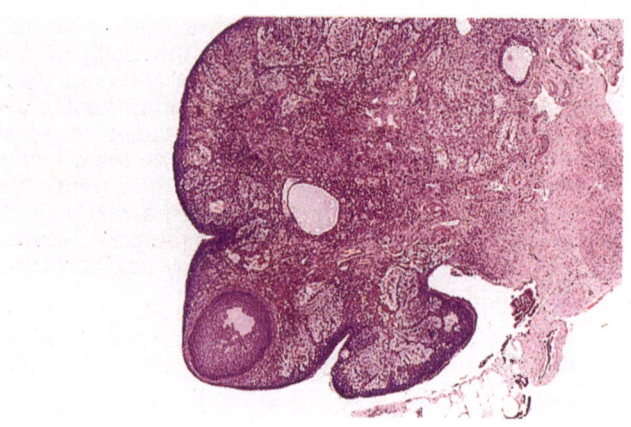

Figure 6.4 Absence of corpora lutea and reduction of follicles in the ovary of a rat. These effects may be produced by prolonged treatment with oestrogenic steroids. H & E

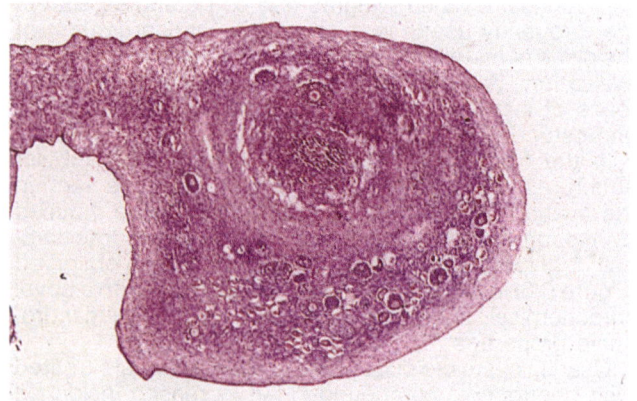

Figure 6.5 Absence of corpora lutea and reduced follicular development in a monkey ovary from a long-term toxicity study with a contraceptive steroid. H & E

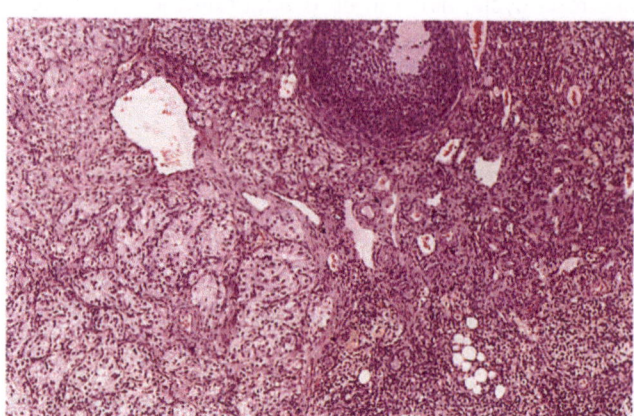

Figure 6.6 Tubules composed of cells like Sertoli's cells in the ovary of a rat treated with a novel agrochemical. These tubules may also develop in the ovaries of aged rats. H & E

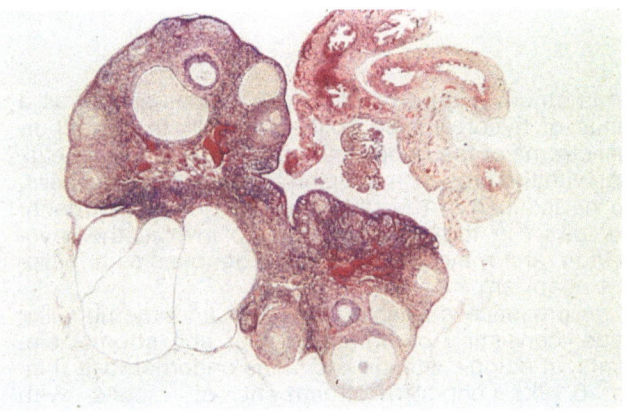

Figure 6.7 Follicular cysts in a rat ovary. The cysts are lined by thin walls. Corpora lutea are absent. Treatment with β-adrenergic agonists, bromocriptine and oestrogenic compounds produced this change.   H & E

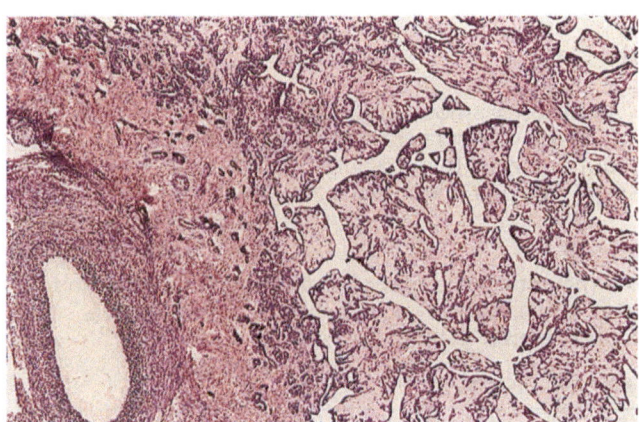

Figure 6.8 Papillary hyperplasia of the mesothelial lining of the ovary in a dog treated with a synthetic oestrogen.   H & E

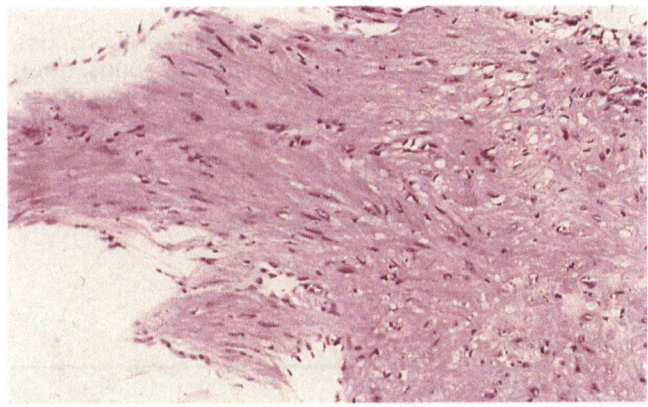

Figure 6.9 Smooth muscle hyperplasia of the mesovarial ligament, adjacent to the ovarian hilus, from a rat given prolonged treatment with a novel β-adrenergic stimulant drug.   H & E

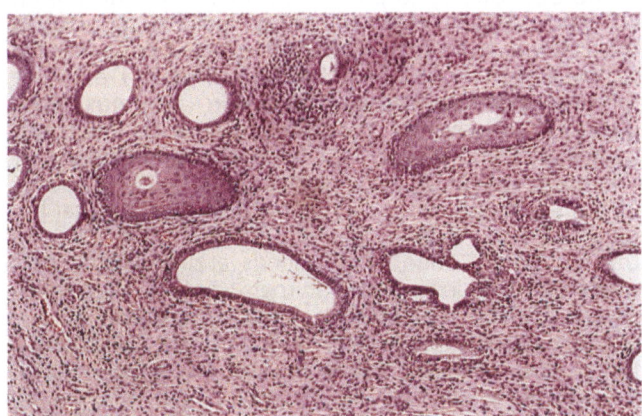

Figure 6.10 Squamous metaplasia of endometrial glands in the uterus of a rat treated with an oestrogenic compound.   H & E

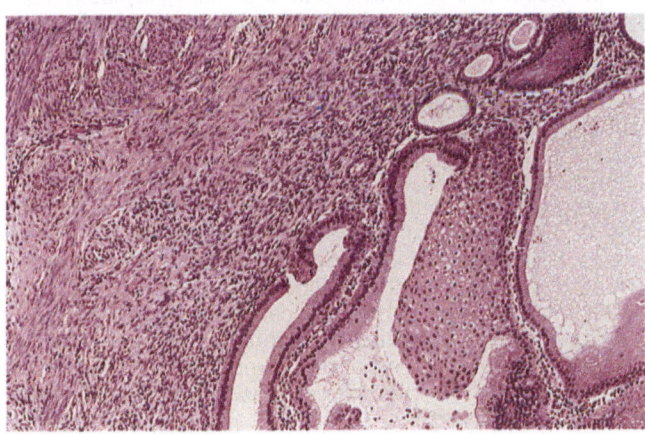

Figure 6.11 Focus of squamous metaplasia of endometrial glands in the uterus of a monkey treated with a synthetic oestrogen.   H & E

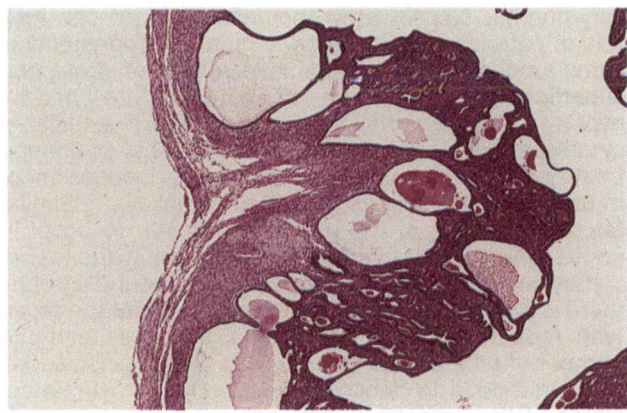

Figure 6.12 Endometrial glandular hyperplasia in a mouse uterus. Endometrial thickening due to glandular proliferation. Occasional cystic glands. This change may be induced by oestrogenic compounds.   H & E

Mesovarial smooth muscle hyperplasia (Figure 6.9) and benign tumours are reported in rats given prolonged treatment with β-stimulants[13,14]. This is a site-specific lesion which is only reported in rats.

Uterus

The majority of the uterine changes encountered in toxicity studies are produced by hormonally active compounds (Table 6.2).

Table 6.2 Induced uterine lesions

Squamous metaplasia of endometrial glands
Myometrial hypertrophy
Mesothelial hyperplasia
Endometrial hyperplasia
Endometritis
Endometrial atrophy
Decidualization
Endometriosis

The oestrous cycle profoundly influences the uterus so again a detailed knowledge of its cyclic morphology in the different species of experimental animals is essential for evaluation of compound-related effects. Treatment with oestrogenic compounds results in squamous metaplasia of endometrial glands (Figures 6.10 and 6.11), hydrometra and pyometra in mice and other species[9]. Vitamin A deficiency also induces squamous metaplasia of the endometrium in many species[1]. Endometrial hyperplasia (Figure 6.12), characterized by an increase in the number of endometrial glands and an increase in uterine size, is described in animals treated with oestrogens[1]. Prolonged oestrogen treatment results in myometrial hypertrophy in rabbits and dogs[15]. The muscle layers are markedly thickened and individual smooth muscle fibres have abundant sarcoplasm. Diethylstilboestrol induces papillary hyperplasia (Figure 6.13) of the serous membrane (mesothelium) in dogs[16]. Progestational compounds also induce endometrial hyperplasia and in dogs (Figure 6.14) the proliferated glands frequently become cystic with abundant mucus[17]. The lesions often progress to purulent endometritis and pyometra[18]. The uterine horns are greatly distended with mucopurulent discharge (Figure 6.15) which is present both in the lumen and in the cystic glands. The endometrial stroma contains plasma cells, lymphocytes and polymorphs. Occasionally the inflammatory cell infiltration extends into the myometrium. In progestational compound-induced glandular hyperplasia of dogs, the superficial glands and surface epithelium are lined by hypertrophic cells with abundant clear, finely vacuolated cytoplasm. However, it is also reported that prolonged treatment with progestational compounds induces endometrial atrophy (Figure 6.16) in monkeys[1]. Similar atrophic changes of the uterus are known to occur in dogs treated with butyrophenones[5] probably due to mediation by gonadotrophic inhibition. In uterine atrophy there is marked reduction in size and weight of the organ with reduction in the endometrial thickness and the number of endometrial glands, which are inconspicuous and embedded in dense compact stroma. The sarcoplasm of the smooth muscle cells is reduced and the myometrium consists of closely packed cells with elongated nuclei and scanty cytoplasm.

Intrauterine devices and intravaginal rings loaded with progestational compounds induce a decidual reaction of the superficial endometrium (Figure 6.17) in monkeys[19]. Prolonged oral administration of certain progestogens to monkeys also causes a focal decidual reaction in the endometrium (Figure 6.18). These lesions appear as a plaque of hypertrophied epithelioid cells in the superficial stroma of the endometrium. A florid decidual reaction, with the presence of pleomorphic and bizarre cells, can be induced in the rat uterus by growth hormone. The lesion in this case extends to involve the myometrium and may be mistakenly diagnosed as a malignant neoplasm.

The presence of viable islands of endometrium-like tissue, consisting of both glandular and stromal elements, at ectopic sites is known as endometriosis (Figure 6.19). Long-term treatment of rabbits with stilboestrol induces this condition[15]. Endometriosis is usually confined to the pelvic cavity affecting the serous surface of the uterus, ovaries, large intestine, urinary bladder and in the mesentery.

A similar condition with extension of hyperplastic endometrial glands into hyperplastic myometrial layers is referred to as adenomyosis which is reported in mice exposed to long term oestrogenic treatment[9].

Vagina and cervix

Sex hormones are known to induce epithelial changes in the vagina and cervix. Oestrogenic compounds, given to dogs and primates, cause hyperkeratosis and hyperplasia of the stratified squamous epithelium of the vagina

Table 6.3 Induced lesions of the vagina and cervix

Vaginal hyperkeratosis and hyperplasia
Vaginal mucification
Atrophy
Endocervical mucoid distension
Os clitoridis
Mucosal inflammation

(Figure 6.20) with oedema of underlying lamina propria[9]. The vaginal mucous membrane appears thick and leathery with several longitudinal folds. Excessive keratinization of vaginal epithelium is recorded in mice treated with stilboestrol[20]. Vaginal keratinization in oophorectomised rats is used as a measure of the oestrogenic activity of compounds[21]. Progestational compounds on the other hand cause mucification of the vaginal (Figure 6.21) and cervical epithelium of rats. The epithelium often becomes columnar and the cell cytoplasm contains mucus. Prolonged treatment with progestational compounds in dogs and primates induces atrophy of vaginal epithelium, reducing it into a thin layer of flattened cells (Figures 6.22 and 6.23). Diminished ovarian function mediated by gonadotrophic inhibition may be a factor in the development of this lesion. Marked mucoid distension of the endocervical canal is seen in monkeys treated with progestogens for prolonged periods (Figure 6.24). Prominent foci of squamous epithelium in the endocervical canal (Figure 6.25) are reported in primates treated with oestrogens[9]. Stilboestrol treatment induces villus proliferation of endocervical epithelium in rabbits[15].

Testosterone injected into female neonate rats induces the development of os clitoridis, which resembles the os penis[22]. Progesterone causes a similar but less pronounced effect[22].

Toxicity studies are performed occasionally with a view to assessing the irritant effects of test substances by studying the responses of vaginal mucosa. In these instances both macroscopic and microscopic features of irritation are recorded and graded. Macroscopic changes include hyperaemia, haemorrhage, erosion and ulceration; microscopic changes which may be detected in-

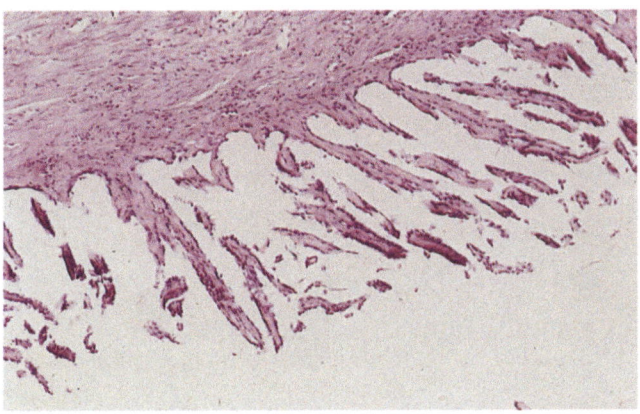

Figure 6.13 Villous and papillary proliferation of the mesothelial lining of the uterus of a dog treated with a synthetic oestrogen. H & E

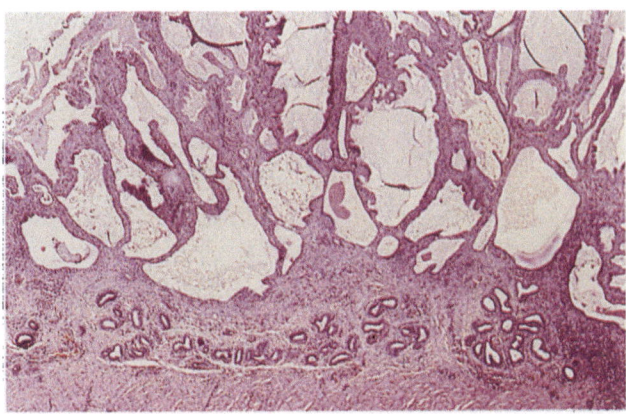

Figure 6.14 Endometrial glandular hyperplasia in the uterus of a dog treated with a progestational compound for a prolonged period. Superficial endometrial glands are distended with mucus. H & E

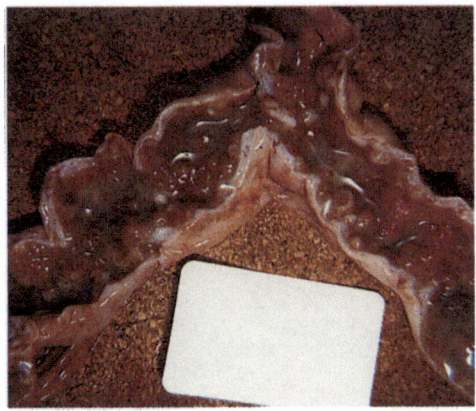

Figure 6.15 Macrophotograph of pyometra in a rat from a chronic toxicity study with bromocriptine. Note the mucopurulent exudate in the lumen

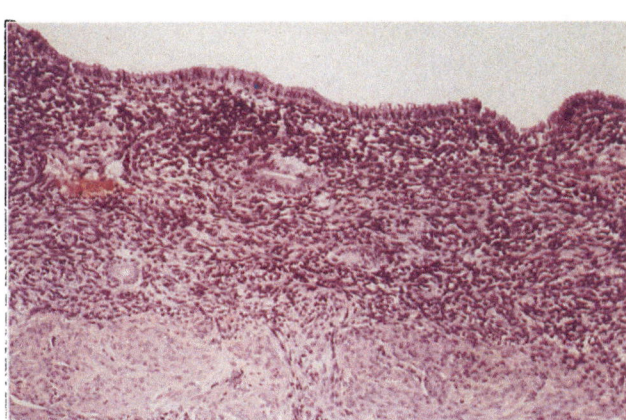

Figure 6.16 Atrophy of the endometrium in the uterus of a monkey from a long-term toxicity study with a contraceptive steroid. The endometrium is thin with reduction of glands and cellular stroma. H & E

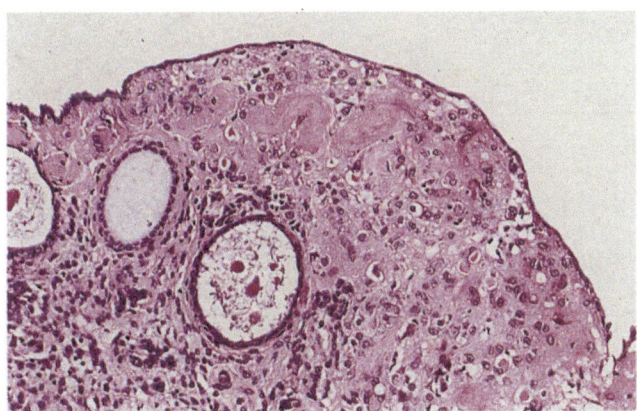

Figure 6.17 A plaque of decidualized cells in the endometrium of a monkey with an implanted intrauterine device. Large, irregularly shaped cells with abundant eosinophilic cytoplasm near the luminal surface, probably where the endometrium was in contact with the device. H & E

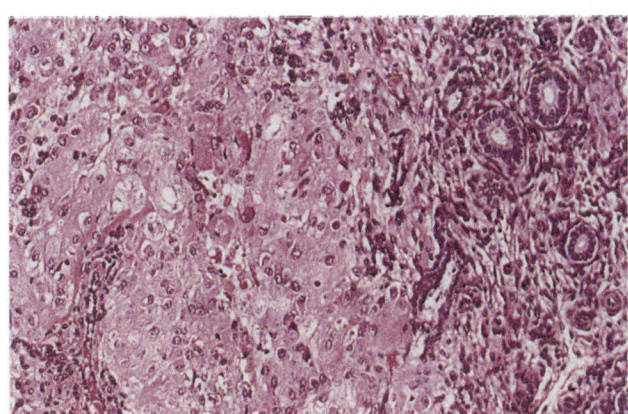

Figure 6.18 Focal decidual reaction in the endometrium of a monkey from a chronic toxicity study with a systemically administered synthetic progestogen. Group of large epithelioid cells with abundant eosinophilic cytoplasm and vesicular nuclei are present within the endometrium. H & E

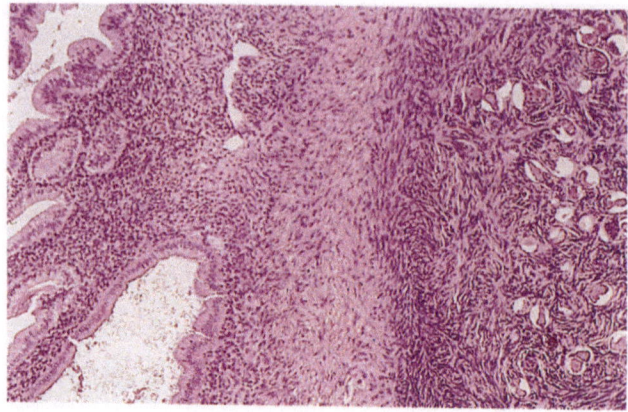

Figure 6.19 Endometriosis on the ovarian surface of a monkey treated for a prolonged period with an oestrogenic compound. The endometrium-like tissue includes both glandular and stromal elements. Endometriosis can also occur spontaneously.   H & E

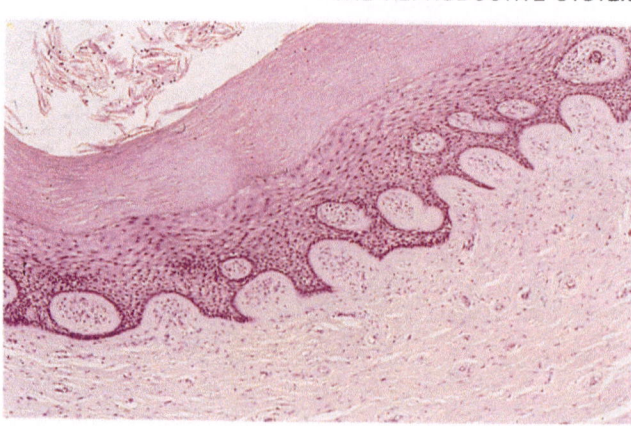

Figure 6.20 Mucosal thickening and hyperkeratosis of vaginal epithelium in a dog treated with an oestrogenic compound. H & E

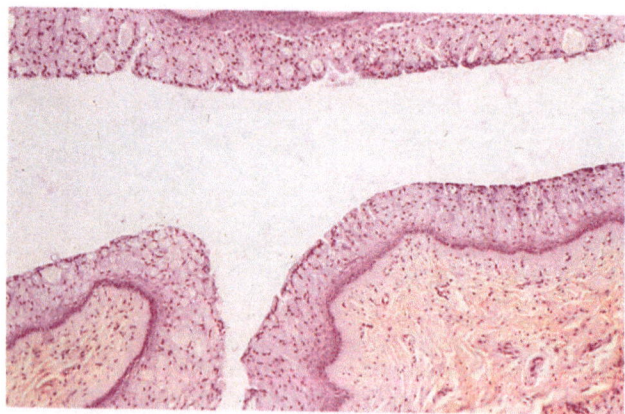

Figure 6.21 Mucification of the vaginal epithelium of a rat treated with a progestational compound. The superficial epithelial cells are columnar with prominent goblet cells.   H & E

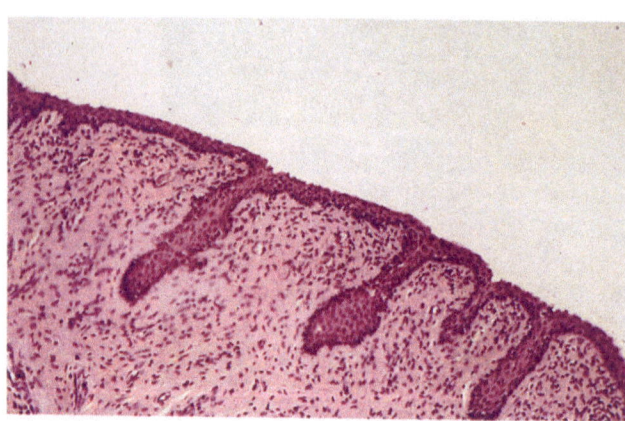

Figure 6.22 Atrophy of the vaginal epithelium in a dog following prolonged treatment with a contraceptive steroid. Keratin layer is absent and the epithelium is thin.   H & E

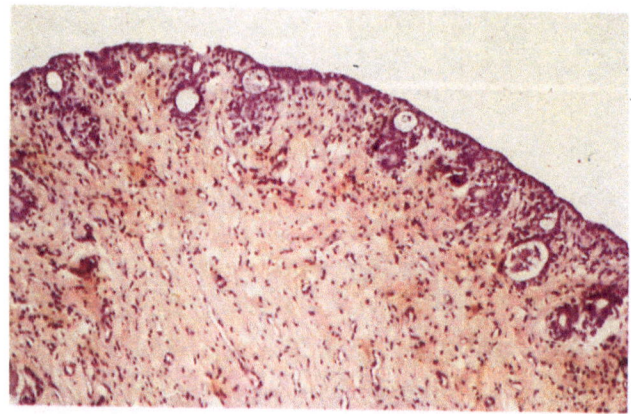

Figure 6.23 Atrophy of the vaginal epithelium in a monkey from a long-term toxicity study with a progestational compound. Epithelium is thin.   H & E

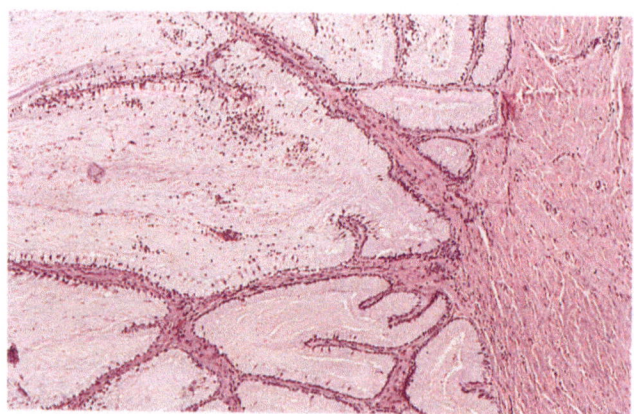

Figure 6.24 Mucoid distension of endocervical glands in the cervix of a monkey following prolonged treatment with a synthetic progestogen. There is no evidence of glandular hyperplasia. The glandular lumina contain laminated mucus.   H & E

clude inflammation, oedema, erosion, necrosis, ulceration, atrophy and hyperplasia.

Mammary glands

The oestrous cycle produces histomorphological changes in the mammary glands, especially of dogs, which are important because features change markedly from one phase of the cycle to another[23]. Although many of the compounds encountered in routine toxicity studies do not provoke any response in the mammary glands several hormonally active agents are known to produce stimulatory or inhibitory effects (Table 6.4).

Table 6.4 Induced lesions of the mammary gland

Glandular development and hyperplasia
Enhanced secretion
Hyperplastic nodules

Contraceptive steroids containing progestational and oestrogenic components induce mammary development and hyperplasia in a number of species of laboratory animals (Figure 6.26 and 6.27). Administration of oestrogens results in mammary hyperplasia which mainly affects the ductular system in mice, primates and dogs[9]. This is often followed by lobular development and formation of cysts. Prolonged administration of oestrogens to rats produces enhanced secretory activity and cystic duct dilation[24]. Marked stimulation of mammary glands in both rats (Figure 6.28) and dogs (affecting both male and females) is reported in repeated dosage studies with dopamine antagonists used as neuroleptics[25]. Here the mammary hyperplasia and excessive secretion is mediated through prolactin (PRL) production. Dopaminergic agonists such as bromocriptine, which lower circulating PRL, inhibit lobulo-alveolar growth and lactation[26]. Florid lobular hyperplasia (Figure 6.29) of the mammary gland is seen in dogs given prolonged doses of progesterone[27].

Long-term administration of progestational compounds, like megestrol acetate or chlormadinone acetate, to female dogs induces nodular hyperplasia of the mammary glands[28]. These mammary nodules involve hyperplasia of various elements of the gland, in varying proportions. Focal proliferative lesions include those with predominantly ductular epithelial cells, acinar epithelial cells or myoepithelial cells (Figures 6.30, 6.31 and 6.32). The proliferative lesions may coexist with sclerosing or degenerative changes. Long-term treatment of rhesus monkeys with contraceptive steroids, such as norlestrin, results in dilation of mammary acini and ducts[29].

Male Reproductive System

Testis and epididymis

Toxic damage to the testes can be due to direct action of the agent on the organ, as in the case of cobalt toxicity or ionizing radiation. Direct action also includes compounds whose toxicity is influenced by metabolic biotransformation at the site[30]. The toxic potential of foreign compounds on the testes, particularly those with large molecular structures may be influenced by the blood-testis barrier. Factors which impede normal cell growth such as ionizing radiation, alkylating agents, antimetabolites and certain antibiotics are known to exert direct damage to the seminiferous epithelium. Elements like cadmium, mercury, lead, cobalt and manganese also produce toxic injury to the germinal epithelium.

In some other instances the testicular effect of an agent is exerted indirectly, for example when the effect is mediated through other endocrine secretions as in the case of the psychopharmacologic compound reserpine. Deprivation of pituitary gonadotrophin, exogenous oestrogens, malnutrition and deficiency of vitamins A and E or zinc also induce testicular inhibition. The induced lesions encountered in the testis are given in Table 6.5.

Table 6.5 Induced lesions of the testis and epididymis

Testicular atrophy
Necrosis of seminiferous tubules
Epididymal atrophy
Spermatic granuloma
Leydig cell hyperplasia

The most frequently seen effect in testicular toxicity is atrophy of the seminiferous epithelium (Figure 6.33). In its milder form this appears merely as an absence of tailed spermatids in the seminiferous tubules of an adult animal. Atrophy can involve deeper layers of spermatids and spermatocytes (secondary and primary spermatocytes) and in marked cases the only discernible cells are a few spermatogonia and Sertoli's cells. In early stages, the lumina of atrophic seminiferous tubules often contain abnormal spermatids and multinucleated giant spermatids (Figures 6.34 and 6.35). In long-standing and extreme cases the tubules are lined only by a few Sertoli's cells (Figure 6.36).

Spermatogenic inhibition due to dietary deficiences is usually reversible upon supplementation. However, testicular atrophy induced by vitamin E deficiency in rats is not reversible[1]. Exogenous oestrogens produce testicular atrophy in dogs, rats and mice[9]. Some of the progestogens are also known to produce testicular atrophy in rats[31]. Dopamine antagonists such as reserpine which stimulate prolactin secretion result in inhibition of spermatogenesis[32]. Dopamine agonists like bromocriptine also induce testicular atrophy in rats[11]. Dietary cobalt induces necrosis of the germinal epithelium and of Sertoli's cells in the seminiferous tubules of rats[33]. Affected tubules contain necrotic debris, spermatogonic and spermatocytic cells with pyknotic nuclei sloughed into the lumina with patchy dystrophic calcification. In the testicular atrophy induced by phthalate esters, early degenerative vacuolation of Sertoli's cells is reported[34]. Vacuolation of ductular epithelium (Figure 6.37) of the epididymis and cyst formation is seen in mice treated with stilboestrol[35]. Butylbenzyl phthalate toxicity in rats is associated with necrosis of the tubular epithelium of the epididymis and also atrophy of the epididymis[36]. Duct atrophy and stromal fibrosis of the epididymis (Figure 6.38) are reported in dogs given oestrogens[3]. In our experience the detection of morphologically abnormal cells in the lumina of epididymal ducts in adult animals is a good indication of testicular malfunction.

There are reported instances of entry of spermatozoa into the interstitium of testes, epididymides or vas deferens provoking granulomata formation[37]. This condition is reported in rats treated with agents such as DL-ethionine and guanethidine[37,38]. With guanethidine, an adrenergic blocker, the spermatic granulomata in the epididymis are attributed to the rupture of the vas deferens. The granulomata are sometimes characterized by central foci of necrotic debris, an outer large zone of spermatozoa and a peripheral zone of macrophages, giant cells and fibroblasts (Figure 6.39).

Seminiferous tubular damage or even oestrogen administration are sometimes associated with Leydig cell hyperplasia[39-41] (Figure 6.36). Leydig cell hyperplasia

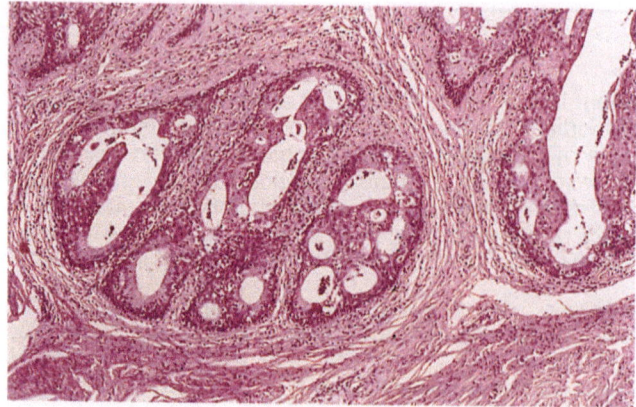

Figure 6.25 Prominent stratified squamous epithelium in the endocervical glands of cervix in a monkey from a toxicity study with an oestrogenic compound.   H & E

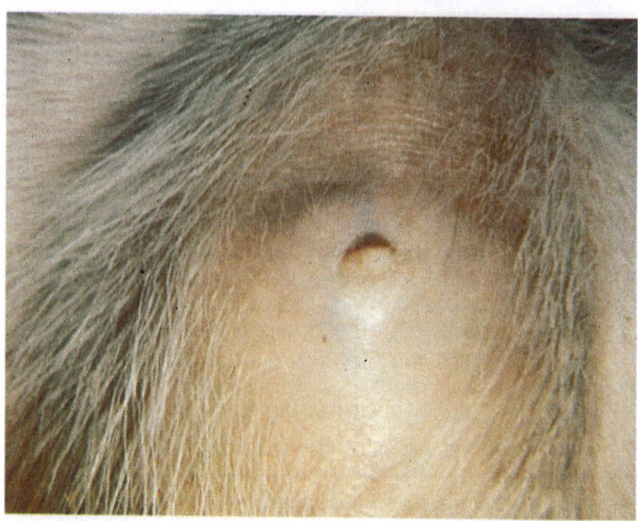

Figure 6.26 Increased mammary gland development in a monkey from a toxicity study with an oestrogenic compound

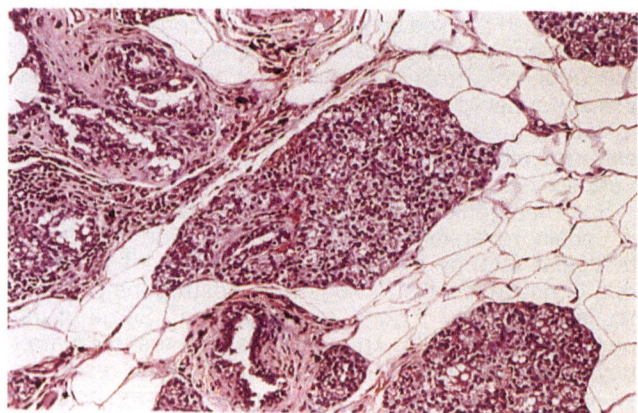

Figure 6.27 Lobular hyperplasia of mammary gland in a rat treated with a progestational compound. Note the proliferation of acinar epithelium but normal duct development.   H & E

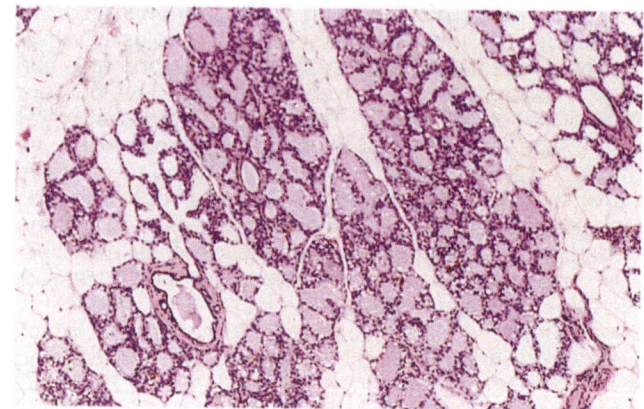

Figure 6.28 Lobular hyperplasia with prominent secretion in the mammary gland of a rat from a toxicity study with a novel neuroleptic compound.   H & E

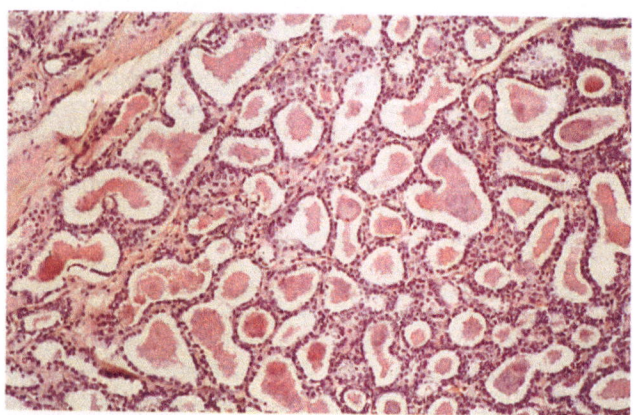

Figure 6.29 Lobular hyperplasia with secretion in the mammary gland of a dog from a toxicity study with a progestational compound.   H & E

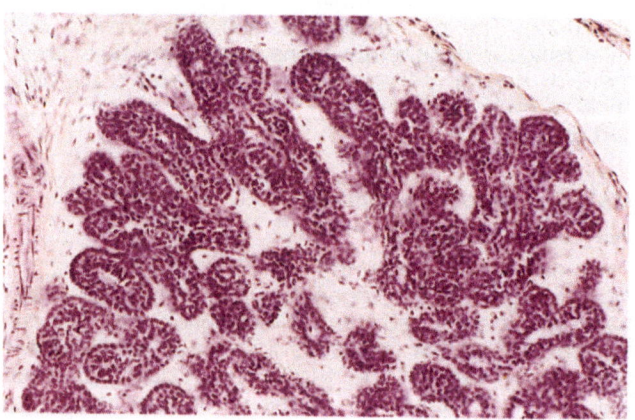

Figure 6.30 Hyperplastic nodule in a mammary gland of a dog following prolonged treatment with a contraceptive steroid. The hyperplastic nodule is mainly composed of ductular epithelial cells.   H & E

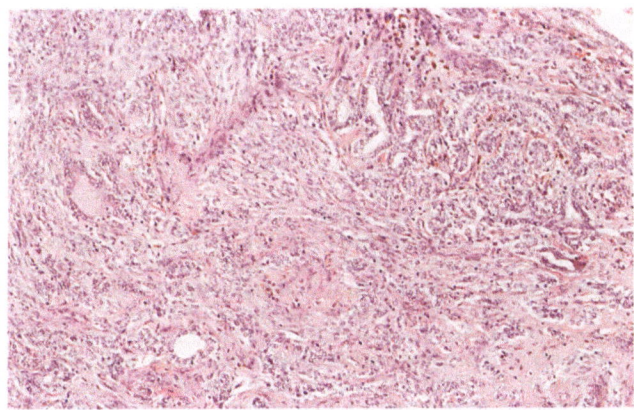

Figure 6.31 A hyperplastic mammary nodule similar to that shown in Figure 6.30 but with hyperplasia of both epithelial and myoepithelial cells. Stromal fibrosis is also seen in this field. H & E

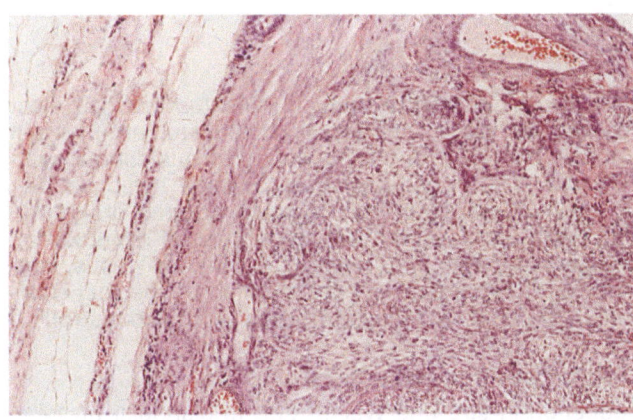

Figure 6.32 A hyperplastic mammary nodule similar to that shown in Figure 6.31. In this case the proliferation is mainly of myoepithelial cells. H & E

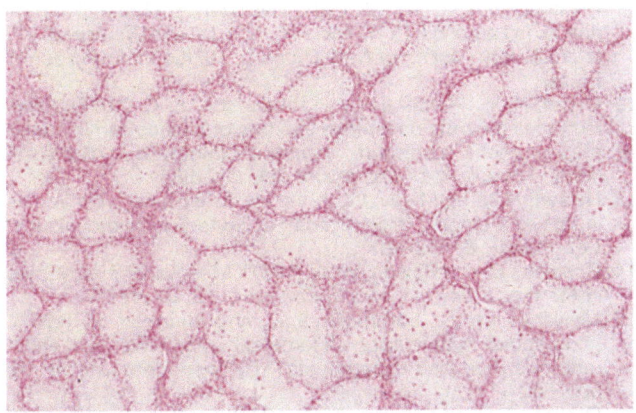

Figure 6.33 Testicular atrophy in a dog treated with an antineoplastic compound. Spermatids and spermatocytes are absent and the seminiferous tubules are lined mainly by Sertoli's cells. H & E

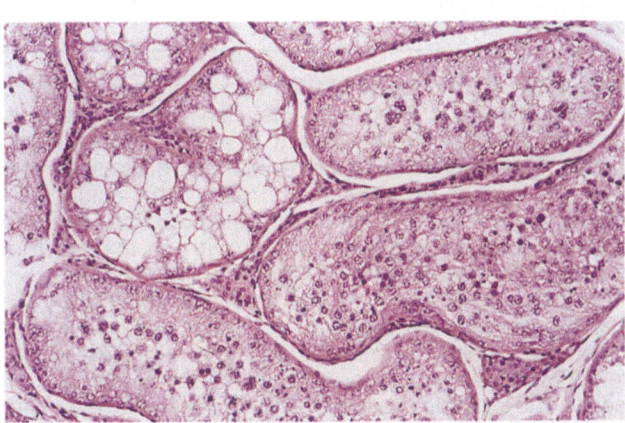

Figure 6.34 Early testicular atrophy in a rat treated with an industrial chemical. Seminiferous tubules show vacuolated cells, reduced numbers of spermatids and occasional abnormal spermatids. H & E

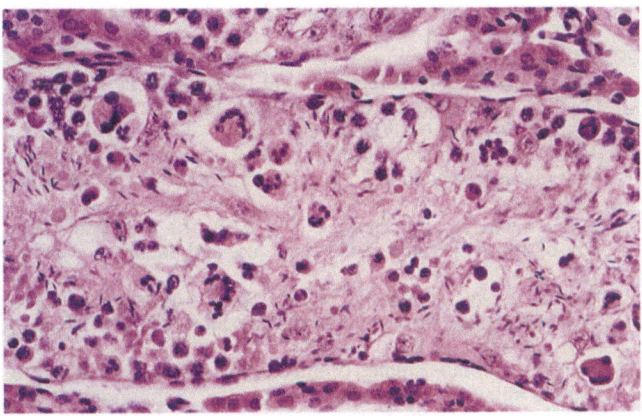

Figure 6.35 Early testicular atrophy in a rat treated with a novel dopamine antagonist. Reduced numbers of spermatids and prominent multinucleated giant spermatids are shown. H & E

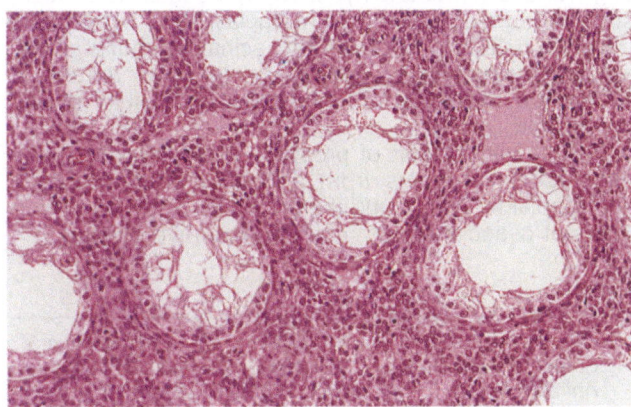

Figure 6.36 Atrophy of the testis in a rat treated with a novel immunostimulant drug. The tubules are lined mainly by Sertoli's cells. Note the marked proliferation of interstitial cells. H & E

without lesions in the seminiferous tubules has also occasionally been detected in rodent studies (Figures 6.40 and 6.41) with certain herbicides in our laboratories. Ethylene dimethane sulphonate causes selective destruction of Leydig cells[42]. In mice, treated prenatally with diethylstilboestrol, varying degrees of hyperplasia, including papillary outgrowths of the rete testis, are reported[43]. Focal papillary proliferation of the testicular serosa is observed in dogs treated with stilboestrol[16].

Prostate and seminal vesicles

Reduction in size and weight due to glandular atrophy are the most common of all changes seen in the prostate and seminal vesicles during toxicity studies. Oestrogens and progestogens produce atrophy (Figures 6.42 and 6.43) in mice and rats[9,24,31]. Phthalates administered to

Table 6.6 Induced lesions of the prostate and seminal vesicles

Atrophy
Hypertrophy and hyperplasia
Squamous metaplasia
Vacuolation

male rats cause atrophy of their accessory sex glands[36]. Certain synthetic progestogens also induce prostatic atrophy in dogs. The treatment of animals with neuroleptics like spiriline also has inhibitory effects on the prostate gland[5]. In prostatic atrophy, the acinar epithelium loses its height, becomes flattened and the acinar lumina collapse and shrink with an apparent increase in connective tissue stroma (Figure 6.44).

Androgen treatment at high dosages can induce hypertrophy and hyperplasia of male accessory sex glands[1]. In dogs hyperplastic prostates are grossly enlarged with a nodular or smooth surface. Microscopically, the glands become irregularly enlarged with multiple papillary projections into the lumina. The glandular spaces are occupied by complex infolding of the epithelium and the lining cells are often hypertrophic (Figure 6.45).

Chronic oestrogen stimulation, vitamin A deficiency and chronic intoxication by certain halogenated hydrocarbons and polychlorinated biphenyl compounds induce squamous metaplasia of prostatic and seminal vesicular epithelium[1]. Prolonged oestrogen treatment of dogs results in prostate hypertrophy, abscess formation, stromal fibrosis, squamous metaplasia and hyperplasia (Figures 6.46 and 6.47) of the acinar epithelium[9]. Diethylstilboestrol given repeatedly to mice results in squamous metaplasia of glandular epithelium of the coagulating gland[44].

Diffuse vacuolation of prostatic epithelium has been observed in primates from a toxicity study using an antineoplastic compound (Figure 6.48). The vacuolation was not associated with any degenerative change.

References

1. King, N. W. (1978). The reproductive tract. In Bernirschke, K., Garner, F. M., Jones, T. C. (eds.) *Pathology of Laboratory Animals.* Vol. 1, p. 524. (New York: Springer-Verlag)
2. Mattison, D. R. (1980). Morphology of oocyte and follicle destruction by polycyclic aromatic hydrocarbons in mice. *Toxicol. Appl. Pharmacol.,* **53**, 249–259
3. Schwartz, E., Tornaben, J. A. and Boxill, G. C. (1969). Effects of chronic oral administration of long acting estrogen, Quinestrol to dogs. *Toxicol. Appl. Pharmacol.,* **14**, 487–494
4. Gibson, J. P., Newberne, J. W., Kuhn, W. L. and Elsen, J. R. (1967). Comparative chronic toxicity of three oral estrogens in rats. *Toxicol. Appl. Pharmacol.,* **11**, 489–510

5. Baker, S. B. de C. and Tucker, M. J. (1968). Changes in the reproductive organs of rats and dogs treated with butyrophenones and related compounds. In Baker, S. B. de C., Boisser, J. R. and Koll, W. (eds.) *Toxicology and Side Effects of Psychotropic Drugs.* Vol. 9, p. 113. Ics no. 145. (Amsterdam: Excerpta Medica Foundation)
6. Heuson, J. C., Waelbroeck-Van Graver, C. and Legros, N. (1970). Growth inhibition of rat mammary carcinoma and endocrine changes produced by 2-Br-α-ergocriptine, a supressor of lactation and nidation. *Eur. J. Cancer,* **6**, 353–356
7. Arias, M. and Aschheim, P. (1974). Hypophysectomy and aging: Primary or secondary ovarian senescence. *Experientia,* **30**, 213
8. Moon, H. D., Simpson, L. E., Li, C. H and Evans, H. M (1950). Neoplasms in rats treated with pituitary growth hormone III. Reproductive organs. *Cancer Res.,* **10**, 549–556
9. Heywood, R. and Wadsworth, P. F. (1981). The experimental toxicology of estrogens. In Chaudhury, R. R. (eds.) *Pharmacology of Estrogens.* p. 68. *International Encyclopedia of Pharmacology and Therapeutics.* Section 106. (New York: Pergamon Press)
10. Nelson, L. W., Kelly, W. A. and Weikel, Jr., J. H. (1972). Mesovarial leiomyomas in rats in a chronic toxicity study of mesuprine hydrochloride. *Toxicol. Appl. Pharmacol.,* **23**, 731–737
11. Richardson, B. P., Turkali, I. and Fluckigen, E. (1984). Bromocriptine. In Laurence, D. R., McLean, A. E. M. and Weatherall. M. (eds.) *Safety Testing of New Drugs.* p. 19. (London: Academic Press)
12. Owen, N. V., Pierce, E. C. and Anderson, R. C. (1972). Papillomatous growths on internal genitalia of bitches administered the synthetic estrogen, *trans*-4,4'-dimethyl-α,α'-diethylstilbene. *Toxicol. Appl. Pharmacol.,* **21**, 582–585
13. Nelson, N. V. and Kelly, W. A. (1971). Mesovarial leiomyomas in rats in a chronic toxicity study of Sorterenol hydrochloride. *Vet. Pathol.,* **8**, 452–457
14. Gopinath, C. and Gibson, W. A. (1987). Mesovarial leiomyomas in the rat. *J. Environ. Health Perspect.,* **73**, (in press)
15. Meissner, W. A., Sommers, S. C. and Sherman, G. (1957). Endometrial hyperplasia, endometrial carcinoma, and endometriosis produced experimentally by oestrogen. *Cancer,* **10**, 500–509
16. O'Shea, J. D. and Jabara, A. G. (1971). Proliferative lesions of serous membranes in ovariectomised female and entire male dogs after stilboesterol administration. *Vet. Pathol.,* **8**, 81–90
17. Anderson, R. K., Gilmore, C. E. and Schnelle, G. B. (1965). Utero-ovarian disorders associated with use of medroxy progesterone in dogs. *J. Am. Vet. Med. Assoc.,* **146**, 1311–1316
18. Nelson, L. W. and Kelly, W. A. (1976). Progestogen-related gross and microscopical changes in female dogs. *Vet. Pathol.,* **13**, 143–156
19. Wadsworth, P. F., Heywood, R., Allen, D. G., Sortwell, R. J. and Walton, R. M. (1979). Treatment of rhesus monkeys (*Macaca mullata*) with intra-uterine devices loaded with levonorgestrel. *Contraception,* **20**, 177–184
20. Greenman, D. L., Highman, T., Kodell, R. L., Morgan, K. T. and Norvell, M. (1984). Neoplastic and non-neoplastic responses to chronic feeding of diethyl stilboesterol in C₃H mice. *J. Toxicol. Environ. Health,* **14**, 551–561
21. Jones, R. C. and Edgren, R. A. (1973). The effects of various steroids on vaginal histology in the rat. *Fertil. Steril.,* **24**, 284–291
22. Glucksmann, A. and Cherry, C. P. (1972). The hormonal induction of an os clitoridis in the neo-natal and adult rat. *J. Anat.,* **112**, 223–231
23. Nelson, L. W. and Kelly, W. A. (1974). Changes in canine mammary gland histology during the oestrous cycle. *Toxicol. Appl. Pharmacol.,* **27**, 113–122
24. Schardein (1980). Studies of the components of an oral contraceptive agent in albino rats, 1. Estrogenic component. *J. Toxicol. Environ. Health,* **6**, 885–894
25. Horowski, R. and Gräf, K-J. (1979). Neuro-endocrine effects of neuropsychotropic drugs and their possible influence on toxic reactions in animals and man. *Arch. Toxicol.,* Suppl. 2. p. 93
26. Gräf, K-J., Friedreich, E., Matties, S., Hassman, S. H. (1977). Homologous radioimmunoassay for canine prolactin and its application in various physiological states. *J. Endocrinol.,* **75**, 93–103
27. Capel-Edwards, K., Hall, D. E., Fellowes, K. P. and Vallance, D.

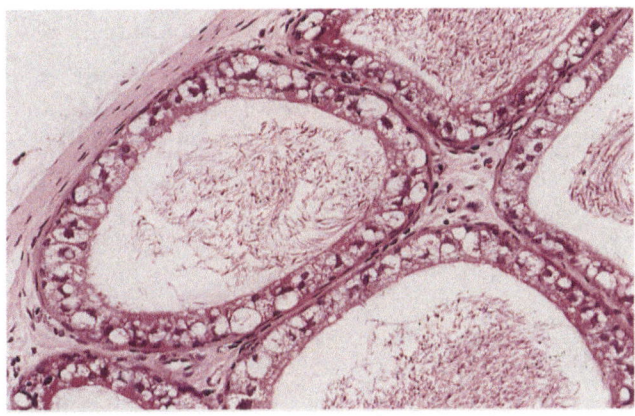

Figure 6.37 Vacuolated epithelium of the epididymal ducts in a dog. Lining cells are vacuolated and distended. Occasional pyknotic nuclei are seen. This type of change may be induced by oestrogenic compounds. H & E

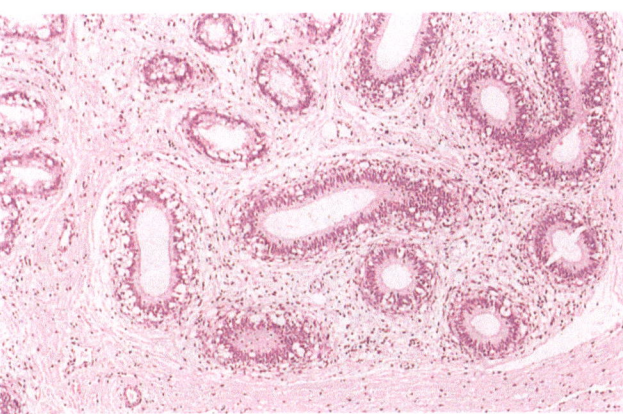

Figure 6.38 Atrophy of the epididymis in a rat treated with an oestrogenic compound. Spermatozoa are absent from the lumina. Note the interstitial fibrosis. H & E

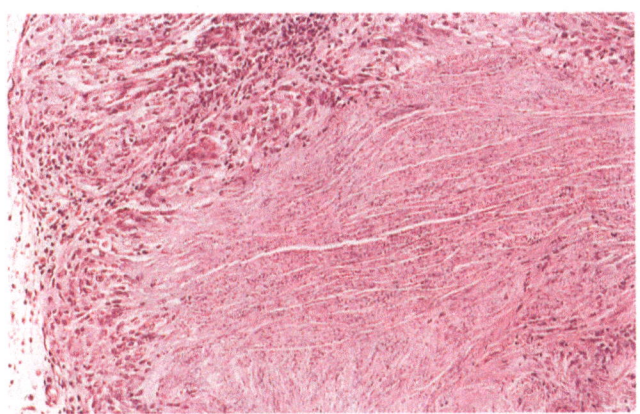

Figure 6.39 Spermatic granuloma in the epididymis of a mouse. Release of spermatozoa into the interstitium has provoked a granulomatous reaction with histiocytes, giant cells and fibroblasts. H & E

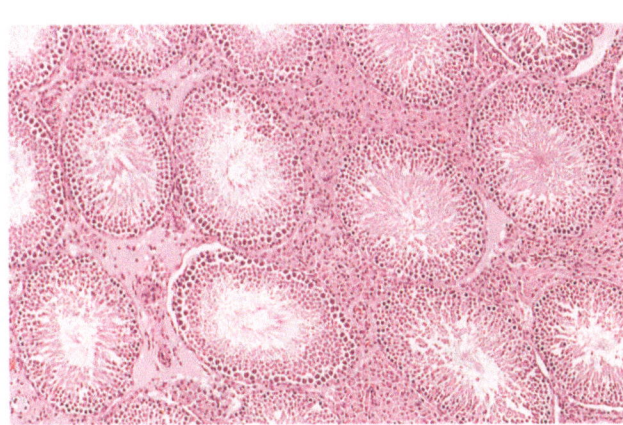

Figure 6.40 Leydig cell hyperplasia in the testis of a rat treated with a novel agrochemical. In this case (in comparison with Figure 6.36) the seminiferous tubules are normal. H & E

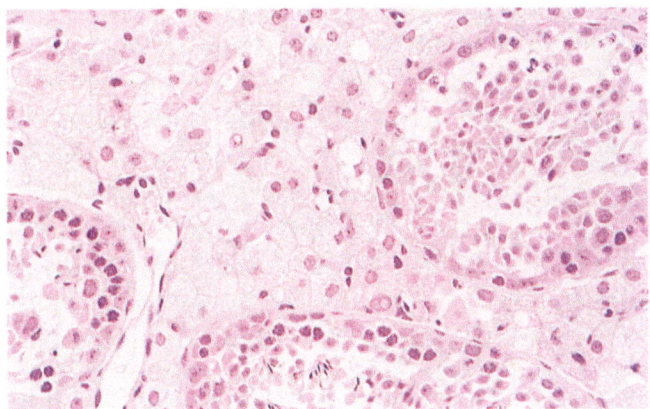

Figure 6.41 Leydig cell hyperplasia in the testis of a mouse treated with a novel herbicide. The interstitial cells have a foamy cytoplasmic appearance. Note the reduction of tailed spermatids in the seminiferous tubules. H & E

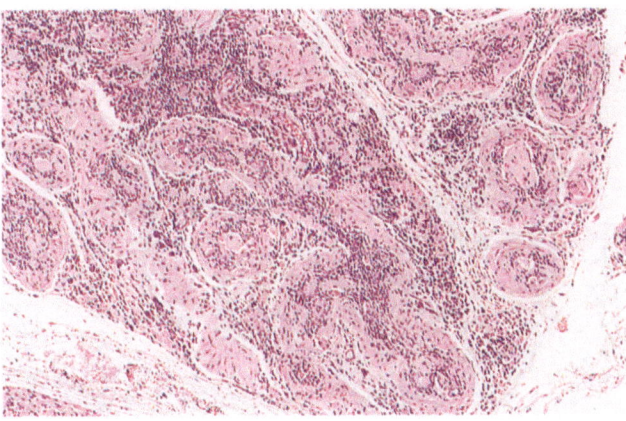

Figure 6.42 Atrophy of the prostate gland in a rat treated with an oestrogenic compound. The acini are collapsed and the interstitial tissue shows fibrosis and inflammation. H & E

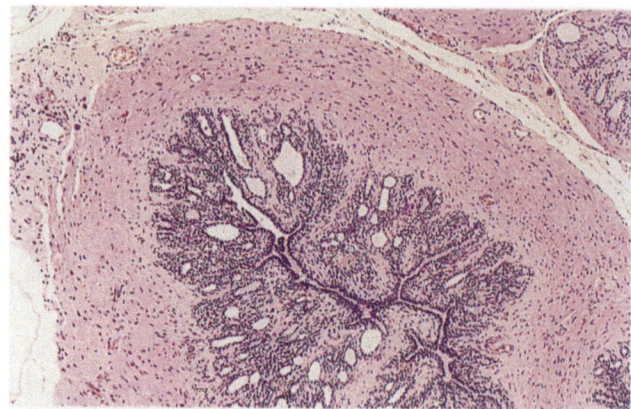

Figure 6.43 Atrophy of a seminal vesicle in a rat treated with an oestrogenic compound. The acini are collapsed and devoid of colloid. The interstitial connective tissue is increased. H & E

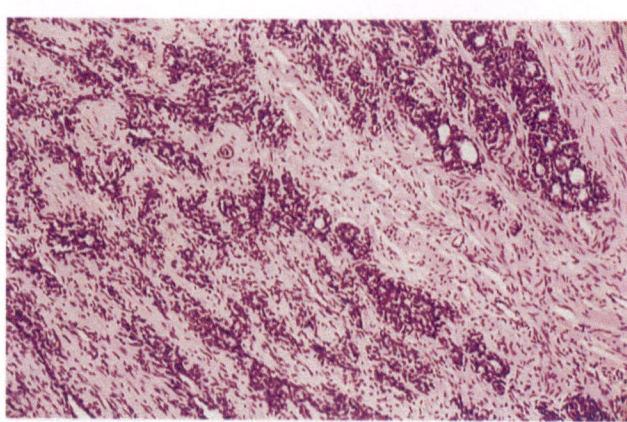

Figure 6.44 Atrophy of the prostate gland in a dog from a toxicity study with a novel neuroleptic drug. The acini are collapsed and lined by low cuboidal epithelium. Interstitial fibrosis is evident. H & E

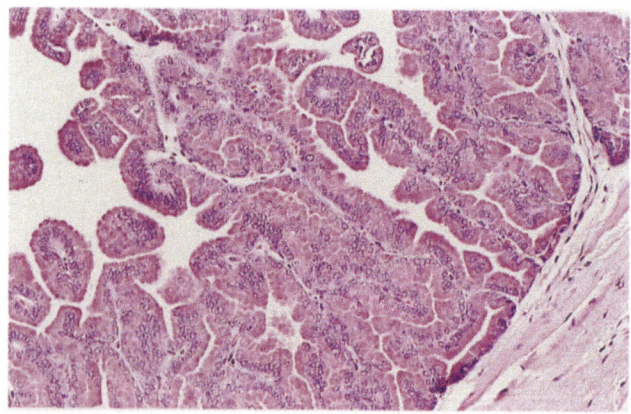

Figure 6.45 Hypertrophy of the prostate in a dog. Note the complex infolding of the epithelium and the dilated lumina. The lining cells are tall columnar. This type of change may be induced by androgenic compounds. H & E

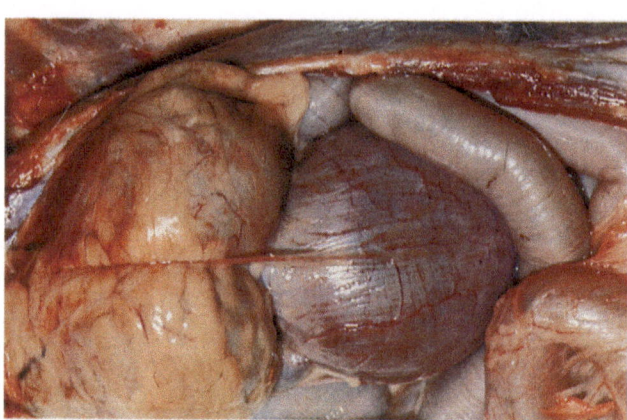

Figure 6.46 Macrophotograph showing prostatic enlargement in a dog treated with an oestrogenic compound

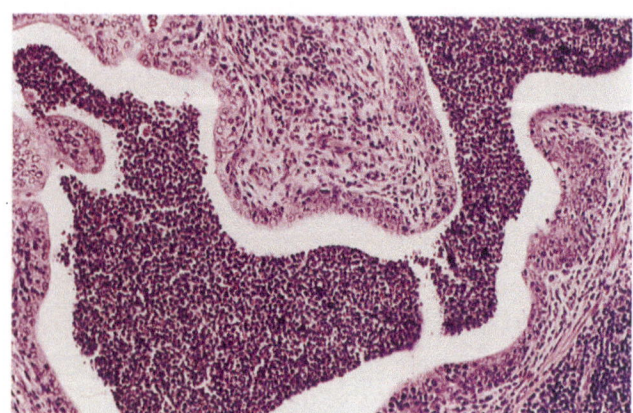

Figure 6.47 Histological appearance of the enlarged prostate shown in Figure 6.46. The acini are distended with purulent exudate and the epithelium shows focal squamous metaplasia. H & E

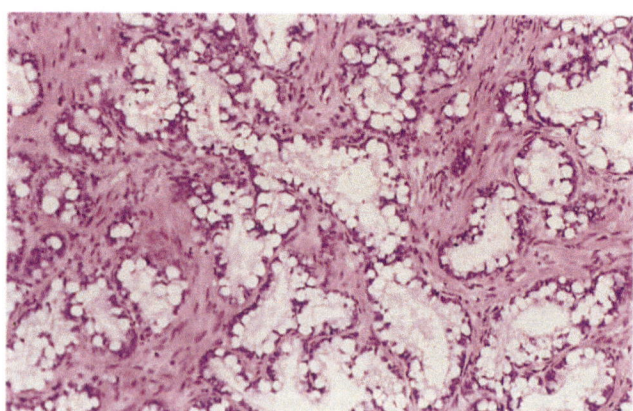

Figure 6.48 Vacuolation of acinar epithelium in the prostate of a monkey from a toxicity study with an antineoplastic compound. Vacuolation of cells from several other organs was also encountered in this study. H & E

K. (1973). Long-term administration of progesterone to female beagle dog. *Toxicol. Appl. Pharmacol.*, **24**, 474–488

28. Nelson, L. W., Weikel, Jr., J. H. and Leno, F. E. (1973). Mammary nodules in dogs during four years treatment with megestrol acetate of chlormadinone acetate. *J. Natl. Cancer Inst.*, **51**, 1303–1311

29. Fitzgerald, J., Iglesia, F. de la and Goldenthal, E. I. (1982). Ten year old oral toxicity study with norlestrin in rhesus monkeys. *J. Toxicol. Environ. Health*, **10**, 879–896

30. Dixon, R. L. (1980). Toxic responses of reproductive system. In Doull, J., Klaassen, C. D. and Amdur, M. O. (eds.) *Casarrett and Doull's Toxicology*. 2nd Ed., p. 332. (New York: Macmillan Publishing Co. Inc.)

31. Schardein, J. L. (1980). Studies of the components of an oral contraceptive agent in albino rats. II. Progestogenic component and comparison of effects of this component and the combined agent. *J. Toxicol. Environ. Health*, **6**, 895–906

32. Neumann, F. (1984). Effects of drugs and chemicals on spermatogenesis. *Arch. Toxicol.*, Suppl. 7, p. 109

33. Corrier, D. E., Mollenhauser, H. H., Clark, D. E., Hare, M. F. and Elissalde, M. H. (1985). Testicular degeneration and necrosis induced by dietary cobalt. *Vet. Pathol.*, **22**, 610–616

34. Creasy, D. M., Foster, J. R. and Foster, P. M. D. (1983). The morphological development of di-N-pentyl phthalate induced testicular atrophy in the rat. *J. Pathol.*, **139**, 309–321

35. Dunn, T. B. and Green, A. W. (1963). Cysts of epididymis, cancer of the cervix, granular cell myoblastoma and other lesions after oestrogen injection in newborn mice. *J. Natl. Cancer Inst.*, **31**, 425–455

36. Agarwal, D. K., Maronpot, R. R., Lamb, J. C. and Kluwe, W. M. (1985). Adverse effects of butylbenzyl phthalate on the reproductive and haemopoetic systems of male rats. *Toxicology*, **35**, 189–206

37. Bhathal, P. S., Gerkens, J. F. and Mashford, M. L. (1974). Spermatic granuloma of the epididymis in rats treated with guanethidine. *J. Pathol.*, **112**, 19–26

38. Benson, W. R. and Clarke, F. S. (1966). Regenerative changes and spermatic granulomas in the rat testes after treatment with DL-ethionine. *Am. J. Pathol.*, **49**, 981–991

39. Rich, K. A., Kerr, J. B. and de Krester, D. M. (1979). Evidence of Leydig cell dysfunction in rats with seminiferous tubule damage. *Mol. Cell. Endocrinol.*, **13**, 123–135

40. Sharpe, R. M. (1982). Cellular aspects of the inhibitory actions of LH–RH on the ovary and testis. *J. Reprod. Fertil.*, **64**, 517–527

41. Bonser, G. M. and Robson, J. M. (1940). The effects of prolonged estrogen administration upon male mice of various strains. Development of testicular tumours in the Strong A Strain. *J. Pathol. Bacteriol.*, **51**, 9–22

42. Molenaar, R., De Rooij, D. G., Rommerts, F. G. and van der Molen, H. J. (1986). Repopulation of Leydig cells in mature rats after selective destruction of the existent Leydig cells with ethylene dimethane sulfonate is dependant in luteinizing hormone and follicle stimulating hormone. *Endocrinology*, **118**, 2546–2554

43. Newbold, R. R., Bullock, B. C. and McLachlan, J. A. (1985). Lesions of the rete testis in mice exposed prenatally to diethylstilbestrol. *Cancer Res.*, **45**, 5145–5150

44. Triche, T. J. and Harkin, J. C. (1971). An ultrastructural study of hormonally induced squamous metaplasia in the coagulating gland of the mouse prostate. *Lab. Invest.*, **25**, 596–605

7

The Endocrine Glands

Many of the induced changes in the endocrine system are a result of interference with feedback control mechanisms and as such are often predictable. However, some lesions also occur which are due to direct toxic effects.

Adrenals

The adrenals are one of the most vulnerable and consequently the most frequently affected of the endocrine tissues in toxicity and safety evaluation studies[1].

Substances may exert toxic effects on the adrenals either directly or via metabolic activation[2]. Adrenal monooxygenases have been shown to be capable of oxidation of many foreign compounds and some xenobiotics are metabolized more rapidly by adrenal than by hepatic microsomal preparations[2]. Adrenal activation is believed to be responsible for the toxicity of 1-(o-chlorophenyl)-1-(p-chlorophenyl)-2,2-dichloroethane (DDD), carbon tetrachloride and chloroform.

Induced lesions of the adrenals in laboratory animals are the subject of two recent detailed reviews[1,3]. The susceptibility of the different zones of the adrenal varies and the most convenient classification (Table 7.1) of induced lesions involves division into: (i) zona glomerulosa; (ii) zona fasciculata/reticularis; and (iii) medulla.

Table 7. Induced lesions of the adrenal

Cortex
Zona glomerulosa:
  Hypertrophy
  Atrophy
  Degeneration

Zona fasciculata/reticularis:
  Hypertrophy
  Atrophy
  Degeneration/necrosis
  Lipidosis
  Intracytoplasmic inclusions
  Inflammation
  Hyperplasia
  Vacuolation of sinusoidal cells

Medulla
  Hyperplasia
  Atrophy
  Intracytoplasmic inclusions
  Vacuolation

Of the three cortical zones, the zona glomerulosa is the least frequently affected by toxic injury. This is probably due in part to its more specialized physiological role and in part because it receives a proportion of its vascular supply from the capsule and thus is not as susceptible to anoxic and infarctive changes as the fasciculata and reticularis[1].

Hypertrophy and altered cytoplasmic staining characteristics, resulting in a more prominent appearance, of the rat zona glomerulosa (Figure 7.1) are detected following administration of high doses of some diuretics such as furosemide. This morphological change is probably a reflection of the electrolyte imbalance caused by these compounds; similar reversible changes are reported following dietary deficiency of sodium and parenteral administration of potassium[4,5]. Conversely, elevation of the sodium/potassium ratio causes a narrowing of the zona glomerulosa with prominent large intracytoplasmic lipid droplets[4].

A frequently studied lesion of the zona glomerulosa is that induced by the diuretic and antihypertensive agent spironolactone[2,3]. This compound exerts its therapeutic action of promoting sodium diuresis, by antagonizing aldosterone and causes hypertrophy of the zona glomerulosa with the formation of intracellular eosinophilic bodies. Ultrastructurally, these 'spironolactone bodies' are composed of hypertrophic concentric arrays of agranular membranes, often with sequestered central lipid droplets[6]. In our laboratories, dogs treated with a spironolactone-like compound also demonstrated a pronounced hypertrophy of the zona glomerulosa. The adrenals were macroscopically enlarged and slightly nodular. The hypertrophy resulted in a highly convoluted arrangement of the pseudoacinar pattern characteristic of the canine zona glomerulosa (Figure 7.2).

Atrophy or condensation of the zona glomerulosa is reported following administration of a sulphated mucopolysaccharide[7]. This change, in rats, is associated with decreased aldosterone production. The renin–angiotensin system stimulates growth of the zona glomerulosa and atrophic changes are induced by timolol maleate which suppresses renin release[8]. Atrophy is also induced by captopril, a specific inhibitor of the angiotensin-converting enzyme[8,9]. Administration of angiotensin II reverses this atrophic effect. In addition, there is some evidence that somatostatin may be involved in the regulation of aldosterone secretion and it inhibits secretion and induces atrophy[10].

Acute degeneration of the zona glomerulosa is induced by hexadimethrine[11]. The necrosis appears to be due to liberation of histamine from mast cells; histamine depletion by pretreatment of rats with compound 48/80 prevents the ischaemic lesions. Simultaneous administration of 5-hydroxytryptamine (5-HT) potentiates the lesion, and prior depletion of 5-HT by reserpine diminishes the severity. Administration of antihistamines reduces the incidence of the lesion and it appears likely that arteriolar spasm with infarction is responsible[1]. Microthrombi are detected ultrastructurally[3].

Following administration of ACTH to rats, the cells of the zona glomerulosa become less differentiated and indistinguishable from the subjacent zona fasciculata. Aldosterone production is correspondingly suppressed[12]. No evidence of cell necrosis is detected and it appears likely that the cells of the zona glomerulosa transform into a fasciculata-like appearance.

The adrenal cortex shows adaptive changes to 'stress'. Any changes in environmental conditions or stressful experimental procedures may cause hypertrophy. The usual histological manifestation (Figure 7.3) of this change is an increase in width of the two zones (ZF/R). Often there is also a corresponding decrease in the number of lipid droplets, giving the cytoplasm a less rarefied and more dense staining intensity. The hypertrophy is caused by increased amounts of ACTH which stimulate release of cortical hormones. Compounds which prevent biosynthesis of corticosteroids also induce hypertrophy in response to increased ACTH secretion in the absence of negative feedback.

Administration of ACTH to rats causes vascular changes in addition to cytoplasmic alterations[12]. A significant proportion of the cortical hypertrophy is attributable to hyperaemia with dilation of the sinusoids and intercellular spaces. The adrenals are amongst the most highly vascularized organs[13], but this is not always appreciated due to collapse of the vasculature in conventional histological preparations. The hyperaemia is followed by extravasation of erythrocytes into intercellular spaces and disruption of the cord-like organization of the cells. This condition may progress to vascular 'pooling' (angiectasis) and haemorrhage due to cell deletion and haemorrhagic infarction. These ACTH-induced changes probably represent pathological reactions to 'over-stimulation' rather than physiological responses.

Enlargement of the adrenal cortex also follows the administration of oestrogens, especially synthetic ones to rats, and may correlate with the known sexual dimorphism of adrenal size. In male rats oestradiol administration leads to an increased cell size[14]. This response is dependent on the integrity of the pituitary and oestrogens probably act by blocking corticosteroid synthesis with increased ACTH release.

Administration of relatively high doses of potent corticosteroids suppresses ACTH release and leads to regression of the adrenal cortex (Figures 7.4 and 7.5), as in the hypophysectomized condition. This atrophic change may be induced in all laboratory animal species. In severe cases the ZF/R becomes virtually absent with only the zona glomerulosa and medulla being clearly identifiable (Figure 7.6). The atrophic changes are accompanied by cell deletion by apoptosis[15]. Ultrastructurally, decreased amounts of smooth endoplasmic reticulum and numbers of lipid droplets in individual cells are the major factors responsible for the cellular atrophy[16]. However, 25 hours after administration of corticosteroids the number of lipid droplets is, in fact, increased due to absence of secretion stimulus by ACTH[13]. The apoptosis phase is initiated and completed rapidly and may be prevented by coincident administration of ACTH[15].

Degrees of cortical atrophy may also be detected in dogs and rats given high doses of some synthetic progestogens and progesterone. These compounds possess some glucocorticoid activity and thus suppress ACTH release[17,18].

Haemorrhagic necrosis may be induced in rats by the heparin antagonist hexadimethrine, acrylonitrile, cysteamine, pyrazole or thioacetamide[19,20]. A possible mechanism suggested to explain the development of this lesion involves an early retrograde embolization of adrenal medullary cells into cortical capillaries. These medullary emboli are believed to cause vascular damage in the cortex followed by epithelial cell necrosis. Evidence for this proposed mechanism is provided by the absence of lesions following a range of pretreatments including: the α-adrenergic antagonist phenoxybenzamine; the α- and β-adrenergic blocker labetalol; the 11-β-hydroxylase inhibitor metyrapone; catecholamine depletion by reserpine; and prior surgical medullectomy. Areas of cortical infarction, similar to those described with hexadimethrine[1], have been observed in our laboratories in rats treated with an industrial chemical. The lesions were inevitably 'wedge-shaped' (Figure 7.7) and confined to the ZF/R.

In addition to its well documented hepatotoxicity, carbon tetrachloride also causes adrenocortical necrosis. This necrosis is generally confined to the inner cortex. Carbon tetrachloride toxicity is mediated via the microsomal cytochrome P-450-dependent mono-oxygenases[2]. The levels of these enzymes are greatest in the inner cortex.

Focal vacuolar degeneration with associated haemorrhage was detected after high doses of a novel cardiotonic agent in baboons in our laboratories (Figure 7.8). Eosinophilic cytoplasmic inclusions similar to spironolactone bodies were also detected (Figure 7.9).

Several compounds produce a selective widespread vacuolar degeneration of the cortex. These compounds include DDD, an insecticide derivative of DDT, and α-(1,4-dioxide-3-methylquinoxalin-2-yl)-N-methylnitrone (DMNM)[3,21–23]. With DMNM, degenerative changes are reported in dogs, rats and monkeys, whereas DDD appears species specific with lesions confined to the dog. A similar lesion was detected in rats, treated with an industrial chemical in our laboratories, and was characterized by vacuolation and swelling of individual cells (Figure 7.10) with eventual rupture causing disruption of the cord-like arrangement. In general, little inflammatory reaction was associated with the condition but pronounced vascular congestion, dilatation, 'pooling' (angiectasis) and haemorrhage (probably secondary to the cell loss) were relatively frequent features (Figure 7.11). In rats exposed to an industrial chemical by inhalation in our laboratories, a form of vacuolar degeneration was detected in the outer zona fasciculata. Focal areas of marked vacuolation and cell swelling, with occasional cholesterol clefts, a mild acute inflammatory cell infiltration, single cell degeneration (with features characteristic of apoptosis) and slight hyperaemia, were observed (Figure 7.12).

Another relatively common form of degenerative change of the adrenal cortex in untreated rats is age-related cystic degeneration of the ZF/R; in our experience this is predominantly, but not exclusively, a condition of the female rat (Figure 7.13). Not unexpectedly, in studies involving administration of high doses of oestrogens, the incidence of the lesion in treated male rats is elevated above the control levels. Conversely, compounds with androgenic activity decrease the incidence in female rats. The zona glomerulosa is usually unaffected except in severe cases. The aetiology of the condition is uncertain but it may be of vascular origin and has been termed adrenal peliosis[24]. Haemorrhagic necrosis of the adrenal gland is reported in rats fed a vitamin B complex deficient diet. Animals subsequently given a synthetic pantothenic acid show repair of the degenerative processes[25].

Although steroids are normally abundant in the adrenal cortex neutral fats are not. The appearance of neutral

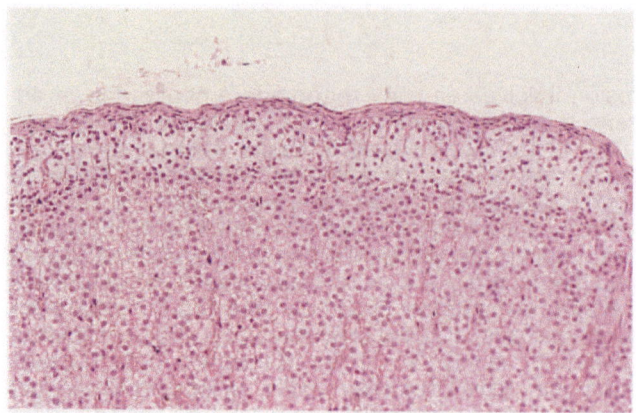

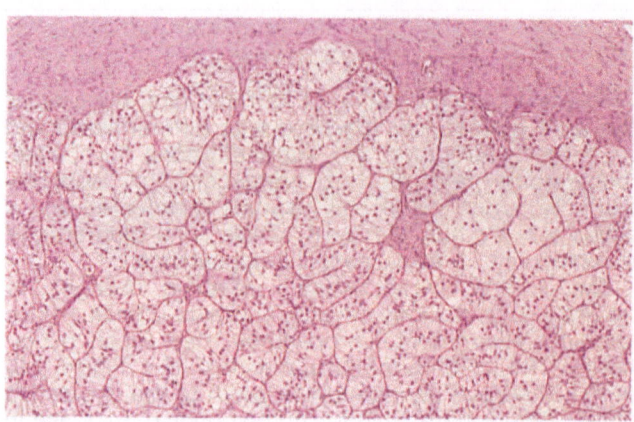

Figure 7.1   Rat adrenal showing hypertrophy of the zona glomeru-losa. The lesion was detected in study with high doses of a diuretic.   H & E

Figure 7.2   Hypertrophy of the zona glomerulosa from a dog treated with a spironolactone-like compound. The zona glomeru-losa is considerably increased in width and the pseudoacinar pat-tern grossly exaggerated. Compare with Figure 7.6 which shows the normal zona glomerulosa.   H & E

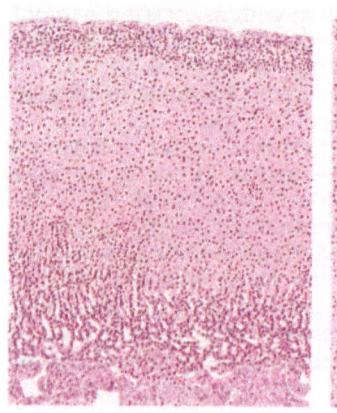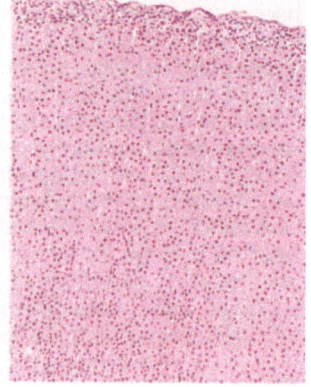

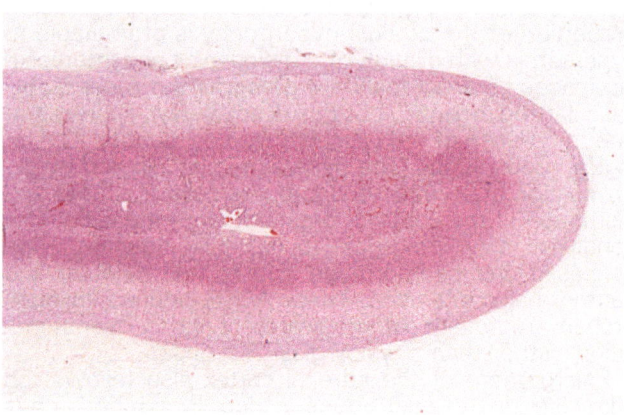

Figure 7.3   Hypertrophy of the zona fasciculata and zona reticu-laris in a rat. Note the homogeneity of cell type. The zona glomeru-losa is unchanged. Section from control rat is included for comparison.   H & E

Figure 7.4   Adrenal from an untreated cynomolgus monkey dem-onstrating the clear distinction between the three cortical zones.   H & E

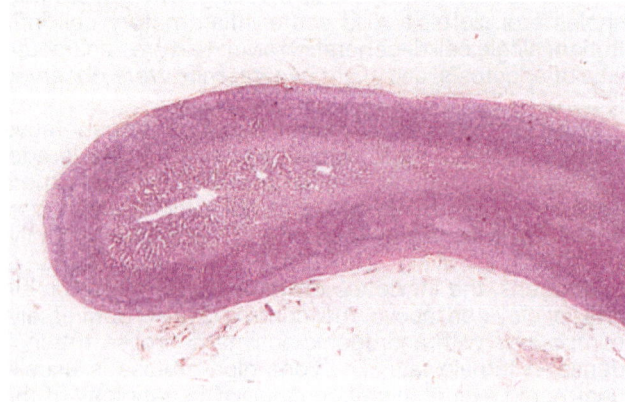

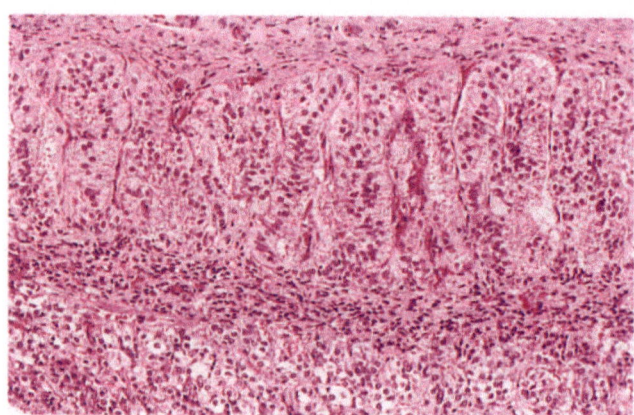

Figure 7.5   Adrenal from a cynomolgus monkey treated with high doses of a novel corticosteroid. In comparison with Figure 7.4 the cortex is decreased in width and more intensely stained.   H & E

Figure 7.6   Adrenal from a dog showing severe cortical atrophy due to administration of high doses of a novel corticosteroid. The zonae fasciculata and reticularis are reduced to a narrow layer between the unaffected characteristic canine glomerulosa and the medulla.   H & E

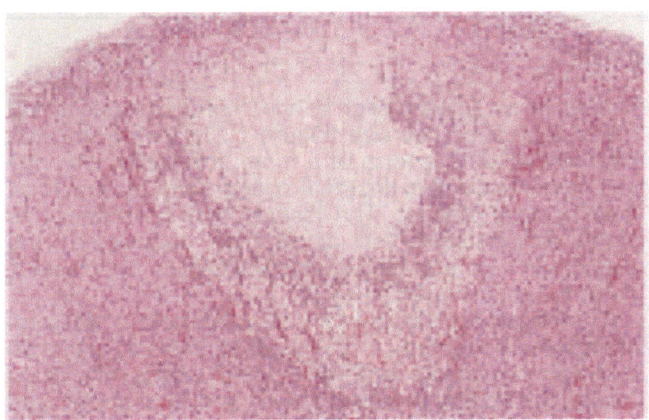

Figure 7.7 Typical 'wedge-shaped' cortical infarct in a rat induced by an industrial chemical. The zona glomerulosa is spared. H & E

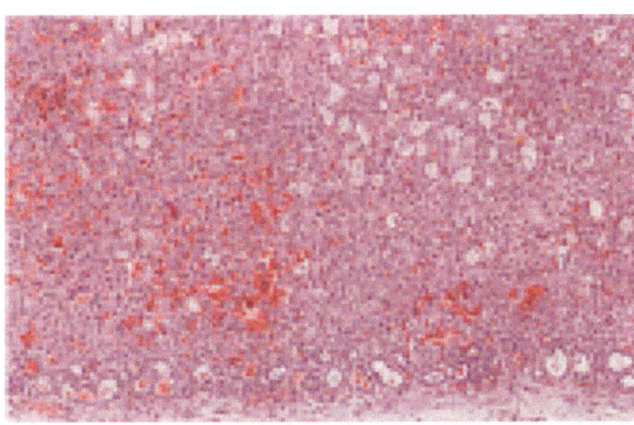

Figure 7.8 Degeneration of single cells in the zona fasciculata of a baboon following administration of a novel cardiotonic agent. The degeneration has led to haemorrhage and vascular pooling. H & E

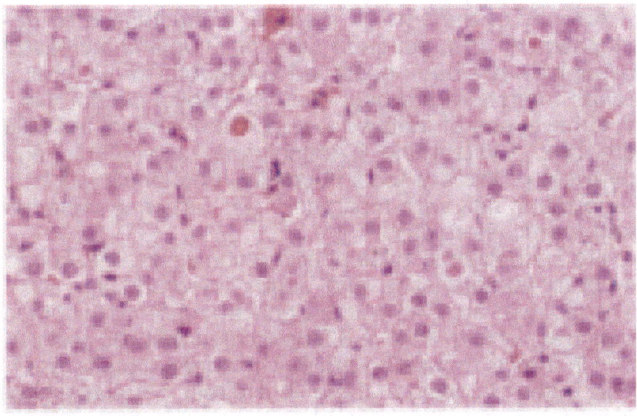

Figure 7.9 Eosinophilic cytoplasmic inclusions in cells of the zona fasciculata from a baboon (from the same study as Figure 7.8). H & E

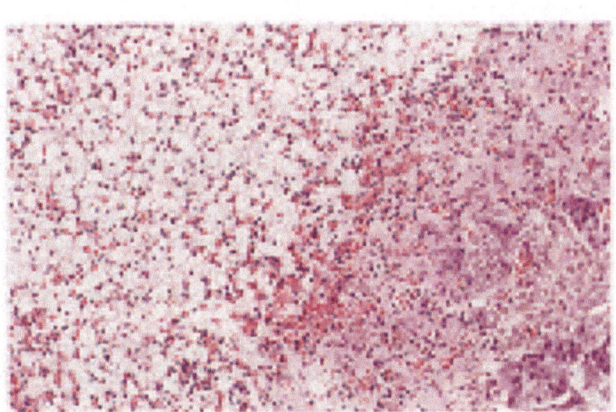

Figure 7.10 Pronounced vacuolar degeneration and congestion in the adrenal cortex of a rat induced by administration of an industrial chemical. H & E

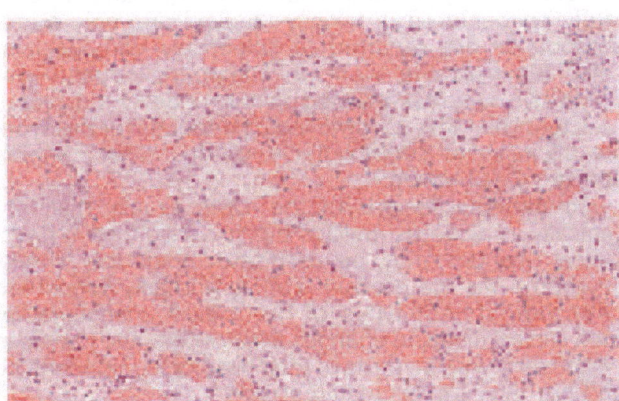

Figure 7.11 Disruption of cords, vacuolar degeneration and vascular pooling in the cortex of an adrenal from a rat treated with an industrial chemical. H & E

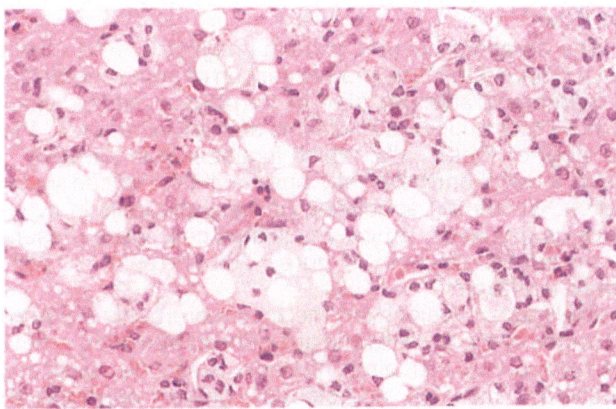

Figure 7.12 Vacuolar degeneration of cells of the zona fasciculata of the adrenal from a rat treated with an industrial chemical by inhalation. H & E

fat droplets indicates a degenerative process[1]. Lipidosis may be induced by a wide range of chemicals, such as aminoglutethimide, which inhibit steroidogenesis and lead to a build up of steroid precursors[3]. The lipidosis appears histologically as fine (Figures 7.14, 7.15 and 7.16) or coarse vacuoles which coalesce, or large 'ballooned cells' and evidence of cell rupture[26].

The so called 'x' zone in the adrenals (Figure 7.17) of some mouse strains may illustrate another form of lipidosis. This zone normally regresses at the onset of sexual maturity in males and at the first pregnancy in females[1]. In a small percentage of animals the normal shrinkage and degeneration of this zone is associated with severe fatty degeneration and replacement. Exacerbation of this fatty change may be induced by some compounds, including thyroxin and methanol[1].

Administration of amphiphilic, cationic compounds such as zimelidine, chlorphentermine, triparanol, chlorcyclizine and iprindole all produce widespread phospholipidosis, including the adrenal cortex[1,27,28]. By light microscopy this is characterized by the presence of inclusions which may be identified with the electron microscope as multilamellar bodies. The change is reported in several species including mice, rats, rabbits and guinea pigs.

Hyaline droplets may be induced in association with several other changes including starvation, thirst and hypertension, as well as with a variety of compounds including the infarction and necrosis induced by hexadimethrine[3] and with the lipidosis induced by aminoglutethimide[26]. Their development following methylandrostenediol administration is described in rats[29] and they are believed to develop from protein-containing absorption vacuoles.

'Brown degeneration' or ceroid deposition in mice is observed with diethylstilboestrol[30] and with propylthiouracil[31].

An unusual cortical lesion has been induced in cynomolgus monkeys treated with thyroid hormones in our laboratories – focal aggregates of lymphocytes in the cortical sinusoids. This focal adrenalitis was assiociated with a few single degenerate cells (Figure 7.18).

Focal nodular hyperplasia (as distinct from generalized cortical hyperplasia) may be a primary event (Figure 7.19) or a secondary regenerative reaction following damage. Induced primary hyperplasia is a rare finding in toxicity studies but nodular hyperplasia is described in rats with DMNM[22].

The adrenal sinusoids contain phagocytic cells which may respond to intravenous injection of some materials. Experimental administration of the polysaccharide zymosan to rats causes stimulation and an increase in the number of these cells, which ingest carbon particles[32]. With a novel antineoplastic agent which induced widespread systemic vacuolation of histocytic cells in cynomolgus monkeys, similar vacuolated cells were present in the adrenal sinusoids (Figure 7.20). The epithelial cells were unaffected.

Proliferative lesions are the most commonly reported changes of the medulla and are induced by a wide variety of compounds including: nicotine, reserpine, synthetic retinoids, thiouracil, neuroleptics, growth hormone, 4-chloro-m-phenylenediamine, 11,2-trichloroethane, an analgesic (Zomepirac), a β-adrenergic blocker (Blocadren), and perhaps most surprisingly lactose and sugar alcohols, such as mannitol, sorbitol, xylitol and lactitol[1,33–35]. These changes are widely reported in rats but there are few reports in other species.

Hyperplastic lesions are usually readily distinguishable from the adjacent normal medullary cells by a more basophilic cytoplasm, slightly hyperchromatic nuclei and often decreased cell size (Figure 7.21). When the proliferation takes the form of a more diffuse hypertrophy and hyperplasia the tinctorial change and anisocytosis may be less distinct. The lesions may be present as single foci, multiple foci or distinctly nodular and the distinction between hyperplasia and benign neoplasm is sometimes difficult[33].

The mechanism behind the development of the proliferative lesions induced by sugar alcohols is uncertain and several factors are suggested[33]: excessive food intake; excessive dietary calcium and phosphate; and excessive intake of other food components such as vitamin D. Poor carbohydrate absorption may also enhance calcium absorption. Roe and Bär[33] suggest calcium homeostasis may be strongly implicated in the aetiology of the lesions. However, changes in serum calcium levels are not detected with xylitol which readily forms complexes with calcium[34]. Xylitol has an inhibitory effect on catecholamine synthesis and this may be a possible mechanism by which a compensatory hypertrophy and hyperplasia are induced.

Atrophy of the adrenal medulla, characterized by decreased cell size, apparent degranulation and increased basophilia, has been observed in baboons in our laboratories treated with a high dose of a novel cardiotonic.

Other types of induced lesion in the adrenal medulla are rare. Cysteamine hydrochloride, acrylonitrile and pyrazole produce a focal necrosis[1]. Phospholipidosis is reported in rats with triparanol[27] and fatty degeneration with corticosteroids.

Intracytoplasmic eosinophilic globules are described in both noradrenaline and adrenaline-producing cells. The globules are PAS positive and are reported in guinea pigs treated with 1,2,3,7,8,9-hexachlorodibenzo-p-dioxin and in rhesus monkeys with polychlorinated biphenyls[36]. The authors consider there is a direct correlation between the development of the globules and adrenal haemorrhage and necrosis.

Extensive vacuolation of medullary cells of cynomolgus monkeys has been found in our laboratories following administration of a novel antineoplastic agent (Figure 7.22)

Islets of Langerhans

Lesions of the pancreatic islets of Langerhans are only rarely encountered in toxicity studies[1] and only a few compounds are reported to selectively damage islet cells. Much of the work on compound-induced islet changes is undertaken using animal models for diabetes mellitus. The most widely used compounds for this work are alloxan and streptozotocin, both of which exhibit specific β-cell action.

Experimental lesions of the islets usually manifest clinically as diabetes mellitus but several different histological changes may be associated with this clinical syndrome. As the present work is primarily concerned with the different types of histological change rather than clinical disease, changes in the endocrine pancreas will be reviewed in terms of their histological appearance and not their clinical manifestation.

Treatment-induced changes are the subject of two relatively detailed reviews[1,2]. Islets contain a mixture of cell types all of which are believed to be derived from the pancreatic duct cells[3]. The development of immunocytochemical techniques has enabled the more precise identification of cell types and their distribution in both normal and pathological islet tissue. In the normal islet the insulin producing β-cells comprise some 80% of the cells and are generally located at the islet centre. The α-cells, which produce glucagon, are located at the periphery. Small numbers of somatostatin producing δ-cells and pancreatic polypeptide-containing cells may also be present at the periphery[4,5]. Somatostatin acts to inhibit the secretion of both glucagon and insulin. The induced lesions of the pancreatic islets are listed in Table 7.2.

Table 7.2 Induced lesions of the islets of Langerhans

Necrosis
Vacuolation
Atrophy
Angiectasis
Hyalinization
Fibrosis
Hypertrophy
Hyperplasia
Oncocytes

Both alloxan and streptozotocin act as specific β-cell toxins in several animal species. Initially, a severe hypoglycaemia occurs due to rapid release of insulin by the damaged cells. Nuclear changes including chromatin aggregation, pyknosis and loss of nucleoli are followed by the loss of secretory granules and vesiculation of the endoplasmic reticulum. No inflammatory response is detected. These compounds are widely used in models for experimental diabetes mellitus[1,2]. Another compound, recently shown to be selectively toxic to β-cells, is the antiprotozoan drug pentamidine[6].

Necrosis may also occur following administration of compounds which bind zinc (found in β-cells in combination with insulin). Some compounds such as oxine and dithizone[1] form zinc complexes and produce this lesion in rats, mice and cats. In addition, although not unexpectedly, a zinc-deficient diet also induces islet lesions.

Reports of compounds inducing necrosis of α-cells are rare, but intra-vascular administration of sodium diethyldithiocarbonate to rabbits causes degeneration of α-cells and capillary lesions[2].

A group of compounds with diverse pharmacological actions are described which selectively induce vacuolation of β-cells of the rat, but not dog, primate, rabbit or mouse[1]. These compounds include a dihydromorphanthridine (EX10-54A), cyproheptadine (an antihistaminic–antiserotonin) and cyclizine (an antihistamine). They all possess a piperidine or piperazine ring substituted at the 4-position. The lesion is characterized at the light microscope level by marked vacuolation of β-cells, often with displacement of the nucleus. Ultrastructurally, loss of secretory granules, dilatation of the rough endoplasmic reticulum with accumulation of granular electron-dense material, and hypertrophy of the Golgi are consistent findings. The changes are reversible and characteristic of hypersecretory activity. A similar vacuolation was noted in cynomolgus monkeys treated with a novel anticancer drug in our laboratories (Figure 7.23).

In beagles, diabetes mellitus associated with pancreatic islet cell vacuolation (Figure 7.24) is found after 4 or 5 years treatment with synthetic progestogens, megestrol acetate[7] and chlormadinone acetate[8].

Vacuolation of β-cells is easily induced in the Sand rat (*Psammomys obesus*) by changing the diet from vegetables to laboratory chow[9].

The administration of growth hormone to dogs causes decreased serum insulin, β-cell degranulation, dilatation of the rough endoplasmic reticulum and Golgi, and cytoplasmic accumulation of glycogen. These changes lead to diabetes and are thought to be the result of sequential

overactivity, exhaustion and consequent atrophy of β-cells[10].

Another form of cellular atrophy characterized by hyposecretion of insulin is described with diazoxide. Secretory granules are present in the β-cells but many are contained within 'multigranular sacs' which probably represent autophagic degradation[1].

Few compounds exert specific effects on the glucagon secreting α-cells. Amongst those reported, cobalt salts, synthalin A and phenylethyldiguamide produce changes suggestive of 'cell exhaustion' due to hyperstimulation of hormone release[1].

Angiectasis may develop in islets and has been detected in our laboratories in cynomolgus monkeys treated with an antineoplastic immunomodulator. Almost all the islets showed dilatation and congestion of the vasculature which led to angiectasis (Figure 7.25). The lesion was believed to have developed as a result of cell degeneration with expansion of the vascular component; animals examined earlier in the study showed evidence of necrosis and in a few cases, peripheral fibroblasts were detected (Figure 7.26). A similar islet lesion described recently was associated with a form of multiple endocrine neoplasm syndrome in man[11]. The blood-filled cavities are not lined by endothelium, suggesting they represent extracellular tissue space. Capillaries show little evidence of damage and the lesion is designated peliosis.

Hyalinization of the islets has been induced in our laboratories in chronic studies with rhesus monkeys treated with two novel pharmaceuticals. The amount of hyaline varied between islets and appeared with H&E stain as eosinophilic homogeneous material. The hyaline was particularly well demonstrated by Heidenhain's azan stain (Figure 7.27), but was negative for amyloid. The lesion was associated with the development of diabetes mellitus. The hyalinization was probably a sequel to degenerative islet changes. Focal islet fibrosis following hydropic degeneration is reported in rats treated with dihydromorphanthridine, however no effect was detected in dogs[12].

The administration of relatively high doses of potent corticosteroids induces hyperglycaemia and the pancreas responds by releasing insulin. This increased demand for insulin induces a hypersecretory state in the β-cells and they become hypertrophic (Figure 7.28). Ultrastructurally, the endoplasmic reticulum is dilated and the Golgi prominent – both consistent with hypersecretion. In severe cases the β-cells may become exhausted due to degranulation by constant insulin release. The hypertrophic cells cause an increase in the size of the islets as a whole and in some cases may be accompanied by a degree of hyperplasia. This change may be induced in most if not all laboratory animal species.

Radioimmunoassay demonstrates the presence of ACTH in isolated rat islets and anti-ACTH immunoreactivity is demonstrated immunocytochemically in cells at the islet periphery, apparently in the α-cells. This distribution is altered in steroid-induced diabetic rats, with increased amounts of immunoreactivity in large central cells but fewer positive cells at the periphery[13].

Hypoinsulinaemia associated with islet hypertrophy, and changes in the tinctorial properties of the cytoplasm, are described in rats following 2,3,7,8-tetrachlorodibenzo-p-dioxin (TCDD) treatment[14].

Although we have been unable to trace reports of specific toxins to δ-cells, pentagastrin and lithium chloride are both reported to increase the nuclear size of these cells[1].

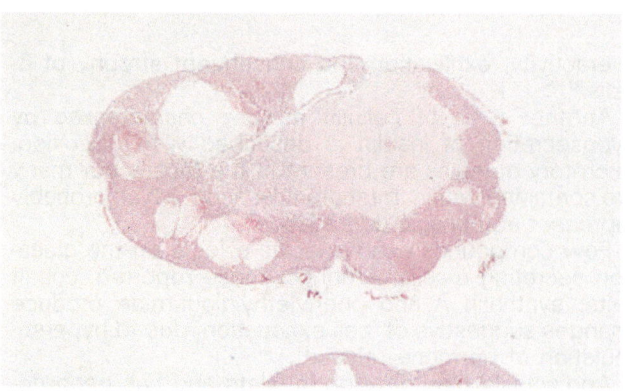

Figure 7.13 Cystic degeneration and haemorrhage of the cortex of a rat adrenal. This lesion is relatively common in aged female rats and the incidence may be increased in males treated with oestrogens. H & E

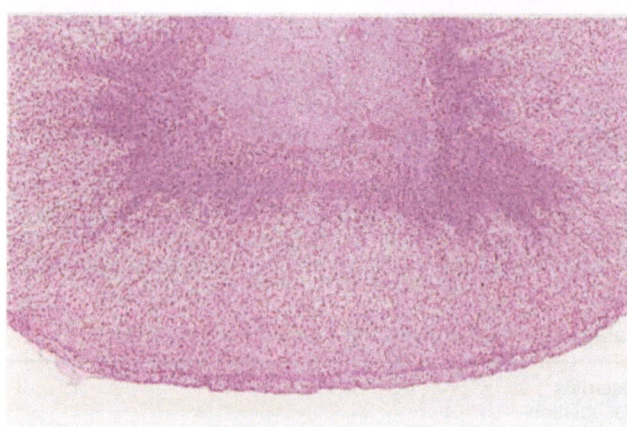

Figure 7.14 Cortical vacuolation of the adrenal of a rat. The lipidosis has caused hypertrophy of the zona fasciculata whilst the glomerulosa and reticularis are unaffected. H & E

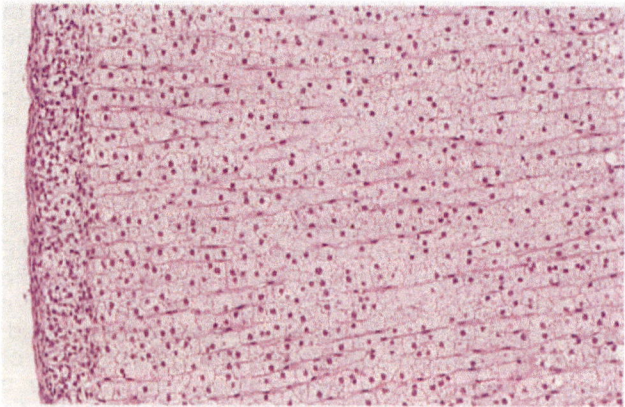

Figure 7.15 Lipidosis demonstrated as fine vacuolation of the zona fasciculata of a rat. H & E

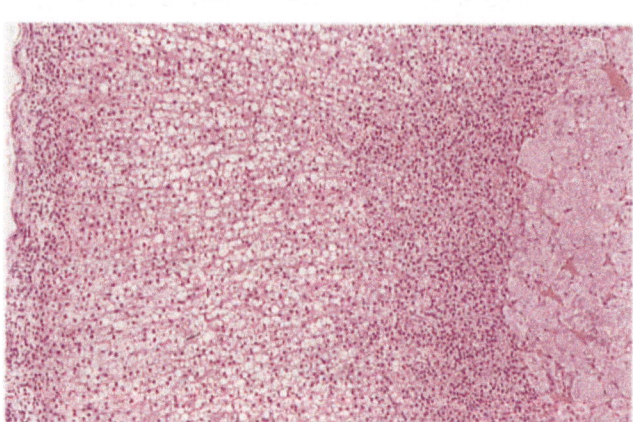

Figure 7.16 Coarse cytoplasmic vacuolation of the adrenal cortex induced in a rat by an industrial chemical. No evidence of degeneration. H & E

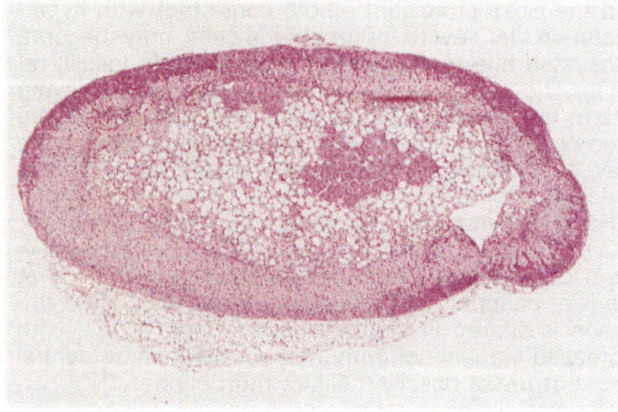

Figure 7.17 The 'x' zone of the mouse adrenal normally regresses, but may undergo fatty degeneration either spontaneously or following treatment with compounds such as methanol. H & E

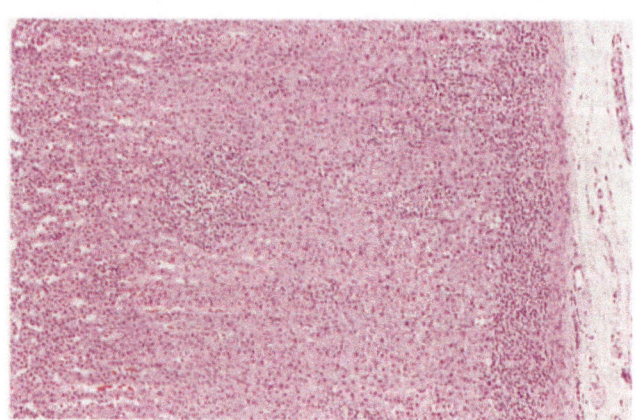

Figure 7.18 Focal adrenalitis in a cynomolgus monkey treated with a thyroid hormone. The inflammatory reaction is associated with a few degenerate cells. H & E

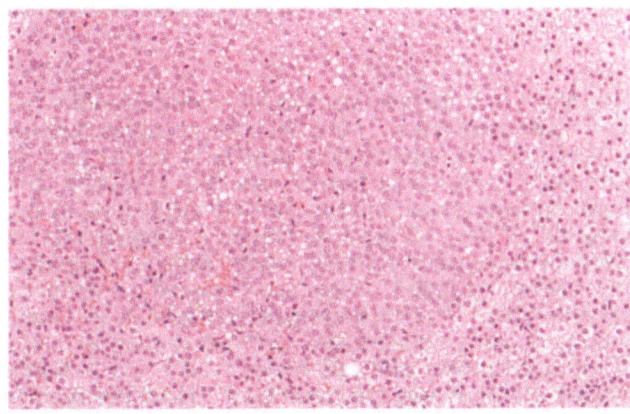

Figure 7.19 Focus of hyperplasia in the cortex of an adrenal of a rat treated with an industrial chemical. The hyperplastic cells appear smaller and more basophilic.   H & E

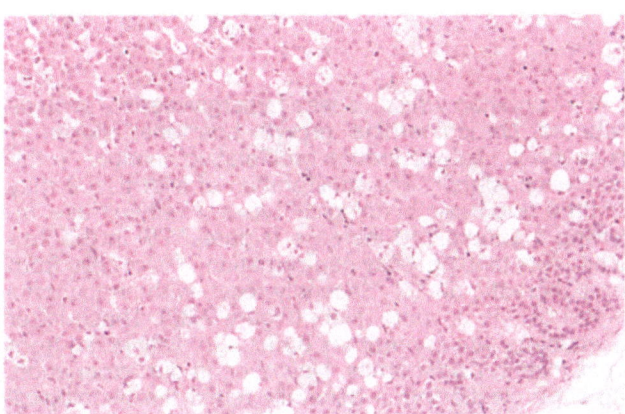

Figure 7.20 Vacuolation of sinusoidal cells in the adrenal cortex of a cynomolgus monkey following administration of a novel antineoplastic agent.   H & E

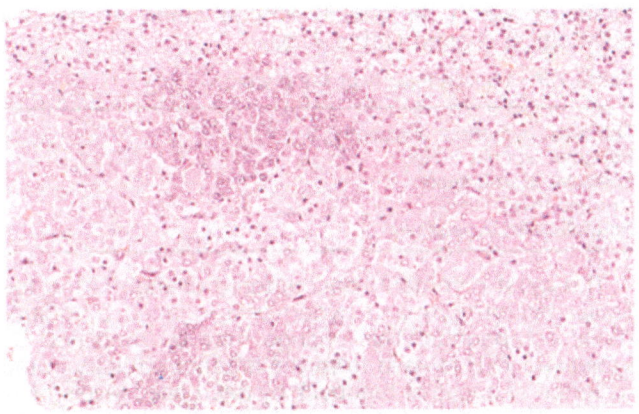

Figure 7.21 Focus of hyperplastic adrenal medullary cells in a rat treated with a novel neuroleptic. The hyperplastic cells are smaller and basophilic.   H & E

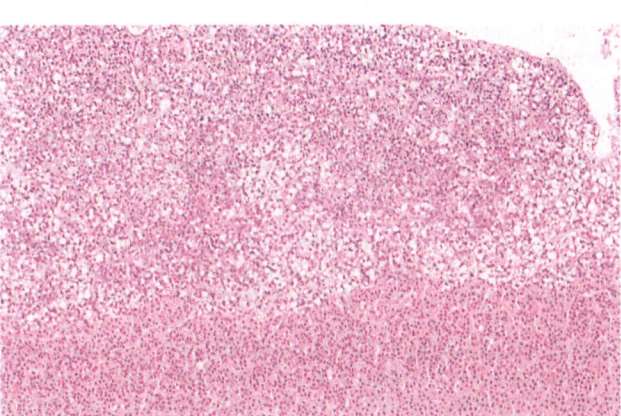

Figure 7.22 Vacuolation of adrenal medullary cells from a cynomolgus monkey treated with an antineoplastic agent.   H & E

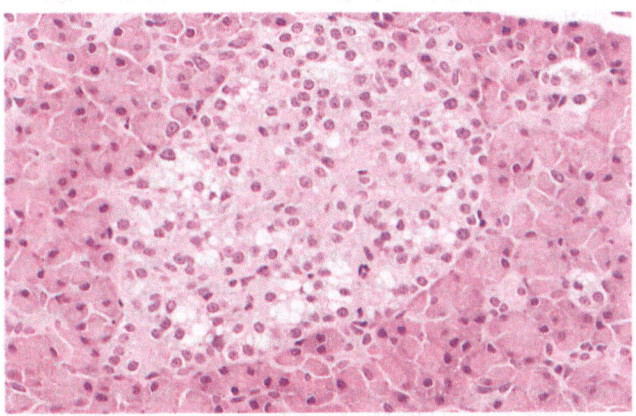

Figure 7.23 Vacuolated pancreatic islet cells in a cynomolgus monkey treated with a novel anticancer drug. The lesion was not associated with diabetes mellitus.   H & E

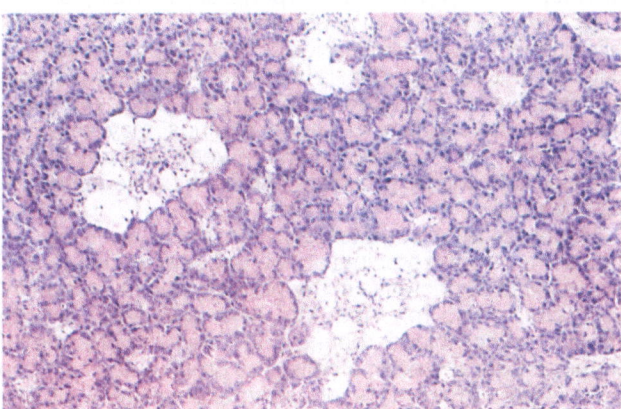

Figure 7.24 Coarse vacuolation and ballooning of pancreatic islet cells in a beagle dog treated with a synthetic progestogen. The lesion was associated with diabetes mellitus.   H & E

Any condition which causes hyperglycaemia, such as diabetes, corticosteroids, growth hormone, alloxan or glucagon is likely to induce proliferative changes in the pancreatic islets[15]. The proliferation of islet tissue may assume two basic histological types. Firstly diffuse, involving a generalized increase (Figure 7.29) in the size of all islets (and possibly neoformation of islet cells from the pancreatic ducts). Secondly focal, with an increase in size of one or more islets (Figure 7.30). These latter 'giant islets' are sometimes difficult to distinguish from small islet cell adenomas. However, in our experience, the hyperplastic forms generally retain the histological pattern and cell type distribution of normal islet tissue and cause no appreciable compression of adjacent exocrine tissue. Immunocytochemical investigations show that, generally, hyperplastic islets are predominently composed of β-cells but the peripheral arrangement of α- and δ-cells is often retained[4].

When interpreting possible islet hyperplasia the effects of tissue sampling should not be ignored, as there are considerable differences in islet frequency between the regions of the pancreas in some species.

Islet β-cell hyperplasia (and neoplasia) may be readily induced in rats by the combined administration of streptozotocin and nicotinamide[16]. Hyperplasia (and neoplasms) are induced by either streptozotocin or alloxan, in combination with several other poly(adenosine diphosphate ribose) synthetase inhibitors[17]. Pyrrolizidine alkaloids are also implicated in the induction of islet tumours[18].

In rabbits, treatment with adrenal steroids initially causes a transient hyperglycaemia. The blood sugar later returns to normal due to the formation of new β-cells probably by neotransformation of small ductules[9]. Glucocorticoid-induced islet hyperplasia is also reported in a subhuman primate. The proliferation is due to β-cell division[19]. No evidence of neotransformation is reported in this study and as increased mitotic activity occurs in the islets, it is likely that β-cells serve as their own progenitor. However, in our experience islet cells may arise both by ductal cell neotransformation and by islet cell mitosis: the mechanism responsible appears to be dependent upon the stimulus involved.

We have observed proliferative islet cell lesions, in rats, following treatment with anabolic steroids and neuroleptic drugs[20]. Androgen therapy is implicated in the development of islet cell hyperplasia in man, and is suggested to be due to abnormalities of glucose metabolism and insulin intolerance[21,22]. Hyperprolactinaemia causes islet cell hyperplasia in mice[15]. Prolactin is known to stimulate insulin secretion and β-cells show prolactin-like immunoreactivity[23]. These findings may offer an explanation for the association between islet cell hyperplasia in rats and neuroleptics known to cause hyperprolactinaemia.

Hyperplasia of somatostatin containing δ-cells is reported in streptozotocin-diabetic rats and guinea pigs[24]. An associated decrease in the number of insulin-containing cells is also reported. We have observed, in both rat and cynomolgus monkey, induced hyperplasia of somatostatin secreting δ-cells, The proliferation of these cells is presumably a response to altered levels of GH.

Variable numbers of large eosinophilic cells, usually located around islets of Langerhans, have been detected in rats from studies with two novel herbicides in our laboratories. On preliminary examination they resembled the hepatocyte-like cells induced in regenerating pancreas of rats and hamsters (see exocrine pancreas for details). However, they were negative for peroxidase and glycogen stains. Ultrastructurally, the cytoplasm was filled with densely packed large mitochondria but few other organelles. The cells bore no ultrastructural resemblance to hepatocytes, islet cells, acinar cells or duct cells; transitional forms were not detected. The ultrastructural characteristics fulfilled the criteria of oncocytes[25]. This cell type is found in several normal glandular organs and epithelial linings including pancreas and salivary glands[25]. They are believed to arise by transformation of normal, mature epithelial cells. Oncocytic pancreatic nodules are reported in man in cases of insulinoma and islet cell hyperplasia[26] and in some tissues oncocytomas are described[25]. No other reports of oncocytic induction are traced in toxicity studies and the toxicological significance is uncertain in view of the sparse physiological data.

Thyroid

In toxicity studies the thyroid is one of the most frequently affected of the endocrine organs, as it is a target for many pharmaceutical, industrial and environmental agents[1]. Despite this frequency of toxic action thyroid tissue shows a remarkably limited range of induced histological change (Table 7.3).

Table 7.3 Induced lesions of the thyroid

Follicular hypertrophy/hyperplasia
Follicular atrophy
Follicular pigmentation
Chronic thyroiditis
Parafollicular hyperplasia

The most commonly encountered change is the follicular hypertrophy and hyperplasia induced by goitrogenic compounds. This change may be mediated by increased TSH release from the anterior pituitary in the absence of negative feedback by decreased levels of T_3 and T_4. The constant, prolonged TSH stimulation causes hypertrophy and hyperplasia of the follicular cells. Goitrogens include aminotriazole, ethylenethiourea, sulphamethazine, spironolactone and its analogue potassium prorenoate, pyridoxine deficiency, propylthiouracil and polychlorinated biphenyls[2-5]. The rat appears particularly susceptible to these compounds; lesions have not been detected in several cases in monkeys and dogs[5,6]. However, in our experience dogs readily develop this lesion following treatment with sulphonamides.

Induction of a goitrogenic effect by antithyroid drugs may be effected by interference with any stage of thyroid hormone formation[5]: transport of iodine into the thyroid; generation of an oxidizing agent; synthesis of thyroglobulin; oxidation of iodine; binding of iodine to the tyrosine in thyroglobulin; formation of iodothyronines in thyroglobulin; deiodination of iodotyrosine; and release of thyroxine and triiodothyronine into the blood.

Histologically, the stimulated glands are composed of diffuse small follicles with hypertrophic epithelium and sparse or no colloid (Figures 7.31 and 7.32). The nuclei are located basally in the vacuolated columnar follicular cells. Increased vascularity may also be a feature. In more severe forms, focally short papillary projections of follicular epithelium are found in the lumina (Figures 7.33 and 7.34). Ultrastructurally, the rough endoplasmic reticulum becomes dilated and surface microvilli become blunted or fuse. In more chronic studies, many goitrogens induce follicular cysts or follicular cystic hyperplasia in addition to the generalized change described above[1].

In cases of severe thyroid hyperplasia and during follicular involution lamellated mineral deposits may be detected in the follicular lumen (Figure 7.32). These deposits resemble corpora amylacea and stain positively with Alizarin Red.

Regression of induced proliferative follicular lesions may occur upon cessation of administration. In rats treated with methimazole, a known antithyroid compound, complete remodelling takes place[7]. In involution of hyperplastic follicles by high doses of iodine, the prominent features are necrosis and inflammation[8]. However, when involution is induced by iodine with T_3 or with T_3 alone, apoptosis is the major mechanism of cell deletion. It may be concluded that excess iodine is directly toxic to iodine-deficient follicular cells. During involution, membrane-bound fragments of epithelial cells are found in the lumen[9]. The authors suggest this may be a mechanism of disposal of excess plasma membrane during the rapid secretion of thyroglobulin into the follicle lumen[9].

A possible relationship between thyroid hyperplasia and liver enzyme induction has been suggested[2]. Enzyme inducers stimulate the uptake of T_4 by the liver and increased levels of UDP-glucuronyltransferase (UDP-GTase) activity, which is involved in the glucuronic acid conjugation of T_4 prior to elimination in the bile, are detected with some goitrogens. Hypothyrodism is frequently associated with hypercholesterolaemia[10] and increased cholesterol biosynthesis is also known to be associated with enzyme inducers such as phenobarbital[11].

Follicular atrophy may be induced by administration of T_3 and T_4. In cynomolgus monkeys this change is characterized by areas of follicular collapse, loss of colloid with atrophy and basophilia of follicular cells (Figure 7.35). In the prolonged absence of TSH the follicular cells in rats become atrophic and flattened[1].

Pigmentation of the follicular epithelial cells is reported following at least five types of treatment: the antibiotic minocycline[12]; synthetic vincamines; vitamin E deficiency; the hair dye component 2,4-diaminoanisole sulphate (2,4-DAA)[13,14]; and UDP-GTase deficiency in the Gunn rat[15]. Considerable interest has been shown in the therapeutic potential of vincamine as a cerebral vasodilator and several derivatives have been synthesized[16]. Toxicity tests with some synthetic vincamines in dogs and rats in our laboratories have identified the thyroid as a target organ. The thyroids appear dark brown at necropsy and microscopically the follicular epithelial cells contain golden-brown pigment granules (Figure 7.36). With the electron microscope the granules correspond to irregular, electron-dense inclusions (Figure 7.37). Some of these compounds also induce (in chronic studies) focal follicular hyperplasia or cystic hyperplasia. The cells comprising these proliferative lesions do not, in our experience, contain pigment.

The tetracycline derivative minocycline causes thyroid pigmentation in laboratory animals and man[12,17]. In rats and dogs, but not in monkeys, follicular hyperplasia is also induced[17]. The pigment may represent forms of lipofuscin, melanin or a metabolic derivative of the compound itself. The pigment remains in the follicular cells of rats 1 year after cessation of treatment. With 2,4-diaminoanisole, brown pigment develops in the thyroids of rats[13,14]. A structurally related compound m-phenylenediamine, when fed simultaneously, prevents the pigmentation[14]. Increased formation of lipofuscin is induced in rats with the aniline analgesics, paracetamol and phenacetin[17]. In the Gunn rat the congenital UDP-GTase deficiency is associated with hyperthyroxinaemia and brownish-black discoloration of the follicular cells[15].

Chronic thyroiditis (Figure 7.38) is induced in mice,

rats and rhesus monkeys with trypan blue, 3-methyl-4-dimethylamino-azobenzene, methylcholanthrene[18,19] and with the immunosuppressive compound frentizole in Wistar rats[19]. With this latter compound the lesion only develops in studies when treatment is initiated during immaturity. The condition is not produced in dogs, rhesus monkeys or mice. The incidence and severity of the lesions are both decreased after a 6-month recovery period.

The parafollicular or 'C' cells arise from the neural crest and contain immunocytochemically demonstrable calcitonin. The cells accumulate calcitonin granules in hypocalcaemia and degranulate in hypercalcaemia[1]. Hyperplasia of parafollicular cells may be induced by increased dietary vitamin D[1]. The hyperplasia in rats may be either diffuse or nodular and the latter is difficult to distinguish from adenoma or even carcinoma.

Parathyroid

Lesions of the parathyroids are rarely induced in routine toxicity studies, those encountered are listed in Table 7.4.

Table 7.4 Induced lesions of the parathyroid

Hyperplasia
Atrophy/degeneration
Parathyroiditis

In chronic studies with treatment-induced severe nephropathies secondary hyperparathyroidism develops associated with hyperplasia of the parathyroid glands (Figure 7.39).

Induced atrophic or degenerative changes of the parathyroid glands are extremely rare[1]. An apparently species specific animal model of hypoparathyroidism is described using intravascular L-asparaginase, in rabbits. By light microscopy, eosinophilic, ovoid cytoplasmic bodies are detected in chief cells. Ultrastructurally, these cells are degranulated, contain lipid droplets and, most significantly, bodies described as autophagic vacuoles[1]. However, the ultrastructural appearance of these bodies suggests possible cell deletion by apoptosis.

Parathyroiditis is induced in dogs and rabbits exposed to ozone[2]. The lesion is characterized by lymphocytic infiltration, lymphoid cell–endothelial interaction and endothelial replication. In addition, microvascular changes including vasculitis, microdestruction of the capillary bed, intravascular platelet aggregation, haemorrhage and fibrin deposition also develop[2]. These changes are likely to represent an immunologically mediated response.

Pituitary

The development of immunocytochemical techniques and particularly immunoperoxidase methods has proved useful in many tissues but in none more so than the pituitary. Previous classification of pituitary cells depended on their tinctorial properties which allowed subdivision into acidophils, basophils and chromophobes. It is now possible to demonstrate intracellular hormones thus allowing confident indentification of different cell types and their histological and functional changes to be monitored.

A quantitative study[1] using immunocytochemical techniques in rats has demonstrated that approximately 51% show PRL reactivity, 21% GH, 5% LH, 4% FSH and 2% TSH. In addition 16% illustrated no reactivity. No major

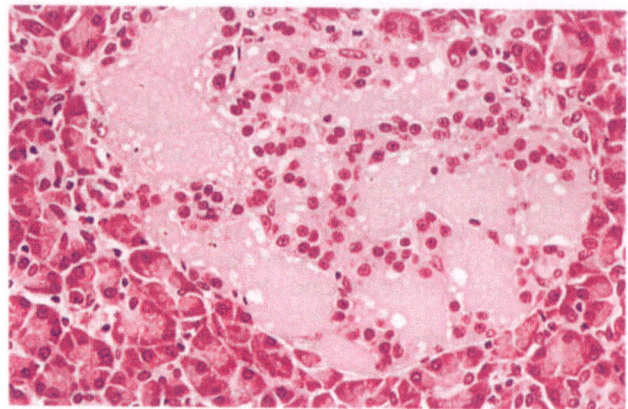

Figure 7.25 Angiectasis of an islet in a cynomolgus monkey treated with a novel immunomodulator. The lesion was preceded by islet cell necrosis (see Figure 7.26). H & E

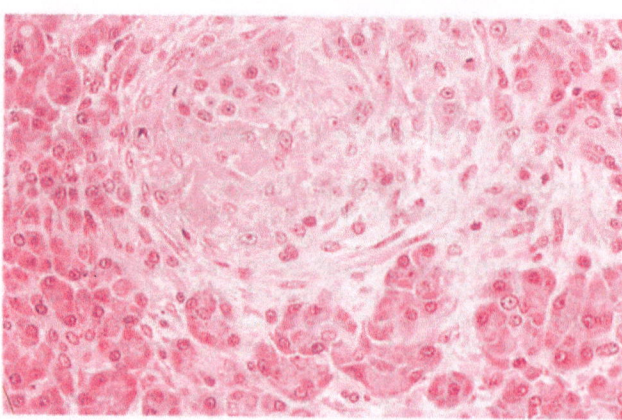

Figure 7.26 Necrosis of islet cells with a few peripheral fibroblasts. This lesion subsequently progressed to a form of angiectasis (shown in Figure 7.25). H & E

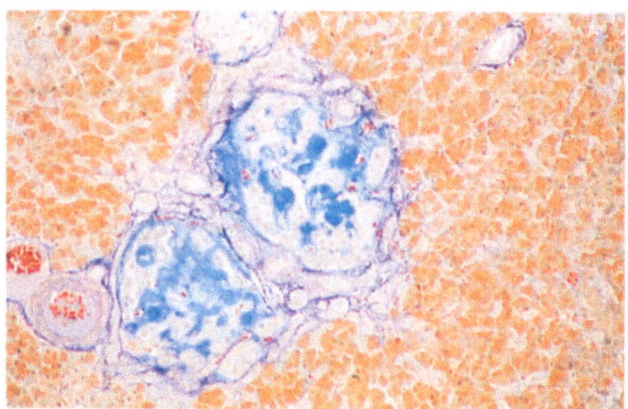

Figure 7.27 Hyalinized islet from a monkey following administration of a novel pharmaceutical. Much of the islet tissue has been replaced by hyalinized connective tissue. The lesion was associated with diabetes mellitus. Heidenhain's Azan

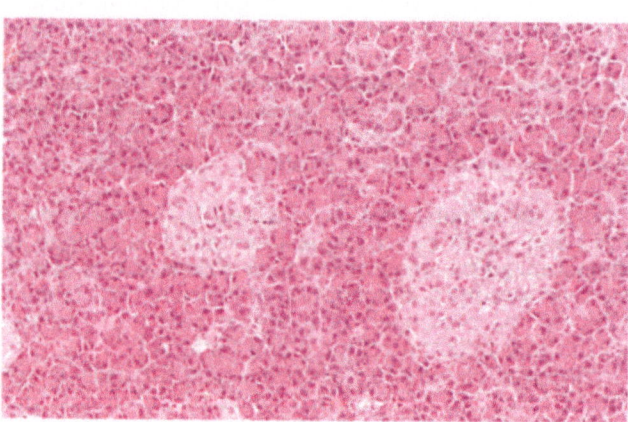

Figure 7.28 Islet cell hypertrophy in a cynomolgus monkey treated with high doses of a novel corticosteroid. 'Haloes' are present in the perinuclear region of most cells which probably represent hypertrophic Golgi bodies. The appearance is consistent with hypersecretion. H & E

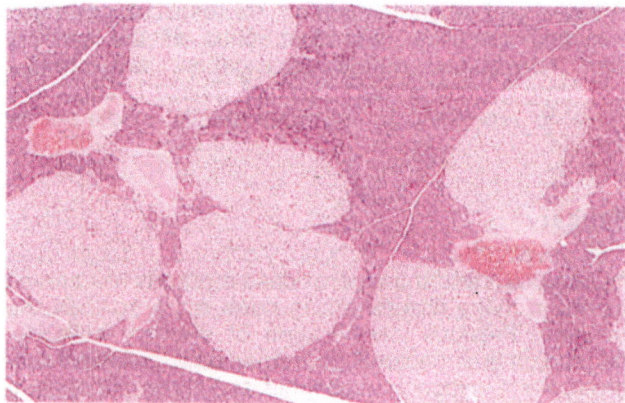

Figure 7.29 Generalized hyperplasia of islets in a young mouse treated with an industrial chemical. All islets are considerably enlarged, but have retained the normal cellular organization. H & E

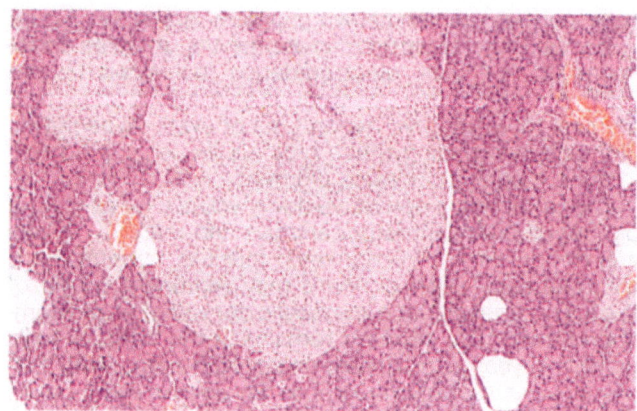

Figure 7.30 Hyperplastic islet in a rat treated with a novel neuroleptic. The islet is grossly enlarged in comparison with the adjacent normal islet. H & E

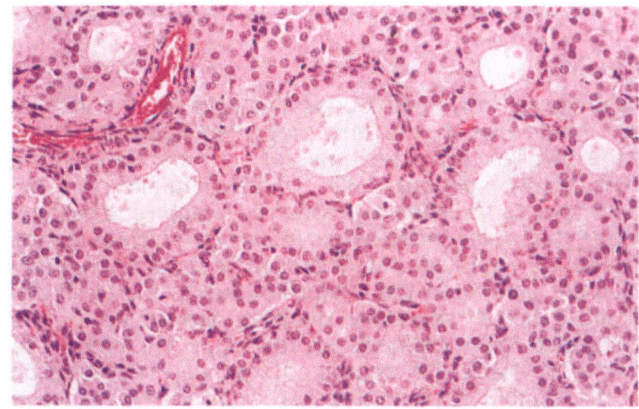

Figure 7.31 Thyroid follicular hyperplasia and hypertrophy in a rat. The follicles are devoid of colloid and the cells hypertrophic, often with a rarefied appearance. H & E

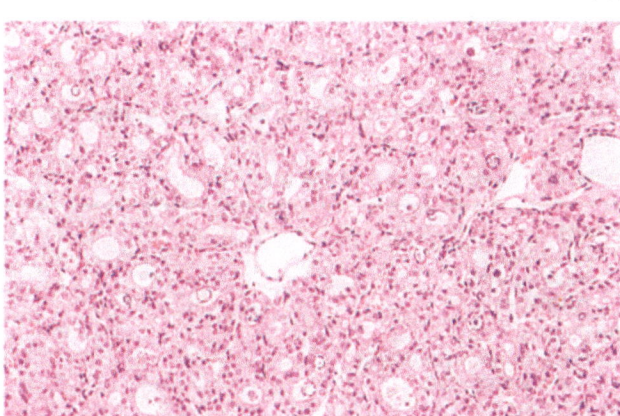

Figure 7.32 Marked follicular hyperplasia and hypertrophy in the thyroid of a rat treated with a sulphonamide. The follicles are small, composed of cuboidal cells and devoid of colloid. Within the lumina small dense lamellated mineral deposits are present. H & E

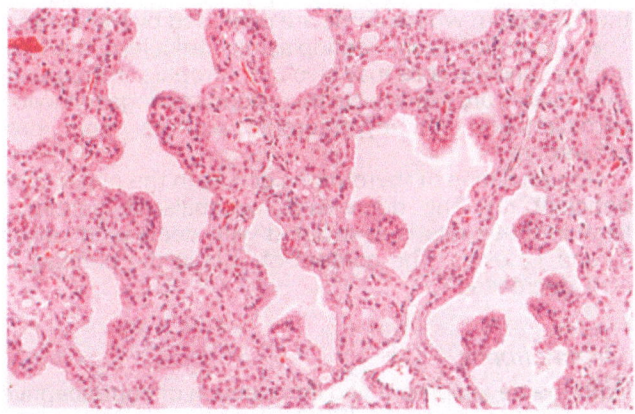

Figure 7.33 Thyroid follicular hyperplasia in a dog treated with a sulphonamide. Short papillary projections are present in the lumina of enlarged follicles. H & E

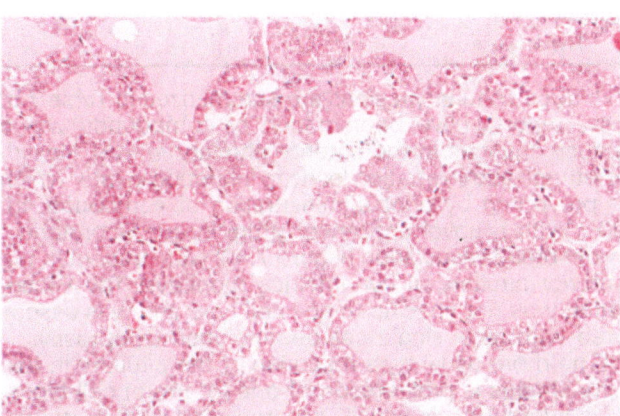

Figure 7.34 Rhesus monkey thyroid showing follicular hyperplasia following administration of a novel immunostimulant. Follicles are slightly irregular and composed of cuboidal cells. In one follicle short papillary projections composed of slightly atypical cells are seen. H & E

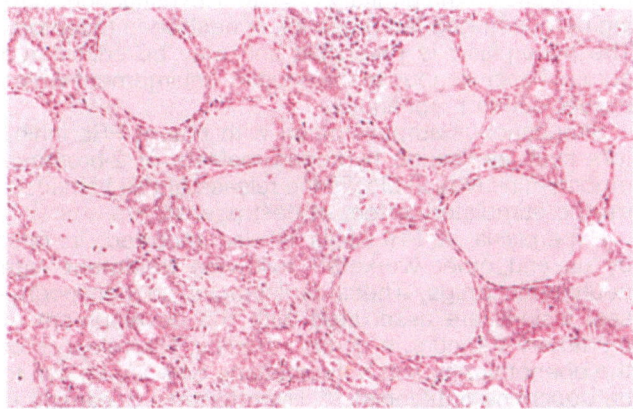

Figure 7.35 Follicular atrophy in the thyroid of a cynomolgus monkey treated with thyroid hormones. The atrophic follicles are collapsed, appear basophilic and are devoid of colloid. H & E

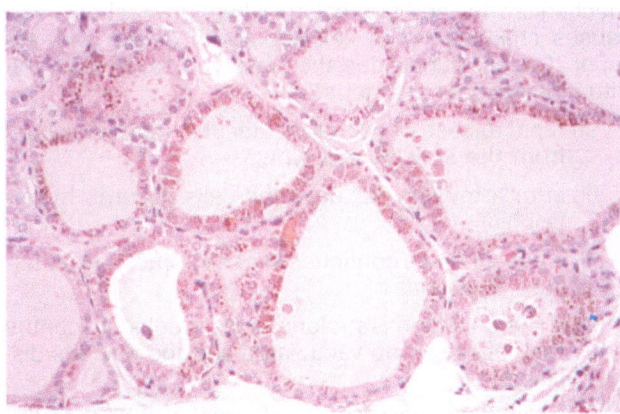

Figure 7.36 Brown pigment in follicular epithelial cells of a dog treated with a synthetic vincamine. No evidence of degeneration. H & E

differences were demonstrated between males and females.

Table 7.5　Induced lesions of the pituitary

General:
    Infarction
    Vacuolation
    Apoptosis
Thyrotrophs
    Hypertrophy/hyperplasia
    'Exhaustion' cells
    Atrophy
Mammotrophs
    Hypertrophy/hyperplasia
    Regression
Somatotrophs
    Hypertrophy/hyperplasia
Gonadotrophs
    'Castration' cells
Corticotrophs
    Hypertrophy
Melanotrophs
    Hyperplasia

Induced pituitary lesions are summarized in Table 7.5. Few reports have been traced of compounds which induce changes in the anterior pituitary *in toto*. Hexadimethrine administration leads to infarction in rats, which is prevented by prior administration of compound 48/80[2]. With a novel anticancer drug, in our laboratories, widespread vacuolation (Figure 7.40) was present in the anterior pituitary of cynomolgus monkeys. The vacuolation was not specific to any cell type and was associated with focal single cell degeneration (apoptosis).

The more usual type response of the pituitary in toxicity studies is proliferation of one (or more) cell types. This hyperplasia is usually accompanied by hypertrophy of the affected cell type.

The most frequently encountered lesions in the pituitary are those which involve changes in a single cell type responsible for the production of a particular hormone (Table 7.5). The changes usually reflect the kind of malfunction of the particular target endocrine gland that results from surgical or chemical ablation. The corresponding reduction in circulating hormone from the endocrine gland removes the negative feedback mechanism to the hypothalamic–hypophyseal axis and causes changes in the cell population of the pars anterior. Capen[3] subdivides the observed reaction in the pituitary into four distinct stages:

    (i) rapid release of secretory granules (degranulation) from the specific cell type;

    (ii) after a few/several days the cells become hypertrophic;

    (iii) if the condition continues the cell population undergoes hyperplasia;

    (iv) if the condition is prolonged for weeks or months the cells become vacuolated and the nucleus displaced.

In view of the consistent, cell specific nature of the pituitary reactions the following review will deal with the individual hormone-producing cell types separately.

Thyrotrophs

Hypertrophy and hyperplasia of the thyrotrophs (Figure 7.41) may be induced by thyroidectomy, radiation or an iodine deficient diet and by antithyroid compounds such as amitrole, ethylenethiourea, thiouracil, methylthiouracil, 2,4-diaminoanisole and propylthiouracil[4–7]. Initially, large swollen 'thyroidectomy' cells are detected in the pars anterior (Figure 7.42). Ultrastructurally, this hypertrophy can be seen to be due to dilatation and ballooning of the rough endoplasmic reticulum which becomes distended with flocculate material. Few secretory granules are present in the cytoplasm due to the rapid discharge. Some secretory granules are found in the distended rough endoplasmic reticulum. The amount of secretory material increases and causes the distension of the rough endoplasmic reticulum. In addition to these hypertrophic changes hyperplasia of thyrotrophs may also occur. This diffuse hyperplasia is reversible[8]. In some cases of severe stimulation 'exhaustion' cells may develop. These appear as grossly vacuolated cells with small shrunken dense nuclei (Figure 7.43). We have observed these cells in dogs treated with sulphonomides.

Administration of thyroxine to hypothyroid animals causes the cells to 'package' some of the 'backed-up' secretory material and secretory granules accumulate in the cytoplasm where some are degraded by lysosomes. The distended rough endoplasmic reticulum then regresses and the cells may involute. Atrophic and regressive changes are reported in thyrotrophs of dogs following administration of cyproterone acetate and progesterone[9].

Degranulation of thyrotrophs occurs in the pyridoxine-deficient rat. The decreased hypothalamic serotonin level in these rats is associated with decreased serum T_3 and T_4 levels. The content of TSH in the pituitary is also decreased[10].

Mammotrophs

With the development and introduction of contraceptive steroids the prolactin (PRL)-secreting mammotrophs have become the subject of many investigations. The administration of oestrogen, synthetic oestrogens such as diethylstilboestrol, and oestrogen-progestogen combinations all cause diffuse hyperplasia (Figures 7.44 and 7.45) of PRL-producing cells[9,11,12]. The PRL hyperplasia and hypertrophy is observed in rats, mice, beagle dogs and non-human primates. It has been suggested that the mechanism for this action could be direct action of oestrogens on the pituitary[11], several investigations having demonstrated the presence of oestrogen receptors. The hyperplasia is reversible and may be considered somewhat analogous to the pituitary enlargement which occurs during pregnancy.

Simultaneous administration with potent PRL inhibitors such as lisuride hydrogen maleate or 2-bromo-α-ergocryptine (which blocks the release of PRL) antagonize the stimulatory effect of oestrogens[9].

Hyperplasia of PRL cells is also reported, in rats, by us and other workers[13] following treatment with neuroleptic drugs. These proliferative adenohypophyseal lesions are associated with the development of mammary tumours in chronic studies. Neuroleptics of the phenothiazine and butyrphenone type are known to be dopamine antagonists[14]. Hypothalamic dopamine is an important inhibitor of PRL release from the pituitary. An increase in dopamine is known to cause reduction of serum PRL levels[15].

In the oestradiol-primed rat a form of autophagy termed 'crinophagy' occurs in mammotrophs 2 minutes after administration of somatostatin[16]. Crinophagy is characterized by rearrangement of the rough endoplasmic reticulum into concentric cisternae with associated intracellular bodies which contain sequestered PRL secretion granules. This sequestration may prevent the release of secretion granules. Somatostatin also inhibits PRL release in men primed with oestrogen and cyproterone acetate[17].

We have observed hyperplasia of PRL cells in dogs treated with an analogue of a pituitary peptide hormone. After a four week withdrawal (recovery) period, pyknosis and karyorrhexis of a proportion of these cells was a prominent feature (Figures 7.46 and 7.47). This cell deletion is presumably due to the cessation of a stimulatory and reflected the return to normal PRL cell numbers. A similar regression of redundant pituitary cells is described in lactotrophs after cessation of lactation[18].

Somatotrophs

The secretion of growth hormone (GH) is controlled by a mechanism different from that of TSH, LH/FSH and ACTH. GH does not act on a target endocrine organ to stimulate secretion of an effector hormone. Thus there is no direct negative feedback by circulating hormone, instead this is achieved by production of a corresponding release-inhibiting neuropeptide (somatostatin) by hypothalamic neurons. Using antisynthetic somatostatin, prominent numbers of immunoreactive neurons have been detected in the anterior hypothalmus of the beagle[9]. The discovery of somatostatin has enabled the development of analogues, which act as receptor agonists, for the treatment of conditions such as acromegaly. These compounds decrease the levels of circulating growth hormone.

Due to the absence of a target organ for GH, changes in somatotrophs are less frequently seen than in other types of pituitary cell. Similarly GH secretion is less readily manipulated than is that of some other pituitary hormones[7]. However, a few days after thyroidectomy or adrenalectomy somatotrophs contain increased numbers of lysosomes which often contain recognizable secretory granules.

Diffuse hyperplasia and hypertrophy of growth hormone (GH) producing cells is described in beagle dogs treated with either oestrogens or progestogens or combinations of both [9,12]. Cyproterone acetate, a synthetic progesterone derivative stimulates GH-cells of ovariectomized beagles[12].

Following castration or compound-induced gonadal atrophy, the number of basophils increases and they become vacuolated and in some instances assume a typical signet-ring appearance characteristic of 'castration cells' (Figure 7.48). This hyperstimulatory condition is due to decreased levels of sex hormones with the corresponding lack of negative feedback on the hypothalamus.

Corticotrophs

Changes are rarely encountered in corticotrophs in routine toxicity studies. The cells demonstrate predictable degranulation with subsequent hypertrophy following adrenalectomy, due to lack of negative feedback.

Melanotrophs

There are few reported toxicological changes in the melanocyte stimulating hormone (MSH) secreting cells of the pituitary. However, in hamsters in contrast to most other species, oestrogens induce hyperplasia of this cell type in the pars intermedia[12,19].

References

Adrenals

1. Ribelin, W. E. (1984). The effects of drugs and chemicals upon the structure of the adrenal gland. *Fundam. Appl. Toxicol.*, **4**, 105–119
2. Colby, H. D. and Eacho, P. I. (1985). Chemical induced adrenal injury: role of metabolic activation. In Thomas, J. A., Korach, K. S. and McLachlan, J. A. (eds.) *Endocrine Toxicology*. pp. 35–66. (New York: Raven)
3. Yarrington, J. T. (1983). Chemically induced adrenocortical lesions. In Jones, T. C., Mohr, U. and Hunt, R. D. (eds.) *Endocrine System. Monographs on Pathology of Laboratory Animals*. pp. 69–75. (Berlin and Heidelberg: Springer-Verlag)
4. Deane, H. W., Shaw, J. H. and Greep, R. O. (1948). The effect of altered sodium or potassium intake on the width and cytochemistry of the zona glomerulosa of the rats adrenal cortex. *Endocrinology*, **43**, 133–153
5. Goldman, M. I., Ronzoni, E. and Schroeder, H. A. (1956). The response of the adrenal cortex of the rat to dietary salt restriction and replacement. *Endocrinology*, **58**, 57–61
6. Davis, D. A. and Medline, N. M. (1970). Spironolactone (Aldactone) bodies: concentric lamellar formations in the adrenal cortices of patients treated with Spironolactone. *Am. J. Clin. Pathol.*, **54**, 22–32
7. Abbott, E. C., Monkhouse, F. C., Steiner, J. W. and Laidlaw, J. C. (1966). Effect of a sulphated mucopolysaccharide (R01-8307) on the zona glomerulosa of the rat adrenal gland. *Endocrinology*, **78**, 651–654
8. Mazzocchi, G. and Nussdorfer, G. G. (1984). Long-term effects of captopril on the morphology of normal rat adrenal zona glomerulosa. *Exp. Clin. Endocrinol.*, **84**, 148–152
9. Robba, C., Mazzocchi, G. and Nussdorfer, G. G. (1986). Further studies on the inhibitory effects of somatostatin on the growth and steroidogenic capacity of rat adrenal zona glomerulosa. *Exp. Pathol.*, **29**, 77–82
10. Rebuffat, P., Robba, C., Mazzocchi, G. and Nussdorfer, G. G. (1984). Inhibitory effect of somatostatin on the growth and steroidogenic capacity of rat adrenal zona glomerulosa. *J. Steroid. Biochem.*, **21**, 387–390
11. Kovács, K., Carroll, R. and Tapp, E.(1966). The pathogenesis of hexadimethrine necrosis of the pituitary and adrenal. *Arzneim.-Forsch.*, **16**, 516–519
12. Pudney, J., Price, G. M., Whitehouse, B. J. and Vinson, G. P. (1984). Effects of chronic ACTH stimulation on the morphology of the rat adrenal cortex. *Anat. Rec.*, **210**, 603–615
13. Rhodin, J. A. G. (1971). The ultrastructure of the adrenal cortex of the rat under normal and experimental conditions. *J. Ultrastruct. Res.*, **34**, 23–71
14. Wernert, N., Antalffy, A. and Dhom, G. (1986). Effects of estradiol on adrenal cortex and medulla of the rat. *Pathol. Res. Pract.*, **181**, 551–557
15. Wyllie, A. H., Kerr, J. F. R., Macaskill, I. A. M. and Currie, A. R. (1973). Adrenocortical cell deletion: the role of ACTH. *J. Pathol.*, **111**, 85–94
16. Nussdorfer, G. G. (1970). Effects of corticosteroid hormones on the smooth endoplasmic reticulum of rat adrenocortical cells. *Z. Zellforsch.*, **106**, 143–154
17. El Etreby, M. F., Gräf, K. J., Günzel, P. and Neumann, F. (1979). Evaluation of effects of sexual steroids on the hypothalmic pituitary system of animals and man. *Arch. Toxicol.*, Suppl. 2, 11–39
18. Nelson, L. W. and Kelly, W. A. (1976). Progestogen-related gross and microscopic changes in female beagles. *Vet. Pathol.*, **13**, 143–156
19. Szabo, S., McComb, D. J., Kovács, K. and Hüttner, I. (1981). Adrenocortical hemorrhagic necrosis. *Arch. Pathol. Lab. Med.*, **105**, 536–539
20. Szabo, S., Hüttner, I., Kovács, K., Horvath, E., Szabo, D. and Horner, H. C. (1980). Pathogenesis of experimental adrenal hemorrhagic necrosis ('apoplexy'). *Lab. Invest.*, **42**, 533–546
21. Yarrington, J. T., Loudy, D. E., Sprinkle, D. J., Gibson, J. P., Wright, C. L. and Johnston, J. O. (1985). Degeneration of the rat and canine adrenal cortex caused by α-(1,4-dioxido-3-methylquinoxalin-2-yl)-N-methylnitrone (DMNM). *Fundam. Appl. Toxicol.*, **5**, 370–381
22. Yarrington, J. T., Huffmann, K. W. and Gibson, J. P. (1981). Adrenocortical degeneration in dogs, monkeys and rats treated with α-(1,4-dioxido-3-methylquinoxalin-2-yl)-N-methylnitrone. *Toxicol. Lett.*, **8**, 229–234
23. Hart, M. M., Reagan, R. L. and Adamson, R. H. (1973). The effect of isomers of DDD on the ACTH-induced steroid output,

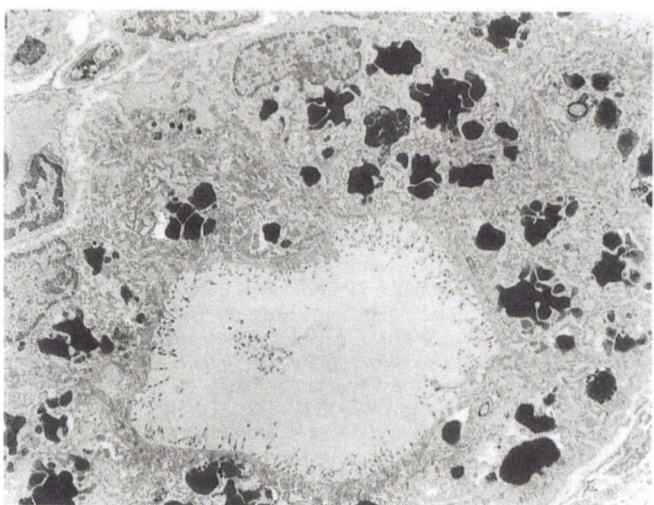

Figure 7.37 Electron-dense inclusions in the follicular epithelial cells of a vincamine-treated dog. These inclusions correspond to the brown granules shown by light microscopy in Figure 7.36. Electron micrograph

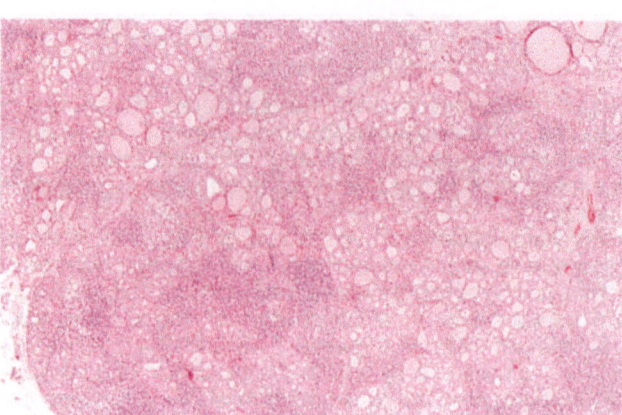

Figure 7.38 Chronic lymphocytic thyroiditis in a rat induced by an industrial chemical. Large areas of the thyroid have been replaced by lymphoid cells. Remaining follicles are small.   H & E

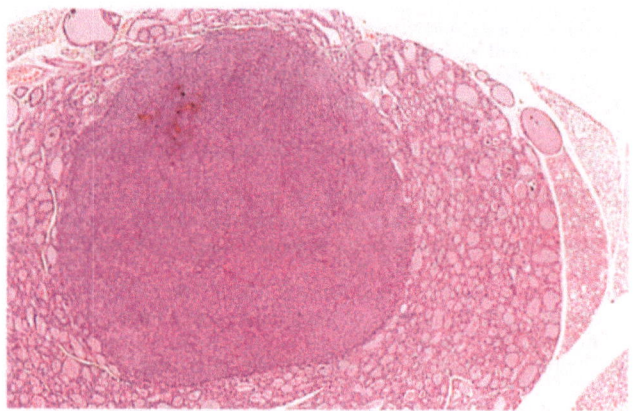

Figure 7.39 Parathyroid hyperplasia secondary to an induced nephropathy in a rat. H & E

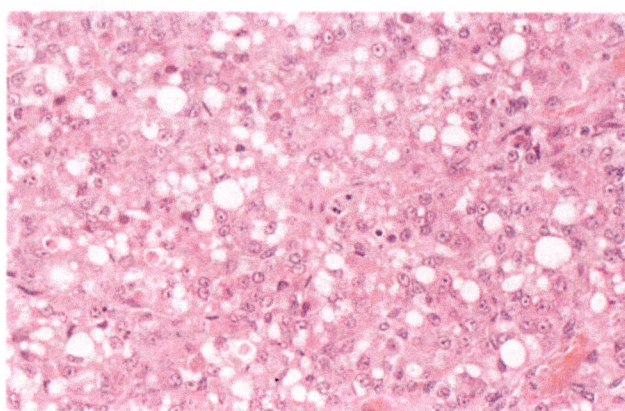

Figure 7.40 Vacuolation of cells in the anterior pituitary of a cynomolgus monkey following administration of a novel anticancer drug. Focal evidence of apoptosis. The lesions showed no evidence of predilection for any single cell type.   H & E

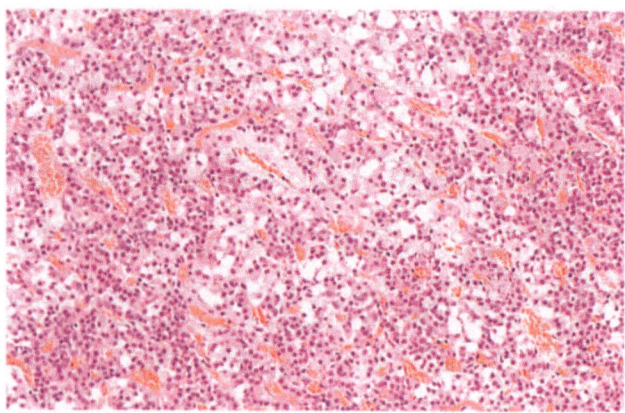

Figure 7.41 Hyperplasia and hypertrophy of thyrotrophs in the anterior pituitary of a rat treated with a sulphonamide. The cells contain large vacuoles. H & E

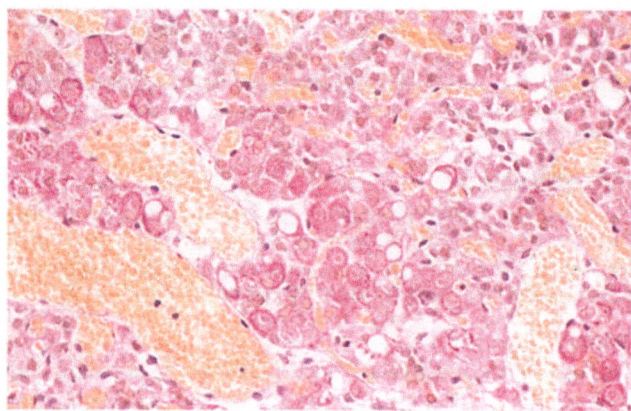

Figure 7.42 Hypertrophic vacuolated thyrotrophs, typical of 'thyroidectomy' cells, from a rat treated with a sulphonamide. PAS–Orange G

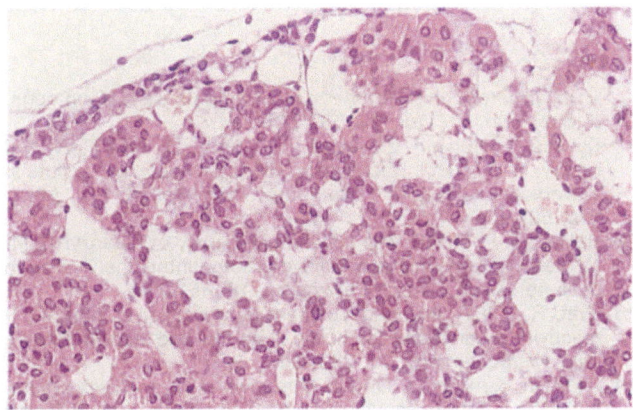

Figure 7.43 In this example, from a dog treated with high doses of a sulphonamide, some thyrotrophs have become grossly vacuolated with little remaining cytoplasm. Nuclei appear small and condensed. These features are characteristic of exhaustion due to intense sustained hypersecretion. H & E

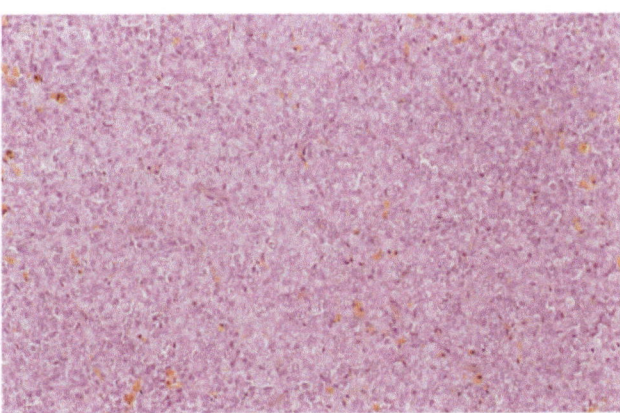

Figure 7.44 Diffuse hyperplasia and hypertrophy of mammotrophs in the anterior pituitary of a rat treated with a novel contraceptive steroid. Note homogeneity of cell type. H & E

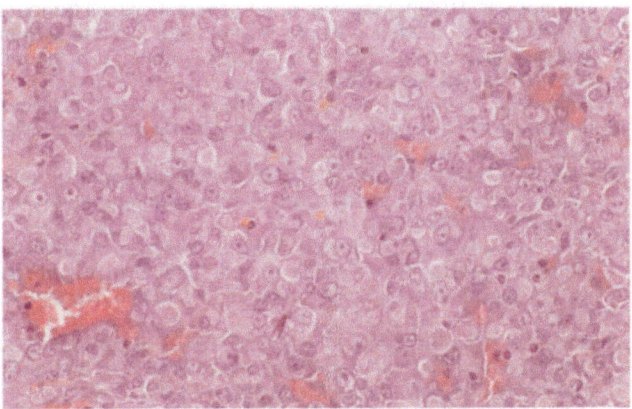

Figure 7.45 Higher power of hyperplastic mammotrophs induced in rat pituitary by a contraceptive steroid. The cells are hypertrophic with characteristic 'haloes' indicative of hypersecretion. H & E

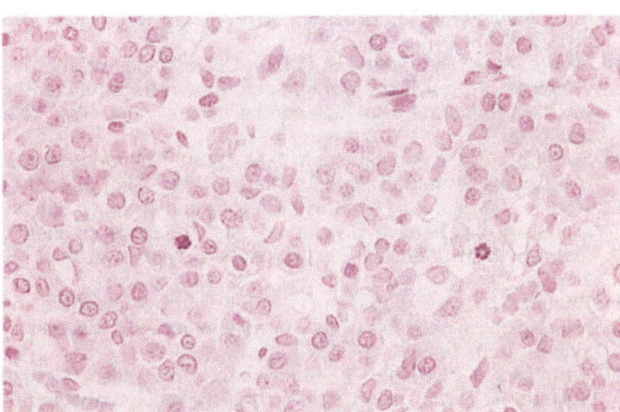

Figure 7.46 Nuclear pyknosis and karyorrhexis of mammotrophs in the anterior pituitary of a dog previously treated with an analogue of a pituitary peptide hormone and then allowed a recovery period. Initially, mammotroph hyperplasia was detected which regressed during the recovery period. H & E

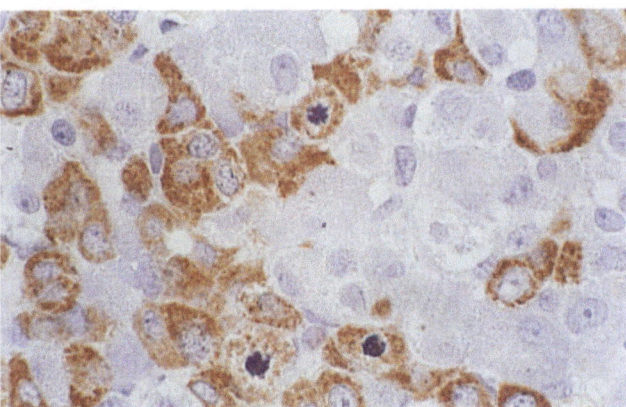

Figure 7.47 From the same study as Figure 7.46. Demonstration of anti-prolactin immunoreactivity shows regressive nuclear changes present in mammotrophs.

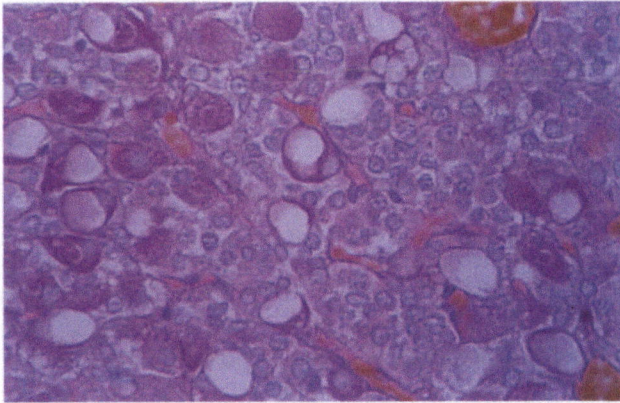

Figure 7.48 'Castration' cells in the anterior pituitary of a rat with induced testicular atrophy. The gonadotrophs demonstrate the typical 'signet ring' appearance associated with the hypersecretory condition. PAS–Orange G

histology and ultrastructure of the dog adrenal cortex. *Toxicol. Appl. Pharmacol.*, **24**, 101–113

24. Dhom, G., Hohbach, Ch., Mäusle, E., Scherr, O. and Ueberberg, H. (1981). Peliosis of the female adrenal cortex of the aging rat. *Virchows Arch. B: Zellpathol.*, **36**, 195–206

25. Daft, F. S., Sebrell, W. H., Babcock, S. H. and Jukes, T. H. (1940). Effect of synthetic pantothenic acid on adrenal hemorrhage, atrophy and necrosis in rats. *Public Health Rep.*, **55**, 1333–1346

26. Zak, F. (1983). Lipid hyperplasia, adrenal cortex, rat. In Jones, T. C., Mohr, U. and Hunt, R. D. (eds.) *Endocrine System. Monographs on Pathology of Laboratory Animals.* pp. 80–84. (Berlin, Heidelberg: Springer-Verlag)

27. Lüllmann-Rauch, R. and Reil, G-H. (1974). Chlorphentermine-induced lipidosis-like ultrastructural alterations in lungs and adrenal glands of several species. *Toxicol. Appl. Pharmacol.*, **30**, 408–421

28. Bockhardt, H. and Lüllmann-Rauch, R. (1980). Zimelidine-induced lipidosis in rats. *Acta Pharmacol. Toxicol.*, **47**, 45–48

29. Motlík, K., Krawczynski, K. and Nowoslawski, A. (1968). Experimental hyaline droplets in the rat adrenal cortex. *Virchows Arch. A: Pathol. Anat.*, **344**, 331–345

30. Greenman, D. L., Highman, B. and Kodell, R. L. (1984). Neoplastic and nonneoplastic responses to chronic feeding of diethylstilbestrol in CBH mice. *J. Toxicol. Environ. Health*, **14**, 551–567

31. Moore, N. A. and Callas, G. (1975). Observations on the fine structure of propylthiouracil induced 'brown degeneration' in the zona reticularis of mouse adrenal cortex. *Anat. Rec.*, **183**, 293–302

32. Surleff, S. V. and Papadimitrion, J. M. (1981). The mononuclear phagocytes of the rat adrenal. *Am. J. Pathol.*, **104**, 258–271

33. Roe, F. J. C. and Bär, A. (1985). Enzootic and epizootic adrenal medullary proliferative disease of rats: influence of dietary factors which affect calcium absorption. *Human Toxicol.*, **4**, 27–52

34. Boelsterli, U. A. and Zbinden, G. (1985). Early biochemical and morphological changes of the rat adrenal medulla induced by xylitol. *Arch. Toxicol.*, **57**, 25–30

35. Kurokawa, Y., Hayashi, Y., Maekawa, A., Takahashi, M. and Kukubo, T. (1985). High incidence of phaeochromocytomas after long term administration of retinol acetate to F344/DuCrj rats. *J. Natl. Cancer Inst.*, **74**, 715–723

36. McConnell, E. E. and Tally, F. A. (1977). Intracytoplasmic hyaline globules in the adrenal medulla of laboratory animals. *Vet. Pathol.*, **14**, 435–440

Islets of Langerhans

1. Fischer, L. J. and Rickert, D. E. (1975). Pancreatic islet-cell toxicity. *CRC. Crit. Rev. Toxicol.*, **4**, 231–262

2. Rerup, C. C. (1970). Drugs producing diabetes through damage of the insulin secreting cells. *Pharmacol. Rev.*, **22**, 484–518

3. Mukai, K. and Rosai, J. (1980). Applications of immunoperoxidase techniques in surgical pathology. In Fenoglio, C. M. and Wolff, M. (eds.) *Progress in Surgical Pathology.* Vol. I, pp. 15–49. (New York: Masson Publ. Inc.)

4. Greaves, P. and Faccini, J. M. (1984). Endocrine glands. In *Rat Histopathology.* pp. 187–210. (Amsterdam: Elsevier)

5. Orci, L. (1984). Patterns of cellular and subcellular organisation in the endocrine pancreas. *J. Endocrinol.*, **102**, 3–11

6. Biollot, D., in't Veld, P., Sai, P., Feutren, G., Gepts, W. and Assan, R. (1985). Functional and morphological modifications induced in rat islets by pentamidine and other diamides *in vitro*. *Diabetologia*, **28**, 359–364

7. Nelson, L. W. and Kelly, W. A. (1976). Progestogen-related gross and microscopic changes in female beagles. *Vet. Pathol.*, **13**, 143–156

8. Tucker, M. J. (1971). Some effects of prolonged administration of a progestogen to dogs. *Proc. Eur. Soc. Study Drug Toxic.*, **12**, 228–238

9. McClure, M. M., Chapman, W. L., Hooper, B. E., Smith, F. G. and Fletcher, O. J. (1978). The digestive system. In Benirschke, K., Garner, F. M. and Jones, T. C. (eds.) *Pathology of Laboratory Animals.* Vol. I, pp. 175–318. (New York: Springer-Verlag)

10. Campbell, J., Pierluissi, J. and Kovács, K. (1981). Pancreatic islet ultrastructure, serum and pancreatic immunoreactive insu-

lin in somatotrophic and metasomatotrophic diabetes in dogs. *J. Submicrosc. Cytol.*, **13**, 599–608

11. Kovács, K., Horvath, E., Asa, S. L., Murray, D., Singer, W. and Reddy, S. S. (1986). Microscopic peliosis of pancreatic islets in a woman with MEN–1 Syndrome. *Arch. Pathol. Lab. Med.*, **110**, 607–610

12. Beliles, R. P. (1971). The subchronic toxicity of 5-benzyl-11-[4-(*N*-methyl-piperidylene)]-5,6-dihydromorphanthridine hydrogen maleate. *Toxicol. Appl. Pharmacol.*, **18**, 451–456

13. Gräf, R. (1981). Immunocytochemical detection of anti-ACTH reactivity in pancreatic islet cells of normal and steroid diabetic rats. *Histochemistry*, **73**, 233–238

14. Rozman, K., Pereira, D. and Iatropoulos, M. J. (1986). Histopathology of interscapular brown adipose tissue, thyroid and pancreas in 2,3,7,8-tetrachlorodibenzo-*p*-dioxin (TCDD)-treated rats. *Toxicol. Appl. Pharmacol.*, **82**, 551–559

15. Mori, T., Nagasawa, H., Namiki, H. and Niki, K. (1986). Development of pancreatic hyperplasia in female SHN mice receiving ectopic pituitary isografts. *J. Natl. Cancer Inst.*, **76**, 1193–1197

16. Rakieten, N., Gordon, B. S., Beaty, A., Cooney, D. A., Davis, R. D. and Schein, P. S. (1971). Pancreatic islet cell tumours produced by the combined action of streptozotocin and nicotinamide. *Proc. Soc. Exp. Biol. Med.*, **137**, 280–283

17. Yamagami, T., Miwa, A., Takasaw, S., Yamamoto, H. and Okamoto, H. (1985). Induction of rat pancreatic β-cell tumours by the combined administration of streptozotocin and alloxan and poly(adenosine diphosphate ribose) synthetase inhibitors. *Cancer Res.*, **45**, 1845–1849

18. Schoental, R., Fowler, M. E. and Coady, A. (1970). Islet cell tumors of the pancreas found in rats given pyrrolizidine alkaloids. *Cancer Res.*, **30**, 2127–2131

19. Like, A. A. and Chick, W. L. (1974). Pancreatic beta cell replication induced by glucocorticoids in subhuman primates. *Am. J. Pathol.*, **75**, 329–341

20. Roe, F. J. C. and Bär, A. (1985). Enzootic and epizootic adrenal medullary proliferative disease of rats: influence of dietary factors which affect calcium absorption. *Human Toxicol.*, **4**, 27–52

21. Novak, R., Wilimas, J. and Johnson, W. (1979). Hypertrophy and hyperplasia of islet of Langerhans associated with androgen therapy. *Arch. Pathol. Lab. Med.*, **103**, 483–485

22. Sale, G. E. and Lerner, K. G. (1977). Multiple tumours after androgen therapy. *Arch. Pathol. Lab. Med.*, **101**, 600–603

23. Meuris, S., Verloes, A. and Robyn, C. (1983). Immunocytochemical localisation of prolactin-like immunoreactivity in rat pancreatic islets. *Endocrinology*, **112**, 2221–2223

24. Orci, L., Beatens, D., Rufener, C., Amherdt, M., Ravazzola, M., Studer, P., Malaisse-Lague, F. and Unger, R. H. (1976). Hypertrophy and hyperplasia of somatostatin-containing D-cells in diabetes. *Proc. Natl. Acad. Sci. USA*, **73**, 1338–1342

25. Tandler, B., Hutter, R. V. P. and Erlandson, R. A. (1970). Ultrastructure of oncocytoma of the parotid gland. *Lab. Invest.*, **23**, 567–580

26. O'Leary, T. J., Costa, J. and Roth, J. (1982). Oncocytic nodules of the pancreas. *Lab. Invest.*, **46**, 63A

Thyroid

1. Stevens, J. T. (1985). Effect of chemicals on the thyroid gland. In Thomas, J. A., Korach, K. S. and McLachlan, J. A. (eds.) *Endocrine Toxicology.* pp. 135–147. (New York: Raven)

2. Lumb, G. D. and Rust, J. H. (1985). The pathologic response of the liver and thyroid of the rat to potassium prorenoate (SC–23992). *Toxicol. Pathol.*, **13**, 315–324

3. Heath, J. E. and Littlefield, N. A. (1984). Morphological effects of subchronic oral sulfamethazine administration on Fischer 344 rats and B6C3F₁ mice. *Toxicol. Pathol.*, **12**, 3–9

4. Collins, W. T., Capen, C. C., Kasza, L., Carter, C. and Dailey, R. E. (1977). Effect of polychlorinated biphenyl (PCB) on the thyroid gland of rats. *Am. J. Pathol.*, **89**, 119–130

5. Takayama, S., Aihara, K., Onodera, T. and Akimoto, T. (1986). Antithyroid effects on propylthiouracil and sulfamonomethoxine in rats and monkeys. *Toxicol. Appl. Pharmacol.*, **82**, 191–199

6. Lumb, G., Newberne, P., Rust, J. H. and Wagner, B. (1978). Effects in animals of chronic administration of spironolactone – a review. *J. Environ. Pathol. Toxicol.*, **1**, 641–660

7. Todd, G. C. (1986). Induction and reversibility of thyroid prolifer-

ative changes in rats given an antithyroid compound. *Vet. Pathol.*, **23**, 110–117

8. Mahmoud, I., Colin, I., Many, M-C., Denef, J-F. (1986). Direct toxic effect of iodine in excess on iodine-deficient thyroid glands: epithelial necrosis and inflammation associated with lipofuscin accumulation. *Exp. Mol. Pathol.*, **44**, 259–271

9. Tachiwaki, O. and Wollman, S. H. (1982). Shedding of dense cell fragments into the follicular lumen early in involution of the hyperplastic thyroid gland. *Lab. Invest.*, **47**, 91–98

10. Kallfelz, F. A. (1977). Thyroid function in the dog. *Vet. Clin. N. Am.*, **7**, 497–512.

11. Jones, A. L. and Armstrong, D. T. (1965). Increased cholesterol biosynthesis following phenobarbital induced hypertrophy of agranular endoplasmic reticulum in liver. *Proc. Soc. Exp. Biol. Med.*, **119**, 1136–1139

12. Tajima, K., Miyagawa, J-I., Nakajima, H., Shimizu, M., Katayama, S., Mashita, K. and Tarui, S. (1985). Morphological and biochemical studies on minocycline-induced black thyroid in rats. *Toxicol. Appl. Pharmacol.*, **81**, 393–400

13. Ward, J. M., Stinson, S. F., Hardisty, J. F., Cockrell, B. Y. and Hayden, D. W. (1979). Neoplasms and pigmentation of thyroid glands in F344 rats exposed to 2,4-diaminoanisole sulfate, a fair dye component. *J. Natl. Cancer Inst.*, **62**, 1067–1073

14. Evarts, R. P. and Brown, C. A. (1981). 2,4-diaminoanisole-induced thyroid pigmentation in rats inhibited by *m*-phenylene-diamine. *Toxicol. Lett.* **8**, 257–264

15. Benathon, M., Lemarchand-Béraud, Th., Gautier, A. and Gardiol, D. (1983). Abnormal iodoprotein distribution and resistance to proteolysis in Gunn rat black thyroid. *Virchows Arch. B: Zellpathol.*, **44**, 323–336

16. Vereczkey, L. (1985). Pharmacokinetics and metabolism of vincamine and related compounds. *Eur. J. Drug Metab. Pharm.*, **10**, 89–103

17. Gordon, G., Sparano, B. M., Kramer, A. W., Kelly, R. G. and Iatropoulos, M. J. (1984). Thyroid gland pigmentation and minocycline therapy. *Am. J. Pathol.*, **117**, 98–109

18. Renber, M. D. and Glover, E. L. (1976). Role of age and sex in chronic thyroiditis in rats fed 3'-methyl-4-dimethylaminoazobenzene. *Vet. Pathol.*, **13**, 295–302

19. Kitchen, D. N., Todd, G. C., Meyers, D. B. and Paget, C. (1979). Rat lymphocytic thyroiditis associated with ingestion of an immunosuppressive compound. *Vet. Pathol.*, **16**, 722–729

Parathyroid

1. Young, D. M., Olson, H. M., Prieur, D. J., Cooney, D. A. and Reagan, R. L. (1973). Clinocopathologic and ultrastructural studies of L-asparaginase-induced hypocalcaemia in rabbits. *Lab. Invest.*, **29**, 374–386

2. Atwal, O. S. and Pemsingh, R. S. (1981). Morphology of microvascular changes and endothelial regeneration in experimental ozone-induced parathyroiditis. *Am. J. Pathol.*, **102**, 297–307

Pituitary

1. Dada, M. O., Campbell, G. T. and Blake, C. A. (1984). Pars distalis cell quantification in normal adult male and female rats. *J. Endocrinol.*, **101**, 87–94

2. Kovács, K., Carroll, R. and Tapp, E. (1966). The pathogenesis of hexadimethrine necrosis of the pituitary and adrenal. *Arzneim.-Forsch.*, **16**, 516–519

3. Capen, C. C. (1983). Functional pathologic interrelationships of the pituitary gland and the hypothalamus. In Jones, T. C., Mohr,

U. and Hunt R. D. (eds.) *Endocrine System. Monographs on Pathology of Laboratory Animals.* pp. 101–120. (Berlin and Heidelberg: Springer-Verlag)

4. Tsuda, H. (1983). Goiter, adenoma and carcinoma of the thyroid induced by amitrole and ethylenthiourea, rat. In Jones, T. C., Mohr, U. and Hunt, R. D. (eds.) *Endocrine System. Monographs on Pathology of Laboratory Animals.* pp. 204–211. (Berlin and Heidelberg: Springer-Verlag)

5. Osamura, R. Y. and Takayama, S. (1983). Histochemical identification of hormones in pituitary tumors, rat. In Jones, T. C., Mohr, U. and Hunt, R. D. (eds.) *Endocrine System. Monographs on Pathology of Laboratory Animals.* pp. 130–134. (Berlin and Heidelberg: Springer-Verlag)

6. Evarts, R. P. and Brown, C. A. (1981). 2,4-diaminoanisole-induced thyroid pigmentation in rats inhibited by *m*-phenylenediamine. *Toxicol. Lett.*, **8**, 257–264

7. Farquahar, M. G. (1969). Lysosome function in regulating secretion: disposal of secretory granules in cells of the anterior pituitary gland. In Dingle, J. T. and Fell, H. B. (eds.) *Lysosomes in Biology and Pathology.* pp. 462–482. (Amsterdam: North Holland)

8. Landolt, A. M. (1979). Pituitary adenomas. *J. Histochem. Cytochem.*, **27**, 1395–1397

9. El Etreby, M. F. (1981). Practical applications of immunocytochemistry of the pharmacology and toxicology of the endocrine system. *Histochem. J.*, **13**, 821–837

10. Dakshinamurti, K., Paulose, C. S. and Vriend, J. (1986). Hypothyroidism of hypothalamic origin in pyridoxine-deficient rats. *J. Endocrinol.*, **109**, 345–349

11. Lloyd, R. V. (1983). Estrogen-induced hyperplasia and neoplasia in the rat anterior pituitary gland. *Am. J. Pathol.*, **113**, 198–206

12. El Etreby, M. F., Gräf, K. J., Günzel, P. and Neumann, F. (1979). Evaluation of effects of sexual steroids on the hypothalamic pituitary system of animals and man. *Arch. Toxicol.*, Suppl. 2, 11–39

13. Roe, F. J. C. and Bär, A. (1985). Enzootic and epizootic adrenal medullary proliferative disease of rats: influence of dietary factors which affect calcium absorption. *Human Toxicol.*, **4**, 27–52

14. Horowski, R. and Gräf, K. J. (1979). Neuroendocrine effects of neurosychotrophic drugs and their possible influence on toxic reactions in animals and man – the role of dopamine-prolactin system. *Arch. Toxicol.*, Suppl. 2, 93–104

15. Meites, J. (1979). Role of neuroendocrine system in regulation of mammary tumors in different species. *Arch. Toxicol.* Suppl. 2, 47–58

16. Saunders, S. L., Reifel, C. W. and Shin, S. H. (1983). Ultrastructural changes rapidly induced by somatostatin may inhibit prolactin release in estrogen-primed rat adenohypophysis. *Cell Tiss. Res.*, **232**, 21–34

17. Gooren, L. J. G., Harmsen-Louman, W. and van Kessel, H. (1984). Somatostatin inhibits prolactin release from the lactotrophs primed with oestrogen and cyproterone acetate in man. *J. Endocrinol.*, **103**, 333–335

18. Haggi, E. S., Torres, A. I., Maldonado, C. A. and Aoki, A. (1986). Regression of redundant lactotrophs in rat pituitary gland after cessation of lactation. *J. Endocrinol.*, **111**, 367–373

19. Saluja, P. G., Hamilton, J. M., Thody, A. J., Ismail, A. A. and Knowles, J. (1979). Ultrastructure of intermediate lobe of the pituitary and melanocyte-stimulating hormone secretion in oestrogen-induced kidney tumors in male hamsters. *Arch. Toxicol.*, Suppl. 2, 41–45

With the greater comprehension of the complexities and mechanisms of the immune response acquired in recent years, the development of compounds intended to modify it has become possible. These immunomodulators may function as immunostimulants or immunosuppressants.

However, in parallel with this deliberate development of immunomodulators has come increasing awareness of the immunotoxic actions of a number of industrial and environmental compounds. Pesticides, metals, drugs and environmental contaminants[1] have been found to bring about changes in immune functions such as: resistance to infections; antibody synthesis; cell mediated immune responses; the phagocytic ability of leukocytes and histiocytes; cytokine production; and cytotoxic responses. Immunotoxicology has thus become the focus of attention for a great deal of work with both pharmaceutical and other chemicals[2,3].

The search for immunomodulators, especially hormonal factors to supplement or replace helper T-cells in the induction of humoral or cell mediated responses, has received considerable attention. Natural mediators such as the thymic hormones thymosin, thymopoietin and thymulin have been shown to be able to restore deficient T-cell functions at least in part[4]. Lymphokines act on a number of different cell types, for example macrophage growth factor promotes macrophage proliferation. Interleukins modulate the activation of lymphocytes[4] and interferons inhibit intracellular viral replication. In addition, xenobiotic immunomodulators have been identified which act on several different facets of the immune defence system.

Corticosteroids have been used for many years to suppress some forms of inflammation and the more recent development of immunosuppressants such as cyclosporin A has brought considerable advances against transplant rejection. During routine toxicity studies immunomodulators, particularly the immunostimulants, may cause histological changes which although often consistent with their therapeutic mechanisms are not normally encountered in toxicity studies with other classes of drugs and chemicals. In addition, in our experience, some such compounds may produce highly undesirable side-effects.

Most pharmacological agents are not immunogenic but there are certain types, such as chlorpromazine, phenacetin and amidopyrene, which if given for long enough to susceptible species may result in the development of drug-induced syndromes[5]. Hypersensitivity reactions due to drugs acting as immunogens, although rare, are difficult to predict and their effects may manifest as anaemia, thrombocytopenia, vasculitis or immune complex deposition.

Numerous highly sensitive *in vitro* assays are available for the assessment of immune functions. However, the investigation of the morphological organization of the immune system remains important in the detection of immunotoxicity[6]. Organ weights and careful macroscopic observations provide valuable supplementary information in the pathological assessment of changes in lymphoid tissues. The histological organization of the lymphoid organs is important in the regulation of immune function and its study provides valuable information as to the significance of changes in immune responses[6]. Lymphoproliferative conditions are known to correlate with cell mediated immunity, and plasma cell hyperplasia and germinal centre formation with antibody mediated reactions[7]. Consequently, histopathological assessment of morphological changes in the thymus, spleen and lymph nodes have been repeatedly recommended in the assessment of immunotoxic compounds[7-9]. Histological examination of tissues other than the lymphoid organs may also give information about immune reactions. For example, perivascular mononuclear inflammatory cell infiltration is considered characteristic of Type IV hypersensitivity reactions[2]. A small number of specifically sensitized T-cells provide the trigger for the tissue response which is subsequently amplified by lymphokine release and leads to chemotaxis, cell death and vascular permeability[2].

During the histopathological interpretation of changes in thymus, spleen and lymph nodes, it should be remembered that many of the cellular populations are best not regarded as permanent architectural structures, but as potentially fluid and dynamic. The cells observed to be resident in the spleen (or lymph nodes) at any one time merely represent a static histological picture of a transient cellularity[6]. The vast majority of lymphocytes are recirculating cells which may be found in the blood, lymph nodes or lymphatics and their distribution (and hence the histological appearance of the tissue) is dependent on physiological and immunological stimuli. The accuracy of microscopic observations is often greatly enhanced by use of a comparison-head microscope, as many induced changes are merely slight shifts in the zonal cellularity of a tissue.

Discussion of the effects of xenobiotics on the lymphoid system will be confined to their morphological manifestations; *in vitro* assays are beyond the scope of this text.

Thymus

Atrophy is by far the most frequently encountered change in the thymus and is a relatively common finding in toxicity studies. Thymic atrophy is reported following administration of a wide variety of industrial and environmental chemicals and pharmaceuticals. While with these the atrophy may be considered completely undesirable, in other cases it is accepted as an inevitable feature of immunosuppressive drugs. The thymus is a sensitive indicator of induced malfunctions of the immune system and also of the general health of the animal. In some cases it may prove impossible to detect thymic tissue, either macroscopically or microscopically, despite multiple sampling. This absence suggests complete atrophy or involution[10].

Table 8.1 Induced lesions of the thymus

Lymphoid atrophy
Epithelial proliferation
Lymphoid hyperplasia
Germinal centre development

Atrophic changes in the thymus may be induced by at least three mechanisms: (i) stress-induced adrenocortical hyperactivity; (ii) decreased levels of growth hormone; and (iii) direct toxicity. It must also be remembered that assessment of thymic atrophy may be complicated by age-related involution. The occurrence of induced thymic atrophy in a toxicity study may therefore have several causes.

Virtually any type of serious stress – whether induced by malnutrition, fighting, overcrowding, disease, trauma, certain experimental procedures or administration of systematically toxic compounds – is capable of inducing thymic atrophy. The effects are all likely to be mediated by glucocorticoid release from the adrenal cortex. These steroids are potent thymolytics[11] and the lesions may be prevented by adrenalectomy.

Hypophysectomy and decreased levels of growth hormone cause an atrophy of the thymus and decreased cellularity of the thymus-dependent areas of the spleen and lymph nodes[12]. The effect is reversible upon administration of growth hormone.

Direct toxic effects on the thymic lymphocytes are classically induced by administration of exogenous adrenocortical steroids, such as dexamethasone, or by alkylating agents such as cyclophosphamide[13]. Study of the sequential histological changes in the thymic cell types during corticosteroid-induced atrophy in rats[13] shows that focal disintegration of cortical thymocytes occurs 4 hours after administration. The disintegration is more prominent after 12 hours, with depletion of the outer zones after 18 hours. By 1 to 3 days, depletion is maximal with only sparse identifiable cortical lymphocytes. Some evidence of repopulation by lymphocytes is observed after 7 days. Phagocytosis of degenerate lymphocytes is a common feature and imparts a typical 'starry sky' appearance (Figures 8.1 and 8.2), this involves features typical of apoptosis (Figures 8.3–8.5), i.e. 'rounding-up' of cells; loss of cytoplasmic projections; condensation with preservation of organelles within inclusions; and nuclear pyknosis and fragmentation[14]. T-lymphocytes are a major target for corticosteroids but there is evidence that some subpopulations are more sensitive than others[15]. It is uncertain whether these steroids also act directly on B-cells, or whether they solely inhibit T-cells which then exert a secondary effect. In toxicity studies in our laboratories, with high doses of synthetic corticosteroids, loss of germinal centres and plasma cells were detected in addition to decreased cellularity of thymus-dependent areas of spleen and lymph nodes. At lower doses however, T-cell depletion was the predominant lesion. A comparison of the activity of different corticosteroids demonstrates that those

which possess marked thymolytic activity also exhibit therapeutic properties[16]. There is some evidence of differential species susceptibility to corticosteroid effects with rabbits and rats being more sensitive than monkeys or guinea pigs[3]. In severe involution the thymus is extremely small (Figure 8.6) and in some cases impossible to detect, either macroscopically or microscopically[10].

An immunosuppressive drug, cyclophosphamide, affects predominantly B-lymphocytes with a relatively minor effect on T-cells[17]. However, thymic atrophy may be induced in rats. Cyclophosphamide causes lymphodepletion by an antiproliferative effect and its greater effect on B-cells rather than T-cells may be attributable to their differing turnover rates[15].

Diethylstilboestrol administration in mice also induces thymic atrophy[7]. In this and some other cases, the lymphocytic depletion is accompanied by thymic epithelial proliferation[18]. The epithelial components are in the form of cords, ducts or cysts (Figure 8.7). They sometimes contain ciliated cells and an eosinophilic, PAS positive intraluminal secretion[19]. Oestrogens promote epithelial cyst formation in rats, whilst testosterone and methylthiouracil inhibit their age-related development. With testosterone, thymic atrophy is independent of the adrenal cortex; it also occurs following adrenalectomy[11]. Organotin compounds are potent inducers of thymic atrophy which is also unrelated to endogenous corticosteroid release[20]. Ultrastructural studies of the thymus in rats following treatment with dioctyltin dichloride reveals extensive vacuolation and increased numbers of secretory granules in the epithelial reticular cells[21].

The induced forms of thymic atrophy described are generally reversible when administration of the injurious compound is ceased. Similarly, the spontaneously occurring thymic involution in aged rats is reversible, in this case upon orchidectomy[22]. The thymus becomes repopulated by thymocytes and reorganized into cortex and medulla but regeneration is inhibited by testosterone implants. Even in severe induced atrophy, with virtual complete loss of thymocytes, the thymus usually displays a remarkable regenerative capacity. However, in some cases despite regeneration taking place evidence of previous degenerative change remains[23]. Following cyclophosphamide-induced atrophy, although the histological structure is essentially restored after 30 days, evidence of fibrosis and foci of metaplastic immature myelopoietic cells remains. It is suggested that the fibrosis is due to the severity of the earlier intense inflammatory reaction[23].

Neonatal thymectomy causes increased numbers of somatotrophs in the anterior pituitary[11]. These cells show features typical of hyperactivity. Thymic hypoplasia is described in Snell–Bagg hypophyseal dwarf mice[12]. This strain has extremely low levels of growth hormone. Treatment with growth hormone restores immune capacity but not in thymectomized animals. Similarly the thymic atrophy caused by hypophysectomy is also reversed by growth hormone administration[11].

The actual effects of thymic involution on clinical immunocompetence have recently been discussed[24]. Despite the often severe histological changes there is evidence that the residual thymic tissue retains some degree of immunocompetence; thymic hormones are still produced and some functions may even be enhanced[24].

Unlike cortical atrophy, hyperplastic changes in the thymic cortex are rarely encountered. However, there are scattered reports of proliferation following antigenic stimulation, such as injections of *B. pertussis*, dansyl

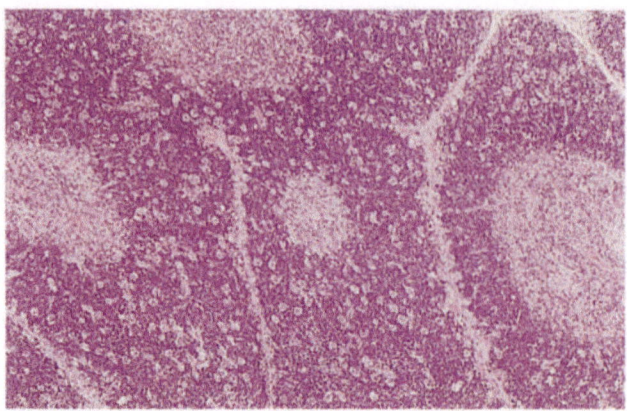

Figure 8.1 Early thymic atrophy in a rat treated with cyclophosphamide. Lymphocytolysis is confined to the cortex and gives a typical 'starry sky' appearance.   H & E

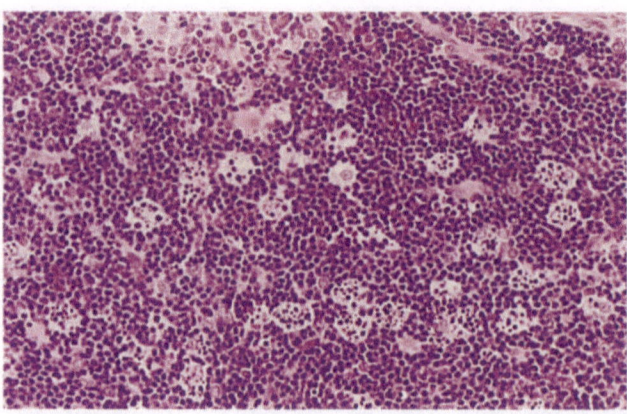

Figure 8.2 Higher magnification of Figure 8.1. Phagocytosis of pyknotic lymphocytes by histiocytes.   H & E

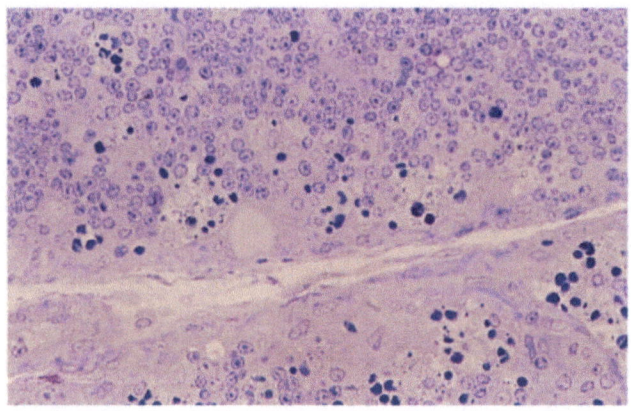

Figure 8.3 Cortical histiocytic cells containing rounded, condensed lymphocytic bodies. From a rat treated with cyclophosphamide. 1 μm section. Toluidine Blue

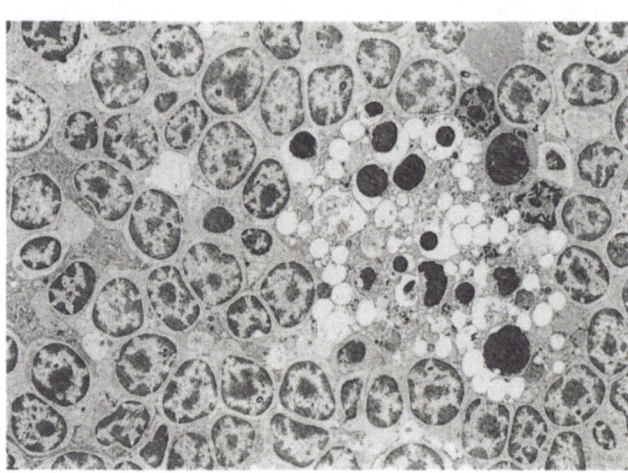

Figure 8.4 Early thymic atrophy in a rat treated with cyclophosphamide. Lymphocytes showing various stages of degeneration including 'rounding up', condensation, nuclear pyknosis and fragmentation. Electron micrograph

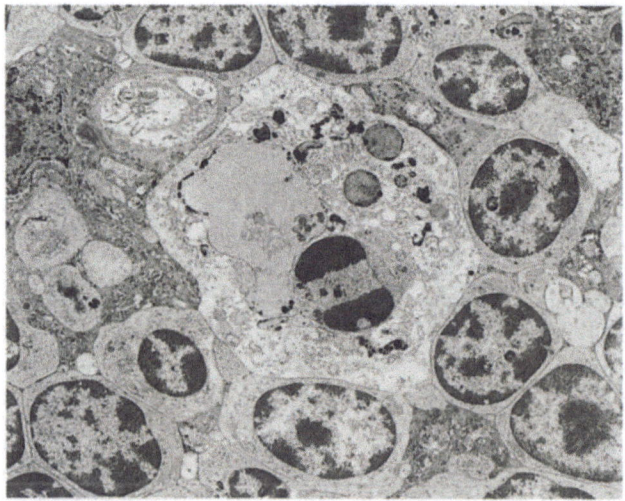

Figure 8.5 Histiocytic cell containing ingested lymphocyte. Electron micrograph

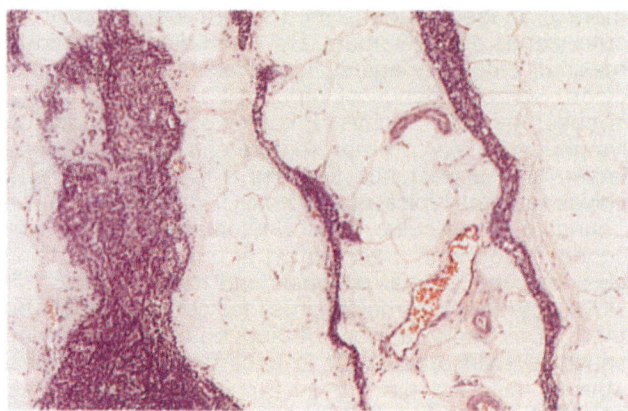

Figure 8.6 Severe thymic atrophy in a cynomolgus monkey treated with high doses of a novel corticosteroid. Cortical and medullary features are completely obscured.   H & E

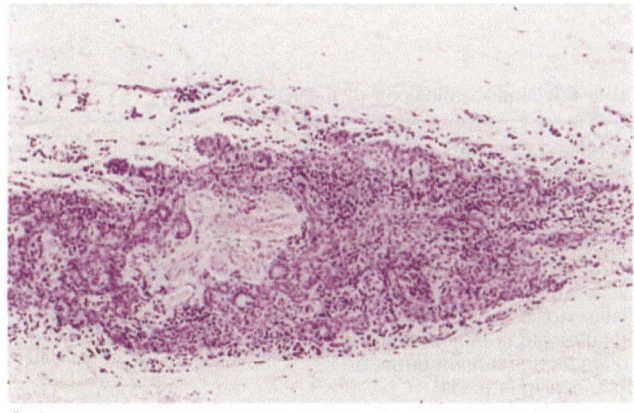

Figure 8.7 Marked thymic atrophy induced by an industrial chemical in a mouse. The thymus is virtually devoid of lymphoid cells and is composed of epithelial cords and acini.   H & E

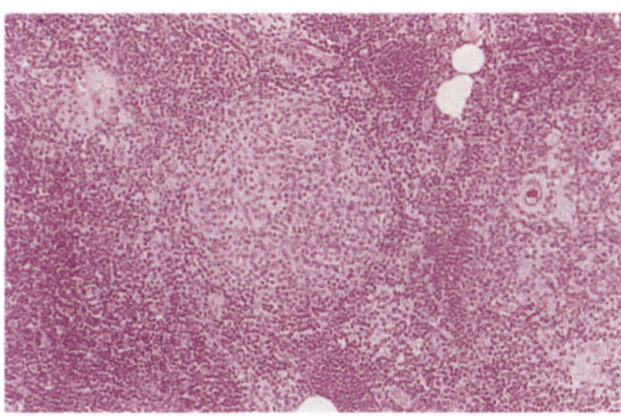

Figure 8.8 Germinal centre development in the thymus of a rhesus monkey following systemic administration of a novel immunostimulant.   H & E

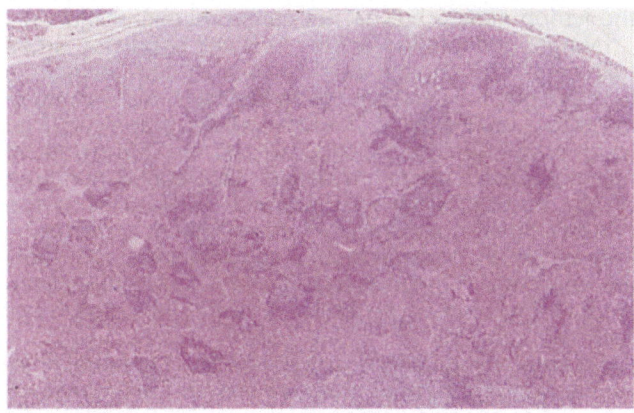

Figure 8.9 Plasmacytosis in a lymph node of rat following antigenic stimulation. Note the displacement of other nodal structures.   H & E

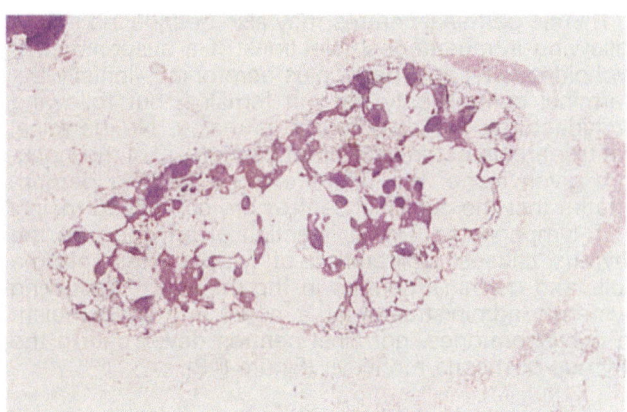

Figure 8.10 Cystic atrophy of a mesenteric lymph node from a rat with ulcerative lesions of the gastrointestinal tract induced by a NSAI. The lesion initially involves sinus dilatation but progresses with eventual lymphoid depletion.   H & E

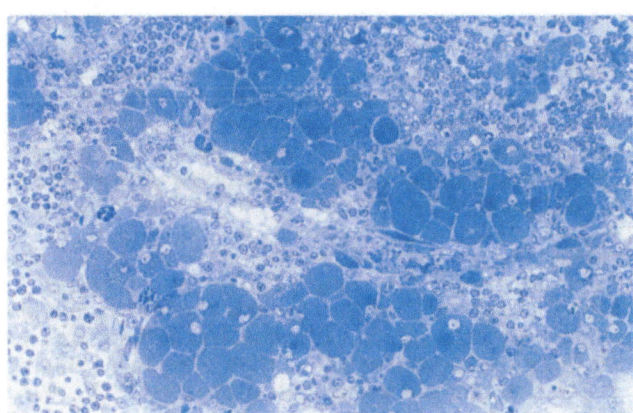

Figure 8.11 Histiocytes in the mesenteric lymph node of a rat following oral administration of a detergent-like compound. The histiocytes are distended and are identical to those found in the lamina propria of the small intestine. 1 µm section. Toluidine Blue

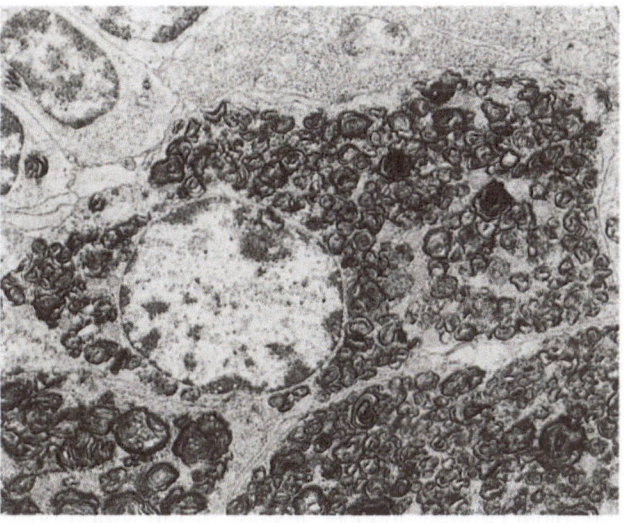

Figure 8.12 From the same study as Figure 8.11. Histiocytes contain numerous multilamellar bodies. A few lymphocytes contain similar bodies. Electron micrograph

chloride and phytohaemagglutinin[25]. Following intraperitoneal injections of *Iscador mali* to mice, the cortical reticular cells become prominent with increased numbers of lymphoblasts and the cortex/medulla ratio is altered[25]. Increased thymic size, due to lymphocyte proliferation, also occurs following adrenalectomy and administration of thyroxine[11].

The thymus, unlike the organs of the peripheral lymphoid tissues, does not ordinarily contain germinal centres nor develop them in response to parenterally injected antigens. However, an unusual form of thymic hyperplasia in which germinal centres are found in the medulla is reported in the thymus in cases of myasthenia gravis[26]. A similar reaction is found in cases of the lupus-like syndrome in NZB mice[25]. An animal model for myasthenia gravis involves guinea pigs immunized with thymus or muscle in Freund's complete adjuvant[27]. Those animals which develop a myasthenic neuromuscular block and antibodies against the thymic epithelial cells show lymphocytic infiltrates in the thymic medulla. The lesion is provisionally interpreted as 'experimental autoimmune thymitis'.

Thymic germinal centres may also be induced in rats following intraperitoneal injections of a suspension of typhoid–paratyphoid bacilli plus serotonin[28]. Initially the germinal centres only form in females, but following orchidectomy are also found in males. No germinal centres are detected with either component of the inoculum given alone. Immunoperoxidase staining demonstrates that the germinal centres are composed mainly of B-lymphocytes. Direct injection of antigen into the thymus causes proliferation of lymphocytes, plasma cells and germinal centres in the medulla[29]. Following systemic administration of a novel immunostimulant in our laboratories, germinal centres developed in the thymus of rhesus monkeys (Figure 8.8).

Lymph Nodes

Careful morphological examination of the cellularity of different zones of lymph nodes provides useful information as to the nature of any induced immunosuppression or immunostimulation. In an attempt to allow correlations between histological findings and changes in immunological function, a standardized system for classification of morphological features as they relate to potential immune capacity has been suggested[30]. Interpretation of changes in lymph nodes involves the assessment of the relative areas and cellularity of the cortex, paracortex, germinal centres, medulla and sinuses[31]. Changes in the cellularity of the paracortex indicates a T-lymphocyte effect, whereas changes in follicles, germinal centres and numbers of medullary plasma cells suggests a B-cell effect.

When assessing changes in the lymph nodes it is important to establish the 'normal' appearance of the control animals from the species under test in a particular experiment. For example, in specific-pathogen-free rodents, maintained under strict barrier conditions, lymph nodes often illustrate a relatively quiescent appearance with little evidence of germinal centres and few medullary plasma cells. However, conventionally derived rodents maintained under non-barrier conditions frequently show a marked plasmacytosis with prominent germinal centres. Similarly, lymph nodes from wild-caught, subhuman primates usually have prominent, well developed germinal centres. Induced lesions of the lymph nodes are listed in Table 8.2.

Following thymectomy, there is a reduction in the number of lymphocytes in the paracortex and similar

Table 8.2 Induced lesions of the lymph nodes

Decreased cellularity of T-cell areas
Decreased cellularity of B-cell areas
Increased cellularity of T-cell areas
Increased cellularity of B-cell areas
Plasmacytosis
Germinal centre development
Cystic atrophy
Histiocytosis
Granulomatous inflammation
Congestion and haemorrhage
Increased mast cells
Extra-medullary haemopoiesis

effects may be seen with thymic atrophy following corticosteroid administration. However, the correlation between thymic atrophy and depletion in T-cell population populated areas does not appear to be absolute as some analogues of tilorone, an interferon-inducer which inhibits cell mediated immunological reactions[32], cause depletion of lymphocytes in thymus-dependent areas of the lymph nodes, but do not cause thymic involution.

Lymphoid depletion occurs in B-cell populated areas following cyclophosphamide administration to guinea pigs and mice[17]. Cyclophosphamide has a relatively sparing effect on T-cells at the dose levels employed. The lymphocytic depletion clearly reveals the framework of spindle-shaped reticulum cells[33]. Decreased numbers of plasma cells with a corresponding decrease in the number of immunologically active cells detected by a fluorescent antibody technique and decreased IgG levels are reported in guinea pigs treated with triphenyltin acetate[34]. However, no effect is detected on germinal centres.

Degenerative changes and depletion of lymphoid elements from germinal centres are seen in cases in which a period of hypoxia precedes death[30].

Several lymphocyte mobilizing agents such as heparin, synthetic polysaccharide sulphates and especially the synthetic polyanion polymethacrylic acid (PMAA) induce lymphocytosis[35]. The lymphocytosis induced by PMAA was shown due to mobilization of cells from the spleen and lymph nodes but not the thymus. All Malpighian corpuscles of the rat spleen illustrate depletion of lymphocytes from the germinal centres and marginal zones. Lymphocytes are also depleted in the mid and deep zones of the lymph node cortex and from the marginal sinuses. PMAA thus mobilizes both T- and B-lymphocytes, whereas synthetic polysaccharide sulphates are believed to mobilize only T-cells[35].

The parathymic lymph nodes are believed to have a specialized role in the local differentiation of T-lymphocytes from the thymus[36]. The lymphocytes show increased proliferative responses to T-cell mitogens and produce increased interleukin II. Cepharanthine increases the numbers of peripheral T-lymphocytes and when administered to mice it causes an increased migration of mature T-cells from the thymus to the parathymic lymph nodes, but has no effect on the cellularity of the mesenteric lymph nodes or spleen[36]. Similar changes are found with decreased PGE_2 levels induced by indomethacin.

In reactive states the cellularity of the various areas of the lymph nodes show selective increases. The particular area affected depends on the nature of the stimulus involved. With the development of cell mediated responses, the thymus-dependent paracortex is the main site of proliferation of lymphocytes and becomes prominent[30]. The paracortex is the site of the so-called 'high endothelial venules'. These specialized vessels (post-capillary venules) play an important role in the translocation of lymphocytes of the recirculating pool between the node itself and vascular and lymphatic compartments[37]. In an inactive lymph node the vessels are inconspicuous, and are poorly developed in 'germ-free' animals, but they become more prominent in reactive nodes. The morphological changes in the high endothelial venules are clearly demonstrated in rats[38]. When the afferent lymphatic vessels of the popliteal lymph nodes are interrupted the macrophages, germinal centres, lymphoblasts and plasma cells are depleted. The high endothelial venules become flattened with a poor affinity for pyronin and no evidence of lymphocyte translocation through the walls is detected. Following the injection of antigen, a reactive hyperplasia is induced and the high endothelial venule cells become cuboidal with evidence of migration by lymphocytes through the walls. It is suggested that antigen-stimulated macrophages activate the venule endothelium and thereby regulate the migration of recirculating lymphocytes into the lymph node[38]. The endothelium is higher in female than in male mice and treatment with oestrogens increases the height of the venule endothelial cells and the Golgi apparatus becomes prominent[39]. It is postulated that oestrogen increases the production of mucopolysaccharides by the endothelial cells which form a cell coat and mediate the passage of lymphocytes.

Following antigenic challenge, the cortical areas of the lymph node involved in humoral immunity undergo reactive hyperplasia. This involves the formation of germinal centres which produce immunocompetent B-cells and are always associated with humoral antibody production[30]. Administration of exogenous lymphokines produces an increased size and mitotic activity of germinal centres in the regional lymph nodes[40]. The number of plasma cells may increase considerably (Figure 8.9) in the medullary cords and under intense antigenic stimulation may extend outwards to the capsule displacing the other nodal components[30].

A chemical sensitizer, oxazolone, when administered subcutaneously to intact and T-cell depleted rabbits causes a marked immunoblast reaction. This reaction commences in the outer cortex and immature plasma cells occupy the depleted paracortical areas in the T-cell depleted animals[41]. This is followed by a germinal centre reaction.

Due to the nature of lymphatic drainage some induced reactions are largely confined to regional lymph nodes. This mechanism is easily demonstrated following the subcutaneous injection of Indian ink into the footpad of guinea pigs[42]. Large numbers of macrophages packed with Indian ink are located in the popliteal lymph nodes. These macrophages initially locate in the marginal (subcapsular) sinus, migrate along the exterior of the follicles and then enter the germinal centres.

Regional lymph nodes may also show lymphoid hyperplasia with plasmacytosis and germinal centre formation in cases of antigen administration. An example of this type of reaction occurs in the popliteal lymph nodes following injection of adjuvant and/or antigen into the rat footpad[38]. In addition to induction of the above typical humoral antibody response (B-lymphocyte reactions), a local reaction may also be seen with a characteristic T-cell response, with increased cellularity of the paracortex. A similar reaction is described with diphenylhydantoin and D-penicillamine[43]. The popliteal lymph node enlargement is primarily due to proliferation of B-lymphocytes with germinal centre development and a slight infiltration by plasma cells.

In studies with non-steroidal anti-inflammatory compounds in our laboratories, ulcerative lesions developed in the gastrointestinal tract and the mesenteric lymph nodes underwent a form of cystic atrophy (Figure 8.10). The lesion was initially characterized by sinus dilatation which became more severe and was associated with lymphoid depletion. In severe cases the lymph nodes were grossly cystic with only a sparse lymphocytic component. In our experience similar changes may develop in the renal lymph nodes following the induction of toxic nephropathies. The pathogenesis of the lesion is uncertain. The lesion does not usually extend to more distant nodes.

The mesenteric lymph nodes also show changes characterized by the accumulation of histiocytes following oral administration of a variety of compounds. These compounds initially induce infiltration of macrophages into the lamina propria of the small intestine ('accumulation enteropathies') and, subsequently, histiocytosis in the mesenteric lymph nodes. Examples of this type of reaction include responses to phospholipids (Figures 8.11 and 8.12), lipids (Figures 8.13 and 8.14), hair dye pigments and other pigmented materials (Figures 8.15 and 8.16). The lesion may initially be considered to be a form of sinus histiocytosis but the macrophages are subsequently found throughout the medulla extending into the paracortex, cortex and occasional germinal centres. The number of macrophages increases with time and they occupy large areas of the node. The macrophages rarely show any degenerative changes and appear to remain for prolonged periods. Presumably the macrophages are unable to degrade their ingested contents and function merely as 'storage' depots.

In rhesus monkeys given a high fat diet in our laboratories, the lymph nodes contained large numbers of macrophages with foamy vacuolated cytoplasm (Figure 8.17). This xanthomatous change was found predominantly in the axillary and inguinal nodes and was associated with the development of atherosclerotic lesions.

The tracheobronchial lymph nodes (and the bronchus associated lymphoid tissue) often show single foci or aggregates of macrophages in inhalation studies with induced pulmonary histiocytosis (Figure 8.18). With materials such as quartz the macrophages show degenerative changes and there are areas of necrosis and giant cells, with the development of granulation tissue (Figures 8.19 and 8.20), fibrosis and hyalinization[44]. In animals exposed to tobacco smoke for prolonged periods, in our laboratories, the tracheobronchial lymph nodes contained macrophages with golden-brown pigment identical to that found in alveolar macrophages.

Congestion and haemorrhage in regional lymph nodes may be an agonal phenomenon. However, in some cases associated erythrophagocytosis and haemosiderosis indicate a more protracted event. These lesions may be seen as secondary effects of induced haemorrhagic visceral lesions.

Interperitoneal injections of metallic tin powder cause a marked enlargement of drainage lymph nodes[45]. A granulomatous inflammatory reaction contributes to this lymphadenopathy but by far the most significant contribution is made by a marked proliferation of plasma cells. It is suggested that the reaction is due to tin acting as a hapten[46] and is associated with increased levels of serum IgG. When tin sulphate or tin chloride are administered in the drinking water of metallic tin treated rats, the plasma cell and Russell body cell responses are eliminated. The granulomatous inflammation, however, persists. The inhibition of the plasma cell reaction may be due to immunological tolerance or a form of metabolic adaptation[46].

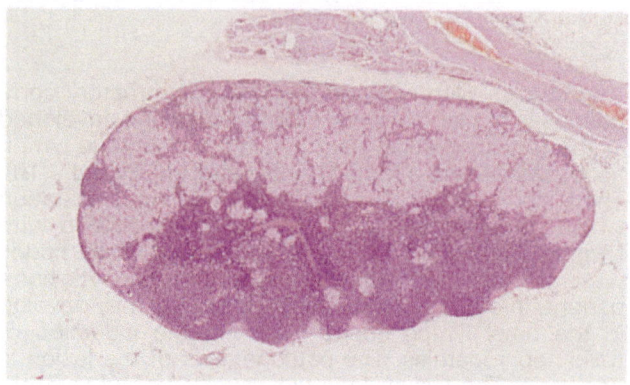

Figure 8.13 Mesenteric lymph node from a rat treated orally with a novel agrochemical. Pronounced numbers of histiocytes. H & E

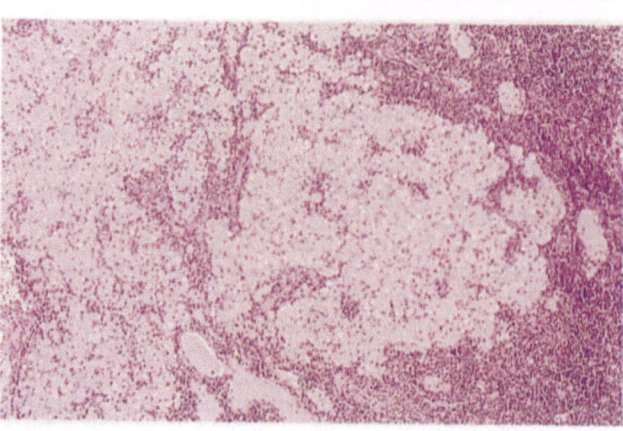

Figure 8.14 From the same study as Figure 8.13. Histiocytes are distended and contain vacuoles. In frozen sections, stained with Oil Red O, abundant fat was present. Similar histiocytes were found in the lamina propria of the small intestine.   H & E

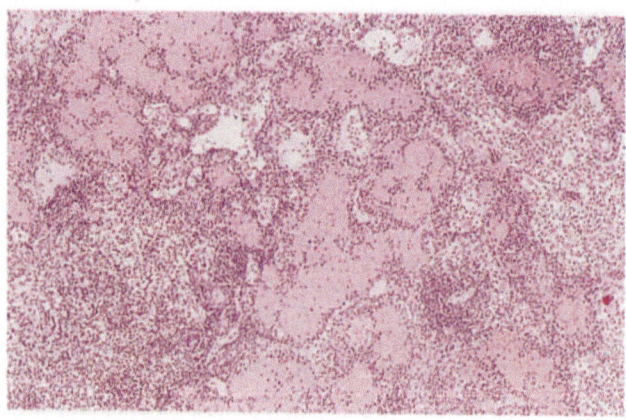

Figure 8.15 Mesenteric lymph nodes from a rat treated orally with pigmented plant extract. Histiocytes are abundant.   H & E

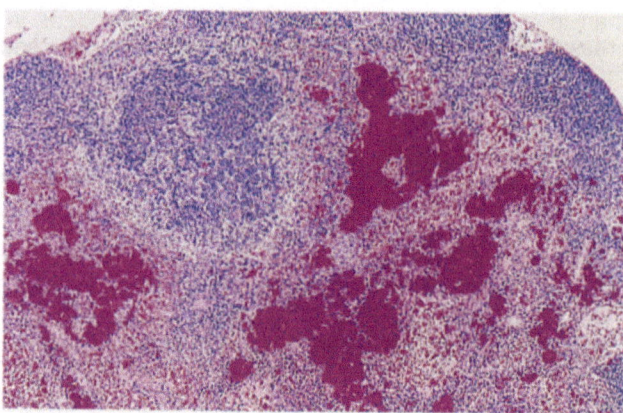

Figure 8.16 From the same study as Figure 8.15. The engulfed plant extract is PAS positive. Similar histiocytes were present in the lamina propria of the small intestine. PAS

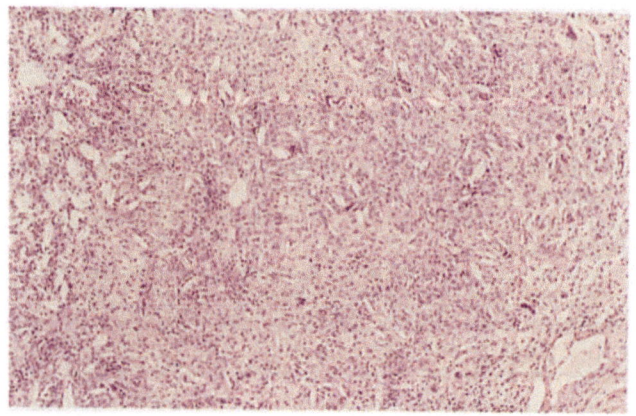

Figure 8.17 Xanthomatous change in the lymph node of a rhesus monkey fed a high fat diet. Note the distended histiocytes and prominent cholesterol clefts. The lesion was associated with the development of atherosclerosis.   H & E

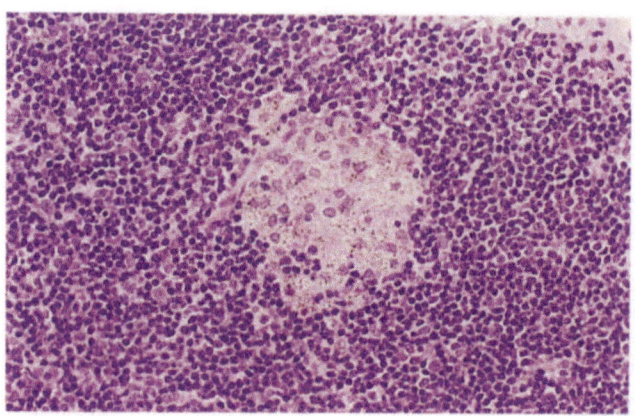

Figure 8.18 Tracheobronchial lymph node from a rat exposed to a dust by inhalation. Histiocytes contain fine dust particles. Similar histiocytes were present in the alveoli and peribronchiolar lymphoid tissue.   H & E

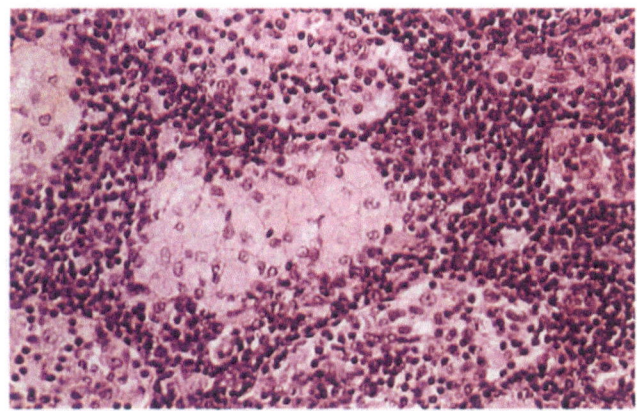

Figure 8.19 Aggregates of histiocytes with early granulomatous inflammation in the tracheobronchial lymph node of a rat exposed to quartz dust by inhalation. H & E

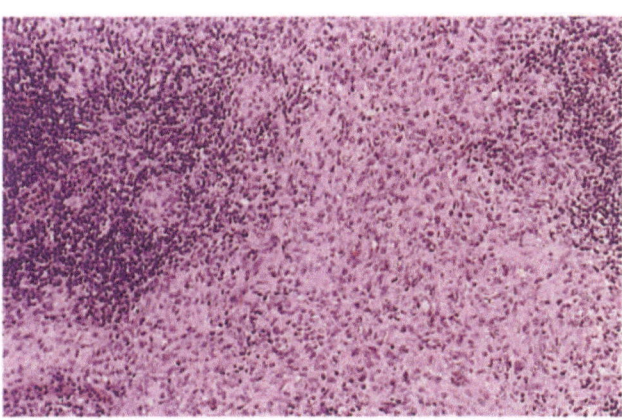

Figure 8.20 From the same study as Figure 8.19. Granulation tissue in the tracheobronchial lymph node. H & E

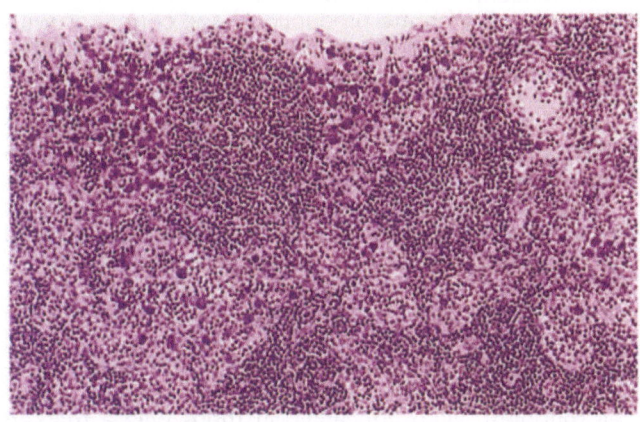

Figure 8.21 Increased numbers of mast cells (identified by basophilic cytoplasmic staining in this preparation), in the sinuses of a mesenteric lymph node of a rat treated with an industrial chemical. H & E

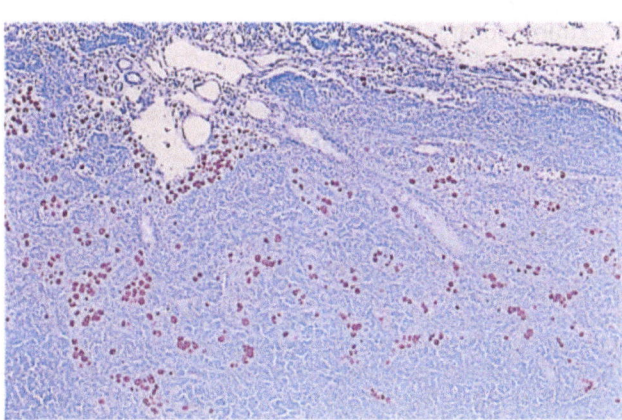

Figure 8.22 From the same study as Figure 8.21. Increased numbers of mast cells. Toluidine Blue

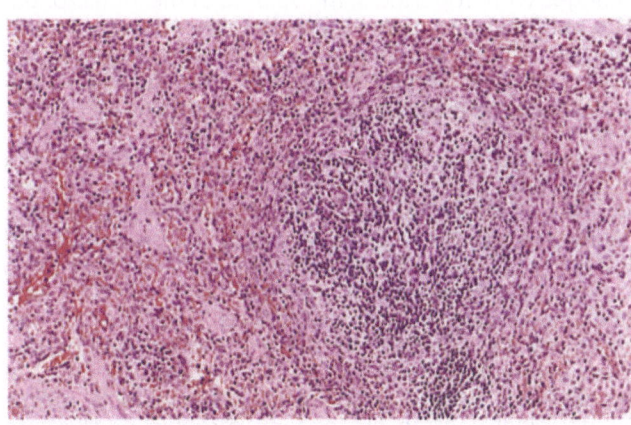

Figure 8.23 Spleen of a rat treated with cyclophosphamide. The marginal zone shows marked lymphoid depletion and the remaining white pulp shows lymphocytolysis. H & E

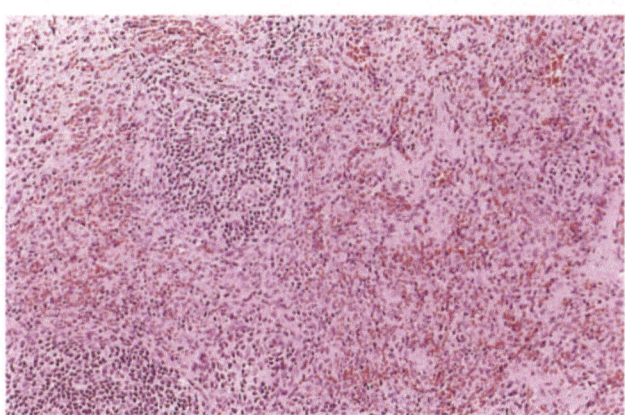

Figure 8.24 From the same study as Figure 8.23. Markedly decreased cellularity of the white pulp. H & E

Changes in the mast cell numbers (Figures 8.21 and 8.22) in lymph nodes are rarely observed in toxicity studies. However, increased numbers are reported following administration of several compounds, including cortisone, in the rat[47]. These reactions are generally confined to regional lymph nodes. Injections of dextran into the thigh increase the numbers of mast cells in the inguinal nodes. *Crotalaria spectabilis* and its alkaloid monocrotaline, fed to rats, cause a marked increase in the mediastinal nodes (and in the lung parenchyma). Oral hydrazine sulphate greatly increases mast cell numbers in the mesenteric nodes[47]. In addition, rats fed hydroxylamine, methylhydrazine or β-aminopropionitrile also contain increased numbers of mast cells in the mesenteric nodes[47]. The mast cells sometimes show mitotic activity and usually occupy the central sinus and medulla. There is also some evidence that mast cells respond in regional lymph nodes following a localized primary antigenic stimulus[48]. With tritiated thymidine, mast cells do not become labelled – suggesting migration into the responding nodes rather than proliferation *in situ*.

Extramedullary haemopoiesis may occasionally be seen as an induced lesion in the lymph nodes of rodents. This haemopoiesis is secondary to other systemic lesions. Granulopoiesis is usually the most common form, with variable numbers of megakaryocytes.

Spleen

The spleen, unlike the lymph nodes, has both lymphoid and non-lymphoid functions, including accommodation of lymphocytes, antigen concentration, antibody production, removal of effete red blood cells and in some species, haemopoiesis. These functions are reflected in the types of induced lesions which may be observed (Table 8.3). As in the lymph nodes, detection of changes in the cellularity of the splenic zones often requires careful comparison with tissue from untreated control animals, as the lesions usually manifest as changes in the size and cellularity of the zones.

Table 8.3   Induced lesions of the spleen

Increased cellularity of T-cell areas
Increased cellularity of B-cell areas
Germinal centre development
Decreased cellularity of T-cell areas
Decreased cellularity of B-cell areas
Hypersplenism
Necrosis/infarction
Extra medullary haemopoiesis
Erythrophagocytosis/haemosiderosis

In common with other parts of the lymphoid system the splenic tissues may be divided into thymus (T)-dependent and T-independent (B cell-predominant) zones. The periarteriolar sheaths of the white pulp are composed of T-cells, whilst the follicles or germinal centres mainly contain B-cells, plus a proportion of T-cells, macrophages and dendritic cells. The marginal zone, which is composed of a sinusoidal network fed by terminal branches of the splenic artery, often contains large numbers of lymphocytes[49].

Assessment of an increase (hyperplasia) or decrease (atrophy) in the cellularity of the histologically distinct zones allows the identification of morphological features which have been found to be consistent with immunostimulation or immunosuppression.

Administration of indomethacin and aspirin to mice causes an increase in the number of T-lymphocytes in the spleen[50]. A corresponding decrease in the number of lymphocytes in the thymus is also reported. In thymectomized mice no change in the splenic lymphocyte count is detected. Prostaglandins inhibit T-cell proliferation but promote their differentiation. The action of indomethacin on splenic T-cell numbers is probably related to its inhibition of prostaglandin synthesis, with reversal of prostaglandin effects. Following exogenous stimulation, immature cortisone-sensitive thymocytes migrate from the thymus to peripheral sites[50] and lymphocyte maturation is believed to involve the differentiation of cortisone-sensitive lymphocytes to cortisone-resistant cells[51].

In intact mice, treatment with thymus extracts causes enlargement of the spleen due to hyperplasia of the white pulp[11]. In previously thymectomized mice the extract causes mitosis and hyperplasia in the depleted areas. This immunomodulatory effect is presumably due to thymic hormones within the extract. Thymosin exerts a similar influence in mice subjected to total body X-irradiation[11].

The reaction to antigenic substances consistently involves germinal centre production[52] and correlates with serum haemagglutinin production. Germinal centres may be induced in the splenic white pulp with endotoxin injections[46]. Following intravenous doses of metallic tin powder, a pronounced increase in the numbers of plasma cells and plasmablasts in both the red and white pulp occurs[45].

Most studies with mitogens involve *in vitro* work. However, an *in vivo* comparison of the effects of several mitogens and adjuvants on mouse spleen is reported[53]. This study compared concanavalin A (a T-cell mitogen); polyadenylic acid (an adjuvant); beryllium sulphate (an adjuvant); a lipopolysaccharide (an adjuvant and B-cell mitogen); a purified tuberculin protein derivative (a B-cell mitogen); and dextran sulphate (an adjuvant and B-cell mitogen). With concanavalin there was a marked enlargement (doubling) of the T-cell zones of the white pulp with numerous blast cells and mitotic figures. No changes were detected in the B-cell zones. Polyadenylic acid and beryllium sulphate both caused enlargement of the T-cell zones by small lymphocytes but the B-cell areas were unaffected. With the lipopolysaccharide changes were largely confined to the B-cell areas which doubled in size due to pronounced blastogenesis. No changes were reported in the volume of the T-cell zones. The purified protein derivative also caused an increased blast activity in the B-cell zones. Dextran sulphate initially caused a marked increase in the cellularity of the white pulp with loss of demarcation between the T- and B-cell zones.

Lymphoid atrophy may readily be produced in the spleen with immunosuppressive compounds. Administration of high doses of cyclophosphamide to rats causes severe loss of lymphocytes (Figures 8.23 and 8.24) from both the T- and B-cell areas[46]. At lower dose levels cyclophosphamide exerts a more selective lymphocyte depletion with decreased cellularity of the lymphoid follicles and germinal centres[9] and at low dose levels selectively depletes T-suppressor cells. In monkeys treated with a polychlorinated biphenyl, follicular germinal centres are absent, atrophic or illustrate proteinosis[10]. Wild-caught, subhuman primates are usually good models for the assessment of atrophy of B-cell areas, as many of these animals have well developed, prominent germinal centres in the white pulp. Conversely, the dog is a poor model as the normal paucity of white pulp in general, and of germinal centres in particular, makes assessment of changes more difficult.

Lymphocyte depletion of thymus-dependent areas occurs with corticosteroids, organo-tins, tilorone and azathioprine[15,32]. After T-cell depletion the reticular framework around the central artery becomes clearly visible. The marginal zone contains both T- and B-cells and this frequently shows depletion with antineoplastic agents (Figure 8.25).

Hypersplenism is induced in rats, monkeys and dogs treated with macromolecular polymers such as polyvinyl alcohol, methyl cellulose[54] and, in our experience, several 'reticuloendothelial system expanders' intended as immunomodulators (Figures 8.26–8.28). In these studies the erythrocyte half-life is sometimes decreased and anaemia develops, presumably due to excessive activity of the spleen[55]. The administered material accumulates in the phagocytic histiocytes causing a 'foamy cell' appearance, predominantly in the red pulp although in some cases the white pulp and germinal centres are also involved. With high doses, the histiocytes accumulate and occupy the majority of the red pulp, distorting the splenic architecture. Ultrastructurally, the histiocytes are distended with large inclusions (Figure 8.28) which sometimes coalesce and distort the eccentric nuclei. Few other organelles are identifiable in the distorted phagocytes. In some cases giant cells develop and in chronic studies fibrosis occurs[54]. Erythrophagocytosis is prominent with the build-up of haemosiderin. Similar lesions are produced in rabbits following infusion of perfluorochemicals[56].

Splenic destruction is reported following administration of ethyl palmitate emulsion to rats. The compound localizes in the red pulp[55]. Focal necrosis is also reported in the red pulp in mice treated with concanavalin A[53]. The necrosis becomes organized with granulation tissue formation and is likely to represent a micro-infarction due to erythrocyte agglutination and consequent plugging of small vessels. Splenic infarcts are induced in rats by vasoconstrictor drugs such as phenylephrine[57]. Multiple necrotic foci in one or several adjacent Malpighian corpuscles develop. Infarction is also produced in rats with hypersplenism due to intravascularly administered powdered metallic tin, and the lymphoid atrophy induced by cyclophosphamide[57].

In haemorrhagic shock the splenic white pulp, and the germinal centres in particular, undergo degeneration and necrosis[58]. These lesions are not considered to be attributable to anoxia or hypoxia, but more likely to release of adrenal cortical hormones which are known to be elevated within an hour post-haemorrhage.

Lesions associated with immune complex disease induced by an antibiotic are described in dogs[59]. In this induced haemolytic anaemia the reticular network (as demonstrated by alkaline phosphatase) becomes highly activated and the monocyte counts (as demonstrated by peroxidase) increase. The condition is associated with raised immunoglobulin and C3 levels and immune complexes on erythrocytes.

In rodents in particular, the spleen often demonstrates extramedullary haemopoiesis (EMH) in response to a variety of induced (and spontaneous) systemic conditions. This haemopoiesis, which predominantly involves granulopoiesis with large numbers of megakaryocytes (Figure 8.29), grossly expands the red pulp. In contrast to rodents, extramedullary haemopoiesis is rarely seen in the normal adult dog, nor is it often seen as an induced event. EMH usually only occurs in the dog in response to impairment of the bone marrow or in conditions of severe blood loss[60]. In dogs given intravascular injections of the synthetic heparin analogue, dextran sulphate, marked haemopoietic activity

is observed in the spleen[60]. The numbers of megakaryocytes and erythroblasts both increase tenfold, but little evidence of increased granulopoiesis is detected. There is no bone marrow impairment in these dogs and no evidence of blood loss. In the spleen of mice treated with diethylstilboestrol a shift in the red pulp/white pulp ratio is described[7]. This change is due to increased erythropoiesis and myelopoiesis in the red pulp.

The red pulp is also the major site of erythrophagocytosis which may be increased in some induced conditions with enhanced erythrocyte degradation. This erythrophagocytosis leads to increased haemosiderin accumulation in macrophages which may be clearly demonstrated with Perl's stain (Figure 8.30).

Following intraperitoneal injections, the splenic capsule may show variable degrees of inflammation and fibrosis (Figure 8.31).

Bone Marrow

The bone marrow is an integral part of both the immune and haemopoietic systems and lesions may result in malfunction of one or both of these. The range of treatment-induced lesions is small and listed in Table 8.4.

Table 8.4 Induced lesions of the bone marrow

Atrophy
Myelofibrosis
Myeloid hyperplasia
Germinal centre development
Mast cell proliferation
Megakaryocyte proliferation

Myeloid atrophy is the most common and frequently investigated lesion. The marrow cavity becomes occupied by adipose tissue (Figures 8.32 and 8.33) with only occasional foci of haemopoietic or lymphopoietic cells. One of the classical methods of marrow atrophy induction is the administration of benzene. In rats, peripheral lymphocytes and differentiating bone marrow precursor cells are the most sensitive cell populations[61]. It is believed that a metabolite is responsible for the myelotoxicity, as partial hepatectomy decreases the severity of the lesion. An animal model of chronic aplastic marrow failure is described with busulfan administration to mice. The mice show atrophy of the bone marrow with significantly decreased numbers of neutrophils and lymphocytes[62]. Bone marrow failure with associated aplastic anaemia is described in dogs treated with phenylbutazone[63].

Cytosine arabinoside causes severe depletion of the erythroid islands of the bone marrow of rats[64]. The depletion is associated with an increased number of small lymphocytes. Myelopoietic elements are unaffected. Nitrogen mustard causes severe widespread changes in the rat bone marrow, with haemorrhage, atrophy and fatty replacement. The administration of the protein synthesis inhibitor cycloheximide exerts a strong protective effect against the cytosine arabinoside changes, but has only limited effect against those induced by nitrogen mustard.

Marked hypocellularity, degeneration and necrosis of all nucleated cells (except megakaryocytes) is produced in dogs treated with chromomycin[65]. Administration of polychlorinated biphenyls to rhesus monkeys causes bone marrow depletion. Individual monkeys show variation in their responses but moderately depressed erythropoiesis is associated with changes in the myeloid series. The haematological findings from the peripheral blood show a corresponding variation, but severe leuco-

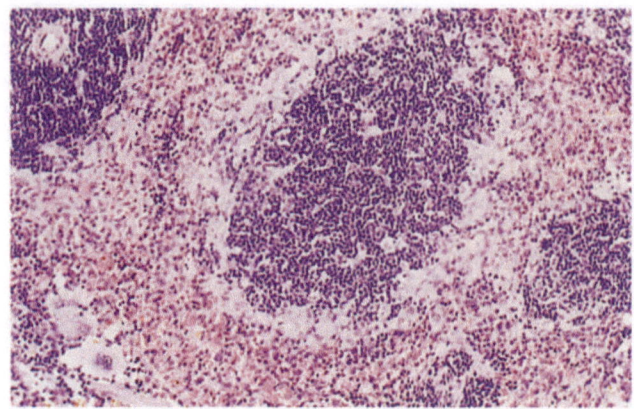

Figure 8.25 Spleen from a mouse treated with an antineoplastic agent. The marginal zone shows virtually complete lymphoid depletion with only histiocytic cells remaining.   H & E

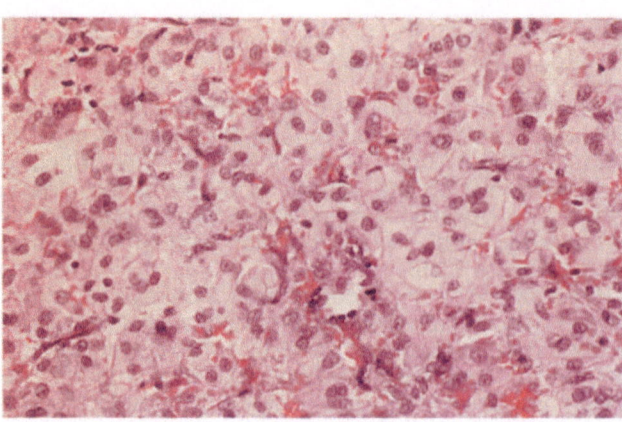

Figure 8.26 Spleen from a rhesus monkey treated with a 'reticuloendothelial system expander'. Large histiocytic cells with amorphous pale cytoplasm in the red pulp.   H & E

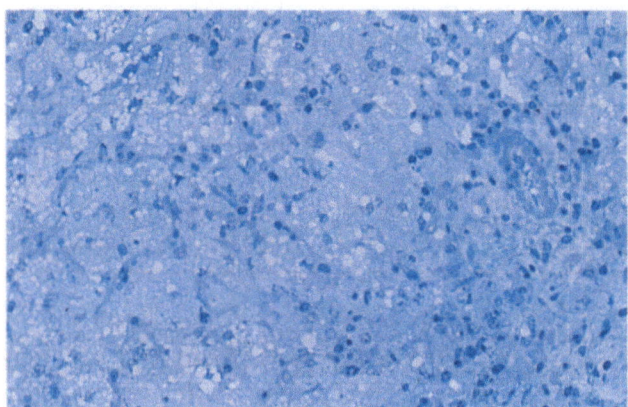

Figure 8.27 From the same study as Figure 8.26. Histiocytic cells filled with irregular vacuoles. 1 μm section. Toluidine Blue

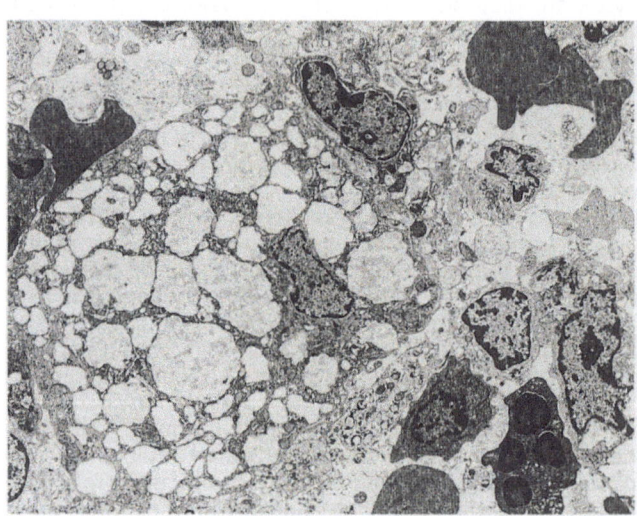

Figure 8.28 From the same study as Figures 8.26 and 8.27. Histiocyte with irregular inclusions. Electron micrograph

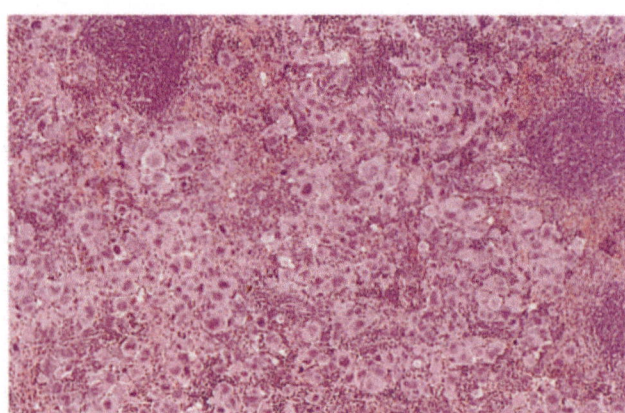

Figure 8.29 Mouse spleen showing numerous megakaryocytes and extramedullary haemopoiesis in the red pulp. The condition was a secondary development to an induced haemorrhagic condition.   H & E

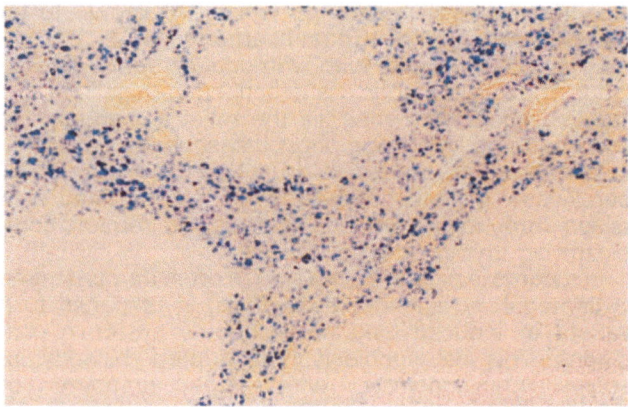

Figure 8.30 Haemosiderosis in the red pulp of the spleen from a rat with induced anaemia. Perl's stain

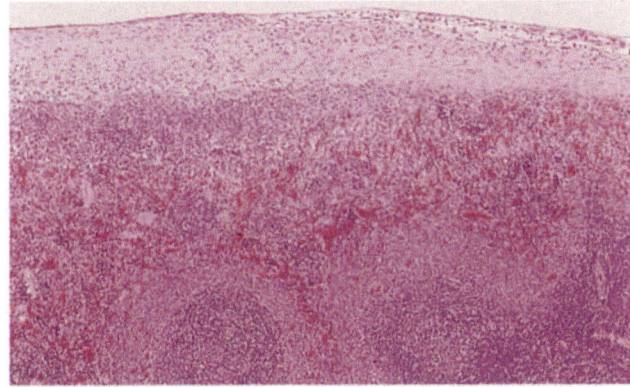

Figure 8.31 Fibrosis of the splenic capsule from a rat treated intraperitoneally with a novel pharmaceutical. The underlying tissue is unaffected. H & E

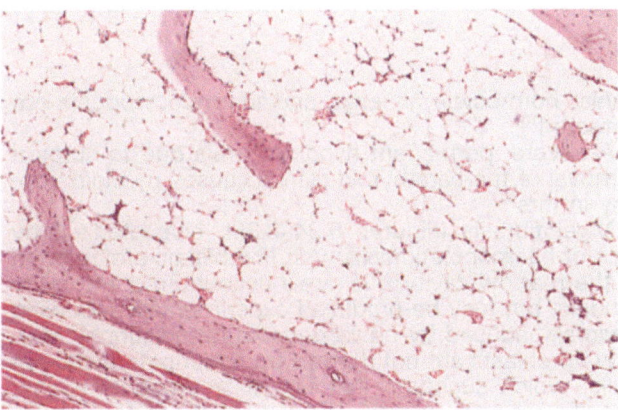

Figure 8.32 Atrophy with adipose replacement of the bone marrow from a mouse treated with a cytotoxic drug. H & E

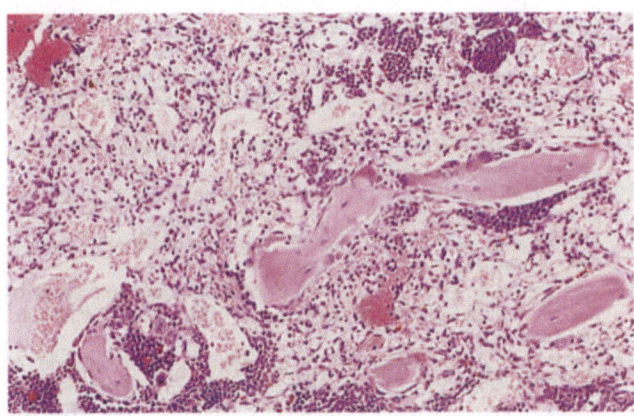

Figure 8.33 Atrophy of the bone marrow in a mouse treated with a cytotoxic drug. Only islands of haemopoietic cells remain. H & E

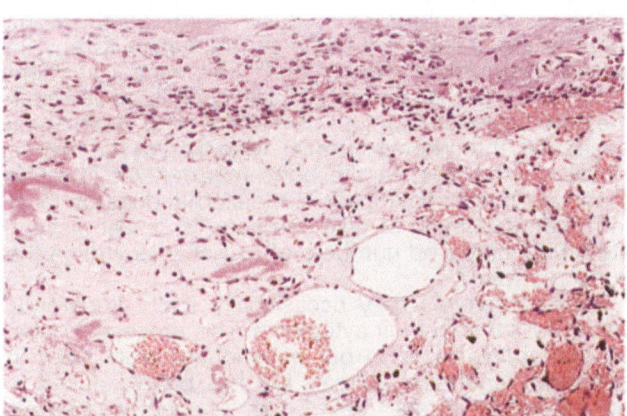

Figure 8.34 Figures 8.34–8.36 show stages in the development of myelofibrosis. Here there is complete depletion of haemopoietic elements with necrosis, hyalinization and early fibrosis in the bone marrow of a mouse treated with an industrial chemical. H & E

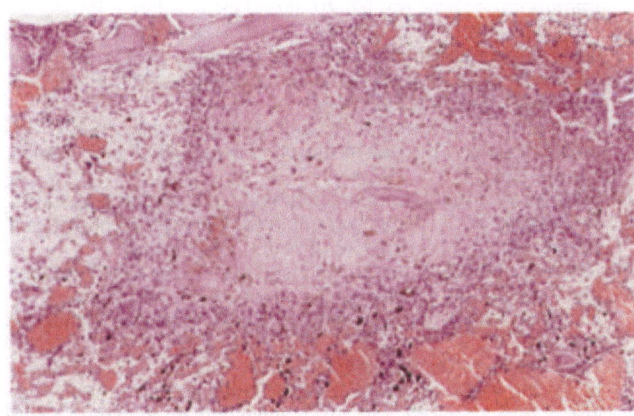

Figure 8.35 Severe atrophy of bone marrow in a mouse treated with an industrial chemical. Necrosis, congestion and fibroblast proliferation. H & E

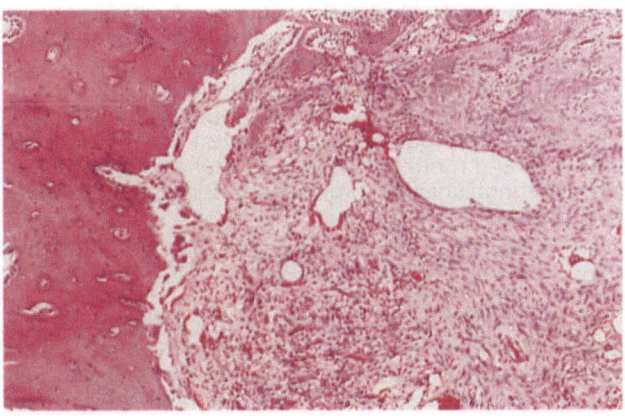

Figure 8.36 Myelofibrosis in the bone marrow of a rat treated with a cytostatic drug. H & E

penia, normocytic anaemia and thrombocytopenia are detected[10].

A severe, permanent hypocalcaemia due to surgical removal of the parathyroid glands causes myeloid atrophy in rats[66].

Myelofibrosis (Figures 8.34–8.36), characterized by loss of haemopoietic cells with fibroblastic proliferation in the marrow cavity[67], is rarely encountered in toxicity studies, but may be produced experimentally following necrosis induced by oestrogens and irradiation[68]. Marrow fibroblasts are not derived from pluripotential stem cells, which suggests that fibrosis represents a nonspecific repair process[67]. The development of saponininduced myelofibrosis in rabbits is described in detail[69]. This work shows that saponin initially damages the marrow vascular sinus walls breaking the barrier between the haemopoietic cells and the circulation. Necrosis and fibrosis of the marrow cavity follows. The fibrosis is often localized around arteries. It is postulated that the functional units of the marrow centre around the intermediate size arterial branches, and are homologous with the splenic periarterial lymphatic sheath[69].

Increased numbers of megakaryocytes in the bone marrow are a common, expected response to any induced haemorrhagic condition[70]. Following treatment of hyperthyroid cats with propylthiouracil, an immune mediated reaction develops[71] which involves severe anaemia and thrombocytopaenia. Megakaryocytic hyperplasia is prominent in the bone marrow. An immune mediated thrombocytopaenia, induced in dogs by longterm administration of gold compounds, is also associated with increased numbers of megakaryocytes in the bone marrow[72].

Megakaryocytes may occasionally show apparently viable cells within their cytoplasm. This process, known as emperipolesis, is in our experience rarely seen in untreated laboratory animals but has been induced in our laboratory in rats treated with a novel β-adrenergic antagonist. In this instance prominent numbers of neutrophils were identified in the majority of megakaryocytes. It has been suggested that emperipolesis represents an early form of apoptosis[73]. However, in our experience little evidence of degenerative changes were detected in the neutrophils.

The number of monocyte–granulocyte precursor cells in the bone marrow of dogs increases following the administration of muramyl peptide, an immunostimulant[59].

Myeloid hyperplasia may occur as a secondary response to induce systemic lesions involving inflammatory and/or haemorrhagic reactions.

Germinal centres are rarely observed in the marrow of untreated animals, but with some novel immunostimulant compounds we have observed their induction in both rats and monkeys. These centres were histologically indistinguishable from those found in lymph nodes and spleen.

Increased numbers of mast cells are induced in the bone marrow of rats fed a calcium-deficient diet or β-aminopropionitrile[47].

In phospholipidosis induced by amphiphilic, cationic drugs, multilamellar bodies develop in a variety of tissues and organs. In the haemopoietic system their presence in lymphocytes enables the diagnosis to be made from peripheral blood samples. The multilamellar inclusions are described in lymphocytes from animals treated with several phospholipidosis-inducing compounds including chloroquinine and chlorphentermine[74].

References

1. Koller, L. D. and Exon, J. H. (1985). The rat as a model for immunotoxicity assessment. In Dean, J., Luster, M. I., Munson, A. E. and Amos, H. (eds.) *Immunotoxicology and Immunopharmacology.* pp. 99–111. (New York: Raven)
2. Lebish, I. J., Hurvitz, A., Lewis, R. M., Cramer, D. V. and Krakowka, S. (1986). Immunopathology of laboratory animals. *Toxicol. Pathol.*, **14**, 129–134
3. Koller, L. D. (1982). Chemical-induced immunomodulation. *J. Am. Vet. Med. Assoc.*, **181**, 1102–1106
4. Hadden, J. W. (1983). Prospects for immunorestoration. In Gibson, G. G., Hubbard, R. and Parke, D. V. (eds.) *Immunotoxicology.* pp. 329–342. (London: Academic Press)
5. Parke, A. L. (1983). Clinical manifestations of drug-induced syndromes. In Gibson, G. G., Hubbard, R. and Parke, D. V. (eds.) *Immunotoxicology.* pp. 27–40. (London: Academic Press)
6. Irons, R. D. (1985). Histology of the immune system: structure and function. In Dean, J., Luster, M. I., Munson, A. E. and Amos, H. (eds.) *Immunotoxicology and Immunopharmacology.* pp. 11–22. (New York: Raven)
7. Dean, J. H., Luster, M. I. and Boorman, G. A. (1982). Methods and approaches for assessing immunotoxicity: an overview. *Environ. Health Perspect.*, **43**, 27–29
8. Vos, J. G. (1977). Immune suppression as related to toxicology. *CRC Crit. Rev. Toxicol.*, **5**, 67–101
9. Luster, M. I., Dean., J. H. and Moore, J. A. (1982). Evaluation of immune functions in toxicology. In Hayes, W. (ed.) *Methods in Toxicology.* (New York: Raven Press)
10. Tryphonas, L., Arnold, D. L., Zawidzka, Z., Mes, J., Charbonneau, S. and Wong, J. (1986). A pilot study in adult rhesus monkeys treated with Aroclor 1254 for two years. *Toxicol. Pathol.*, **14**, 1–10
11. Trainin, N. (1974). Thymic hormones and the immune response. *Physiol. Rev.*, **54**, 272–315
12. Roth, J. A., Lomax, L. G., Altszuter, N., Hampshire, J., Kaeberle, M. L., Shelton, M., Draper, D. D. and Ledet, A. E. (1980). Thymic abnormalities and growth hormone deficiency in dogs. *Am. J. Vet. Res.*, **41**, 1256–1262
13. van Haelst, U. (1967). Light and electron microscopic study of the normal and pathological thymus of the rat. *Z. Zellforsch.*, **80**, 153–182
14. Robertson, A. M. G., Bird, C. C., Waddell, A. W. and Currie, A. R. (1978). Morphological aspects of glucocorticoid-induced cell death in human lymphoblastoid cells. *J. Pathol.*, **126**, 181–187
15. Spreafico, F., Allegrucci, M., Merendino, A. and Luini, W. (1985). Chemical immunodepressive drugs: Their action on the cells of the immune system and immune mediators. In Dean, J., Luster, M. I., Munson, A. E. and Amos, H. (eds.) *Immunotoxicology and Immunopharmacology.* pp. 179–192. (New York: Raven)
16. Shewell, J. (1957). The activity of different steroids in producing thymic involution. *Br. J. Pharmacol.*, **12**, 133–139
17. Parker, D. and Turk, J. L. (1983). Regulation of hypersensitivity reactions. In Gibson, G. G., Hubbard, R. and Parke, D. V. (eds.) *Immunotoxicology.* pp. 57–70. (London: Academic Press)
18. Ebbesen, P. and Doenhoff, M. J. (1971). Abrogated thymoma development and increased amyloid development in estrogenized mice grafted spleen and bone marrow cells. *Proc. Soc. Exp. Biol. Med.*, **138**, 850–855
19. Cherry, C. P., Eisenstein, R. and Glücksman, A. (1967). Epithelial cords and tubules of the rat thymus. *Br. J. Exp. Pathol.*, **48**, 90–106
20. Seimen, W. (1981). Immunotoxicology of alkyl tin compounds. In Sharma, R. P. (ed.) *Immunologic Considerations in Toxicology.* Vol. 1, pp. 103–120. (Florida: CRC Press)
21. Miller, K. (1983). Various mechanisms in chemically-induced thymic injury. In Gibson, G. G., Hubbard, R. and Parke, D. V. (eds.) *Immunotoxicology.* pp. 193–204. (London: Academic Press)
22. Greenstein, B. D., Fitzpatrick, F. T. A., Adcock, I. M., Kendall, M. D. and Wheeler, M. J. (1986). Reappearance of the thymus in old rats after orchidectomy: inhibition of regeneration by testosterone. *J. Endocrinol.*, **110**, 417–422
23. Milicevic, N. M., Millicevic, Z., Piletic, O., Ninkov, V. and Mujovic, S. (1984). Restriction of regenerative capacity of the rat thymus after the application of cyclophosphamide. *J. Comp. Pathol.*, **94**, 425–431
24. Clarke, A. G. and MacLennan, K. A. (1986). The many facets of thymic involution. *Immunol. Today*, **7**, 202–205
25. Rentea, R., Lyon, E. and Hunter, R. (1981). Biologic properties

of Iscador: a Viscum album preparation. *Lab. Invest.*, **44**, 43–48

26. Grody, W. W., Jobst, S., Keesey, J., Herrmann, C. and Naeim, F. (1986). Pathologic evaluation of thymic hyperplasia in myasthenia gravis and Lambert-Eaton syndrome. *Arch. Pathol. Lab. Med.*, **110**, 843–846

27. Goldstein, G. and Whittingham, S. (1966). Experimental autoimmune thymitis. *Lancet*, **2**, 315–317

28. Matsuno, K., Eking, S. and Kotani, M. (1982). Formation of germinal centres in the rat thymus. In Nieuwenhuis, P., van der Broek, A. A. and Hanna, M. G. (eds.) *In vivo Immunology.* pp. 843–844. (New York: Plenum)

29. Sherman, J. D., Adner, M. M. and Dameshek, K. W. (1964). Direct injection of the thymus with antigenic substances. *Proc. Soc. Exp. Biol. Med.*, **115**, 866–872

30. Cottier, H., Turk, J. and Sobin, L. (1972). A proposal for a standardised system of reporting human lymph node morphology in relation to immunological function. *WHO Bull.*, **47**, 375–385

31. Taylor, C. R. (1976). Immuno-histological observations upon the development of reticulum cell sarcoma in the mouse. *J. Pathol.*, **118**, 201–219

32. Levine, S., Sowinski, R. and Albrecht, W. L. (1977). T-lymphocyte depletion induced in rats by analogs of tilorone hydrochloride. *Toxicol. Appl. Pharmacol.*, **40**, 137–145

33. Turk, J. L. and Poulter, L. W. (1972). Selective depletion of lymphoid tissue by cyclophosphamide. *Clin. Exp. Immunol.*, **10**, 285–296

34. Verschauren, H. G., Ruitenberg, E. J., Peetoom, F., Helleman, P. W. and van Esch, G. J. (1970). Influence of triphenyl tin acetate on lymphatic tissue and immune responses in guinea pigs. *Toxicol. Appl. Pharmacol.*, **16**, 400–410

35. Ormai, S., Hagenbeck, A., Palkovits, M. and van Bekkum, D. W. (1973). Changes of lymphocyte kinetics in the normal rat, induced by the lymphocyte mobilizing agent polymethacrylic acid. *Cell Tissue Kinet.*, **6**, 407–423

36. Nihashi, Y., Koga, Y., Gondo, H., Taniguchi, K. and Nomoto, K. (1985). Thymus-dependent increase in number of T-cells in parathymic lymph nodes induced by the biscoclaurine alkaloid, cepharanthine. *Immunobiology*, **170**, 351–364

37. Anderson, A. O. and Anderson, N. D. (1976). Lymphocyte emigration from high endothelial venules in rat lymph nodes. *Immunology*, **31**, 731–748

38. Hendricks, H. R., van Hemert, H. A. B. and van der Heijden, M. (1982). The effect of stimulated macrophages on high endothelial venules and germinal centres in lymph nodes of rat. In Nieuwenhuis, P., van den Broek, A. A. and Hanna, M. G. (eds.) *In vivo Immunology.* pp. 207–212. (New York: Plenum)

39. Kittas, C. and Henry, L. (1980). An electron microscopic study of the changes induced by oestrogens on the lymph node post-capillary venules. *J. Pathol.*, **129**, 21–28

40. Kelly, R. H., Harvey, V. S., Sadler, T. E. and Dumond, D. C. (1975). Accelerated cytodifferentiation of antibody-secreting cells in guinea pig lymph nodes stimulated by sheep erythrocytes and lymphokines. *Clin.. Exp. Immunol.*, **21**, 141–154

41. Veldman, J. E., Keuning, F. J. and Molenaar, I. (1978). Site of initiation of the plasma cell reaction in the rabbit lymph node. *Virchows Arch. B: Zellpathol.*, **28**, 187–202

42. Kotani, M., Ezaki, T., Ekino, S., Matsuno, K., Fujii, H. and Nawa, Y. (1982). Lymph macrophages enter the germinal centre of regional lymph nodes. In Nieuwenhius. P., van den Broek, A. A. and Hanna, M. G. (eds.) *In vivo Immunology.* pp. 837–842. (New York: Plenum)

43. Gleichmann, H., Pals, S., Radaszkiewicz, T. and Wasser, M. (1982). T cell-dependent B cell lymphoproliferation and activation induced by the drug diphenyl-hydantoin. In Nieuwenhuis, P., van den Broek, A. A. and Hanna, M. G. (eds.) *In vivo Immunology.* pp. 617–622. (New York: Plenum)

44. Dauber, J. H., Rossman, M. D., Pietra, G. G., Jimenez, S. A. and Daniele, R. P. (1980). Experimental silicosis. *Am. J. Pathol.*, **101**, 595–612

45. Levine, S., Sowinski, R. and Koulish, S. (1983). Plasma cellular and granulomatous splenomegaly produced in rats by tin. *Exp. Mol. Pathol.*, **39**, 364–376

46. Levine, S. and Sowinski, R. (1983). Tin salts prevent the plasma cell response to metallic tin in Lewis rats. *Toxicol. Appl. Pharmacol.*, **68**, 110–115

47. Takeoka, O., Angevine, M. and Lalich, J. J. (1962). Stimulation

of mast cells in rats fed various chemicals. *Am. J. Pathol.*, **40**, 545–554

48. Roberts, A. N. (1970). Early mast cell responses in mouse popliteal lymph nodes to localised primary antigenic stimuli. *J. Immunol.*, **105**, 187–192

49. Kumararatne, D. S., MacLennan, I. C. M., Bazin, H. and Gray, D. (1982). Marginal zones: the largest B cell compartment of the rat spleen. In Nieuwenhuis, P., van den Broek, A. A. and Hanna, M. G. (eds.) *In vivo Immunology.* pp. 67–74. (New York: Plenum)

50. Koga, Y., Taniguchi, K., Kubo, C. and Nomoto, K. (1983). Thymus-dependent increases in splenic T-cell population by indomethacin. *Cell. Immunol.*, **75**, 43–51

51. Ihle, J. N., Pepersack, L. and Rebar, L. (1981). Regulation of T cell differentiation: *in vitro* induction of 20α-hydroxysteroid dehydrogenase in splenic lymphocytes from athymic mice by a unique lymphokine. *J. Immunol.*, **126**, 2184–2189

52. Hanna, M. G., Congdon, C. C. and Wust, C. J. (1965). Effect of antigen dose on lymphatic tissue germinal center changes. *Proc. Soc. Exp. Biol. Med.*, **121**, 286–290

53. Moatamed, H., Karnovsky, M. J. and Unanue, E. R. (1975). Early cellular responses to mitogens and adjuvants in the mouse spleen. *Lab. Invest.*, **32**, 303–312

54. Weisman, S. M., Waldman, T. A., Levin, E. and Berlin, N. I. (1961). An attempt to produce hypersplenism in the dog, using methylcellulose. *Blood*, **17**, 632–642

55. Gralla, E. J. (1975). Adverse drug reactions. *Vet. Clin. N. Am.*, **5**, 699–715

56. Nanney, L., Fink, L. M. and Virmani, R. (1984). Perfluorochemicals. *Arch. Pathol. Lab. Med.*, **108**, 631–637

57. Levine, S. and Sowinsky, R. (1985). Splenic infarcts produced in rats by vasoconstrictor drugs. *Exp. Pathol.*, **28**, 13–19

58. Kajihara, H., Yasui, W., Nakagawa, H. and Maeda, H. (1986). Light and electron microscopic observations of the white pulp of the dog spleen during haemorrhagic shock. *Pathol. Res. Pract.*, **181**, 586–595

59. Wachsmuth, E. D. (1983). Evaluating immuno-pathological effects of new drugs. In Gibson, G. G., Hubbard, R. and Parke, D. V. (eds.) *Immunotoxicology*, pp. 237–250. (London: Academic Press)

60. Calvo, W., Ross, W. M. and Flieder, T. M. (1983). Stimulation of extramedullary haemopoiesis by dextran sulfate. *Blut*, **46**, 39–45

61. Irons, R. D., Heck, H. d'A., Moore, B. J. and Muirhead, K. A. (1979). Effects of short-term benzene administration on bone marrow cell cycle kinetics in the rat. *Toxicol. Appl. Pharmacol.*, **51**, 399–409

62. Morley, A. and Blake, J. (1974). An animal model of chronic aplastic marrow failure. I. Late marrow failure after busulfan. *Blood*, **44**, 49–56

63. Watson, A. D. J., Wilson, J. T., Turner, D. M. and Culvenor, J. A. (1980). Phenylbutazone-induced blood dyscrasias suspected in three dogs. *Vet. Rec.*, **107**, 239–241

64. Ben-Ishay, Z. and Farber, E. (1975). Protective effects of an inhibitor of protein synthesis, cycloheximide, on bone marrow damaged induced by cytosine arabinoside or nitrogen mustard. *Lab. Invest.*, **33**, 478–490

65. Fleischman, R. W., Schaeppi, U., Heyman, I. A., Phelan, R. S., Rosenkrantz, H. and Ilievski, V. (1974). Preclinical toxicologic evaluation of chromomycin A3 in mice, dogs and monkeys. *Toxicol. Appl. Pharmacol.*, **27**, 259–270

66. Rixon, R. H. and Whitfield, J. F. (1972). Hypoplasia of the bone marrow in rats following removal of the parathyroid glands. *J. Cell. Physiol.*, **79**, 343–352

67. Dunn, J. K., Doige, C. E., Searcy, G. P. and Tamke, P. (1986). Myelofibrosis-osteosclerosis syndrome associated with erythroid hypoplasia in a dog. *J. Small Anim. Pract.*, **27**, 799–806

68. Weiss, D. J. and Armstrong, P. J. (1985). Secondary myelofibrosis in three dogs. *J. Am. Vet. Med. Assoc.*, **187**, 423–425

69. Hoshi, H. and Weiss, L. (1978). Rabbit bone marrow after administration of saponin. *Lab. Invest.*, **38**, 67–80

70. Krizsa, F., Gergely, G. and Rak, K. (1968). Megakaryocyte response in posthaemorrhagic thrombocytosis of mice. *Acta Haematol.*, **39**, 112–117

71. Peterson, M. E., Hurvitz, A. I., Leib, M. S., Cavanagh, P. G. and Dutton, R. E. (1984). Propylthiouracil-associated haemolytic anaemia, thrombocytopenia, and antinuclear antibodies in cats with hyperthyroidism. *J. Am. Vet. Med. Assoc.*, **184**, 806–808

72. Bloom, J. C., Blackmer, S. A., Bugelski, P. J., Sowinski, J. M. and Saunders, L. Z. (1985). Gold-induced immune thrombocytopenia in the dog. *Vet. Pathol.*, **22**, 492–499

73. Burns, E. R., Zucker-Franklin, D. and Valentine, F. (1982). Cytotoxicity of natural killer cells. Correlation with emperipolesis and surface enzymes. *Lab. Invest.*, **47**, 99–107

74. Payne, B. J., Merril, T. G. and Tousimas, A. J. (1971). Lymphocytic vacuolation and membranous cytoplasmic bodies in rats dosed with an acridan. *Vet. Pathol.*, **8**, 433–444

In routine toxicological studies with laboratory animals histological examination of the nervous system is often limited to a few H&E stained sections of the brain and spinal cord and perhaps one or two sections of a major peripheral nerve. However, in safety assessment the toxicologist does not only rely on the detection of morphological alterations in the nervous system but places much reliance on sound neurological and behavioural examinations during the course of the toxicological investigation. If such 'in-life' investigations reveal or suggest a disorder, then the level of histological surveillance of the nervous system is increased. The 'in-life' investigations may even indicate the probable site of the lesion within the nervous system. Good clinical observations detect the majority of chemically induced nervous lesions. On the other hand, many induced disorders of the nervous system are not accompanied by morphological change, e.g. chemicals which interfere with or modify synaptic transmission rarely cause histopathological changes but may have profound neurological effects.

Good tissue fixation and preparation are of paramount importance in routine toxicological studies. In the histology laboratory, where multiple tissues from many animals are processed together, the nervous system is notoriously susceptible to the induction of histological artefacts which may resemble actual lesions (Figures 9.1 and 9.2). In order to avoid this situation it may be advisable to fix a small proportion of animals by vascular perfusion rather than by immersion.

The choice of stains for the routine examination of paraffin sections evokes much discussion among toxicological pathologists. In our experience well prepared, haemotoxylin and eosin stained preparations are adequate for screening for the presence of lesions. Once a lesion is detected, then it is frequently beneficial to use specific stains for the various components of the nervous system to determine more precisely the nature of the lesion. In addition to special stains, other specialized techniques of pathological investigation, such as electron microscopy, teased nerve fibre preparations, use of resin sections, morphometry, histochemistry and immunocytochemistry also have a place in elucidating neurotoxicological problems but usually in specially designated studies. The use of resin sections, with their increased resolution, has become especially popular amongst neuropathologists.

As neurotoxins tend to affect one cell type in the nervous system the most convenient classification of neurotoxic disorders involves reference to the particular cell type affected (Table 9.1). However, it is important to recognize that the initial damage can proceed to a secondary or even a tertiary cellular effect. Factors which influence the precise anatomical location of lesions within the nervous system are on the whole unknown.

Table 9.1 Induced lesions of the nervous system

Neuronopathies
Axonopathies
Myelinopathies
Gliopathies
Vasculopathies
Choroid plexus vacuolation

However, the state of the vasculature, the ability of the chemical to pass through the blood–brain and blood–nerve barriers and the affinity of the chemical for neuronal receptor sites, appear in some instances to be crucial. In spite of the heterogeneous cell population within the nervous system, the system can react to toxic insult only in a limited number of ways – the most common being degeneration. So many dissimilar neurotoxic chemicals appear to act in a similar fashion and for convenience these chemicals can be grouped together under their morphological manifestations.

Neuronopathies

Neuronopathies involve damage to the nerve body itself which proceeds to axonal and dendritic degeneration. Subsequent removal of the degenerating axon's myelin sheath is a tertiary effect. In the CNS loss of nerve fibres stimulates astrocyte proliferation to fill the potential void. Histologically, damaged neurones usually appear shrunken, darkly stained with indistinct Nissl substance and may contain lipofuscin. Adjacent glial cells may be conspicuous. At this stage of degeneration there is only a fine distinction in appearance between the damaged cell and artefactual dark neurones[1]. Satellitosis and neurone removal by glial cells confirm the degeneration. Neuronal vacuolation may be found as part of reversible change or also as part of the degenerative process, particularly following ischemia.

In our experience neuronopathies are encountered only rarely in the routine toxicological testing of many differing chemical compounds. However, there are several well known examples of chemically induced neuronopathies which may be subdivided into cytoplasmic, nuclear and postsynaptic[2]. Mercury is an example of a chemical which causes cytoplasmic neuronopathy. Human exposure to both organic and inorganic forms of mercury results in neurotoxicity. The organic forms, particularly methyl mercury, tend to be more toxic than the inorganic forms. The human disasters in Japan and Iraq resulted from the ingestion of organic forms of mercury[3,4].

Animal models of mercury poisoning closely reflect the human situation[5]. Atrophy and loss of the cerebellar

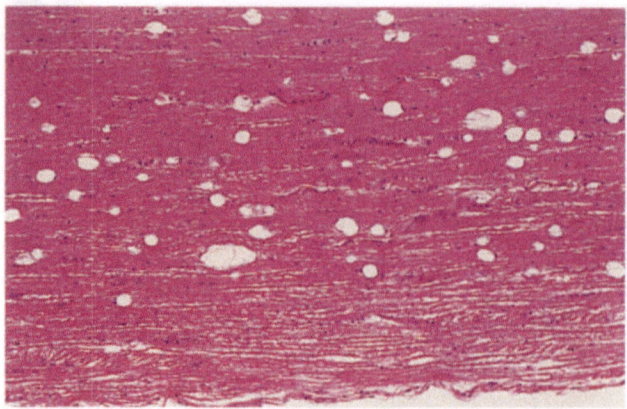

Figure 9.1 Extensive artefactual vacuolation of spinal cord white matter. The 'holes' in this longitudinal section of the cervical region of a beagle dog are the result of inadequate fixation.   H & E

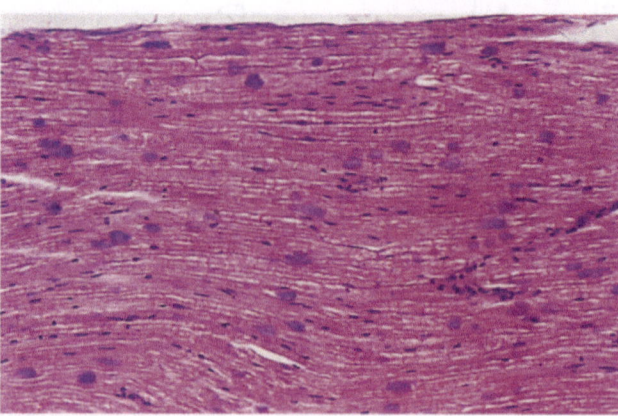

Figure 9.2 Artefactual 'degeneration' of axons in longitudinal section of sciatic nerve of a dog, caused by excessive handling and stretching of specimen at postmortem examination.   H & E

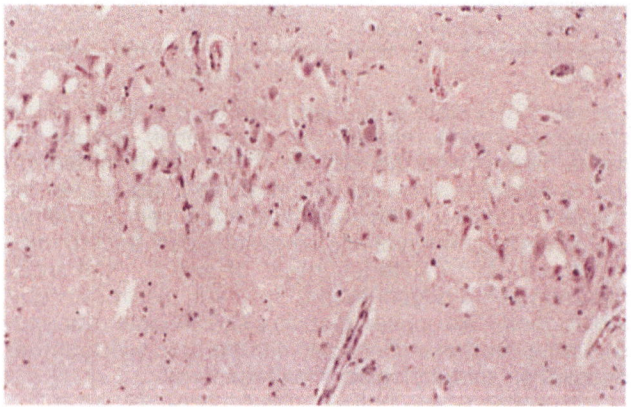

Figure 9.3 Neuronal degeneration and vacuolation in the hippocampus of a dog treated with a novel pharmaceutical preparation. Similar lesions are described following treatment with some hydroxyquinoline derivatives.   H & E

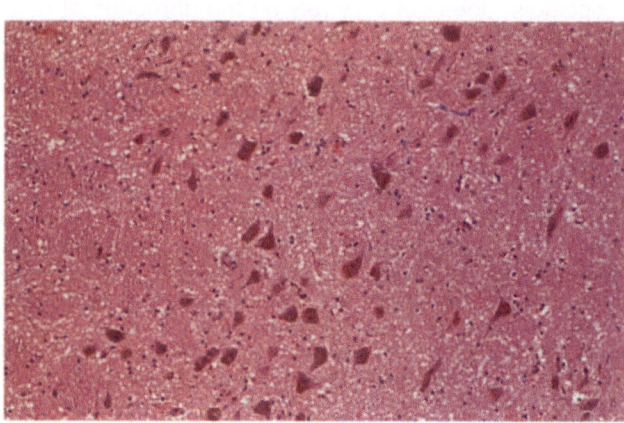

Figure 9.4 Neuronal pigmentation in a rat brain. Numerous neurones throughout the CNS show intense brown staining. The pigment stained positively for lipofuscin. Similar changes are occasionally found in untreated cynomolgus monkeys.   H & E

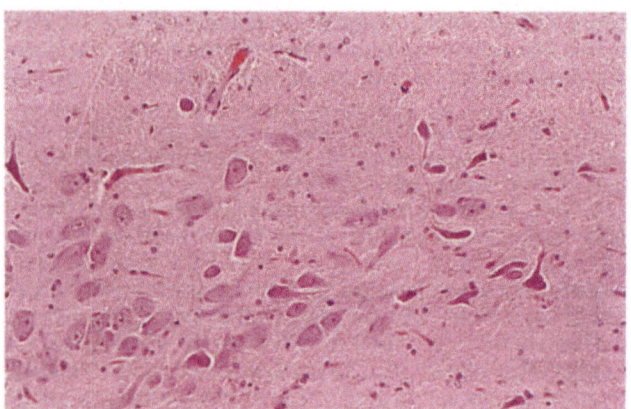

Figure 9.5 Shrunken eosinophilic neurones with pyknotic nuclei in the substantia nigra of a monkey with an induced Parkinsonian-like syndrome. As shrunken eosinophilic neurones can occur artefactually in paraffin preparations[1], careful evaluation is necessary. H & E

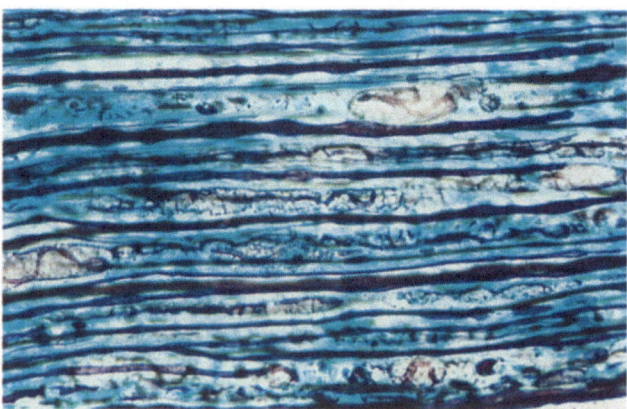

Figure 9.6 Longitudinal section of a tibial nerve of a young rat showing extensive axonal degeneration. The silver impregnation stain shows axonal disruption and fragmentation. Myelin density is reduced in areas of axonal degeneration. This animal had been treated with an organophosphorous compound and exhibited delayed neurotoxicity. Bodian's stain with Luxol fast blue

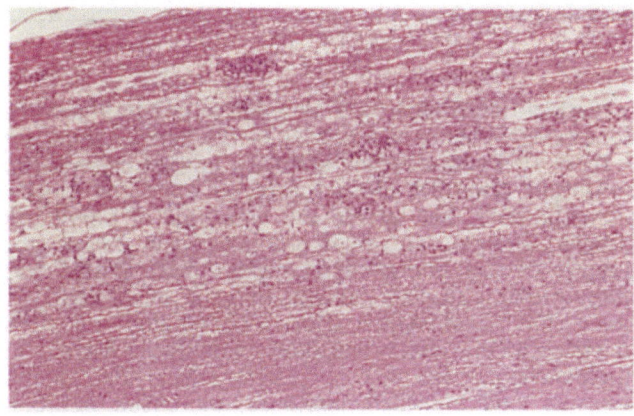

Figure 9.7 Acute delayed neurotoxicity in the hen. Extensive degeneration of spinal cord white matter in a hen, 21 days after a single oral dose of 500 mg kg⁻¹ tri-*ortho*-cresyl phosphate. The longitudinal section shows widespread secondary demyelination and increased cellularity due to reactive glial cells. A few swollen fragmenting axons are discernable.   H & E

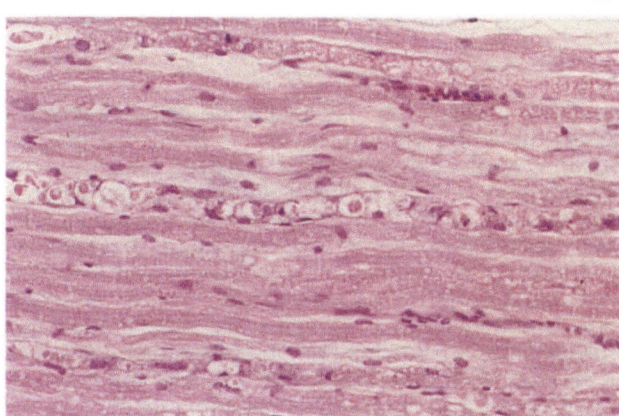

Figure 9.8 Acute delayed neurotoxicity in the hen. This bird received 500 mg kg⁻¹ TOCP orally. Swollen and degenerating axons together with secondary myelin breakdown and digestion chambers are present in this photomicrograph of sciatic nerve.   H & E

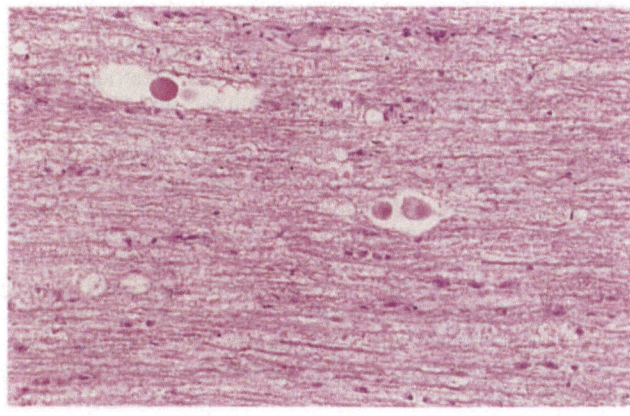

Figure 9.9 Axonal swelling in a longitudinal section of spinal cord of a rat following administration of an organophosphorous compound. Similar degenerative changes are encountered with carbon disulphide and acrylamide and are due to accumulation of neurofilaments.   H & E

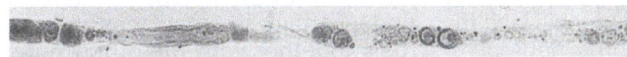

Figure 9.10 Axonal degeneration in the sciatic nerve of a hen treated with TOCP showing myelin fragmentation. Teased nerve fibre preparation

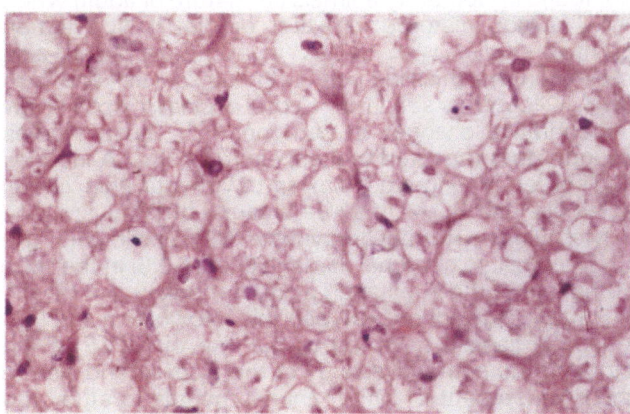

Figure 9.11 Myelinophages in a transverse section of the dorsal columns of the spinal cord of a dog. At least two myelinophages with hyperchromatic nuclei and ill-defined 'fluffy' cytoplasm are present within small digestion chambers. The myelin degeneration in this case is secondary to a distal axonopathy.   H & E

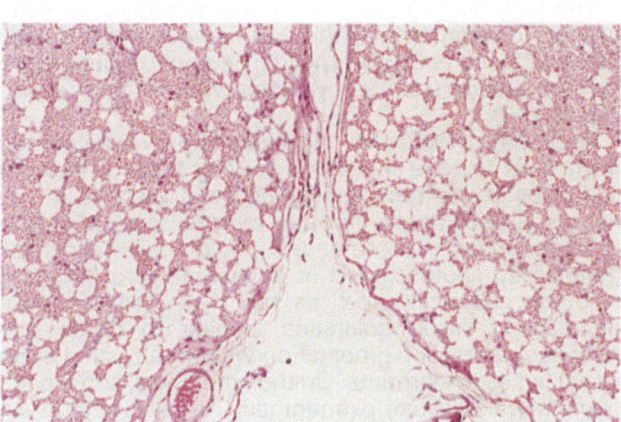

Figure 9.12 Marked spongiform myelinopathy in the spinal cord of a dog treated with hexachlorophene. This transverse section shows the oedematous appearance of the myelin in the ventral columns of the cervical region. Generally, if the toxic insult is not extensive segmental demyelination does not occur and on cessation of treatment recovery may be complete.   H & E

granular cell layer with loss of granule cells are characteristic, the sensory neurones of the dorsal root ganglia appearing particularly sensitive. However, the pattern of degeneration in the dorsal root differs between organic and inorganic mercury. With methyl mercury, early changes show the formation of intracytoplasmic hyaloid material leading to cytoplasmic vacuolation and eventual disintegration of the neurone. With chronic mercuric chloride administration, vacuoles are seen around the neurone prior to its destruction. Ultrastructurally, the vacuoles are found extracellularly between the neurone and satellite cells. Relatively small amounts of mercury can cause signs of neurotoxicity[6]. This may be due in part to the ability of mercury ions to impair the blood–brain barrier and thus to allow circulating mercury direct access to susceptible neurones[7].

Administration of soluble aluminium salts to laboratory animals is associated with neurofibrillary degeneration when the brain aluminium concentrations are greatly elevated[8]. The importance of aluminium remains unknown in the processes associated with neurofibrillary degeneration in humans, including senile dementia of the Alzheimer type.

Trimethyl and tetramethyl tin cause neurone damage and death in selected areas of the brain in rats, gerbils, hamsters and marmosets[9]. This is in contrast to the neuropathological changes brought about by the administration of other organic tin compounds which are characterized principally by oedema of the nervous system[10]. Inorganic lead may, under certain circumstances, induce some neuronal necrosis together with the other more pronounced features (peripheral nerve degeneration and generalized encephalopathy) of lead poisoning[11]. Organic lead compounds induce lesions in the rat nervous system like those caused by trimethyl tin[12]. The susceptibility of the monkey's nervous system to organic lead appears to be variable[13].

High doses of pyridoxine, a water-soluble vitamin (B$_6$), induce neuronal degeneration in dogs in dorsal root and Gasserian ganglia. This sensory neuronopathy first appears histologically as cytoplasmic clearing and vacuolation. The process is followed by cell death and Wallerian-like demyelination[14]. However, there is some evidence that damage to annulo-spiral endings may contribute to the sensory dysfunction seen with B$_6$ hypervitaminosis[15].

The high oxygen requirements of neurones, in comparison to other cells within the nervous system, lead to the induction of a non-specific neuronal degeneration by compounds such as cyanides, which cause anoxia (Figure 9.3).

Neuronal cytoplasmic pigmentation is encountered from time to time in routine toxicity testing. In most instances the pigment deposition is not associated with neurological disorders or other morphological changes. In our experience some neuroleptic drugs which cause generalized lipofuscinosis in animals (Figure 9.4), and coloured chemicals such as hair dyes, which induce generalized tissue coloration, appear to cause pronounced neuronal pigmentation without affecting other nervous tissue elements. On the other hand, some compounds which cause pigmentation are associated with neurological disorders and degenerative change. A well known example is the fragrance compound acetylethyltetramethyl tetralin (AETT) which causes neuronal lipopigmentation and also neuronal degeneration and myelin degradation in rats[16]. It is worthwhile noting that there were no reports of human nervous disorders following exposure to the fragrance up to the time its use was discontinued.

Nuclear neuronopathy is recorded in rats treated with doxorubicin[17] but similar lesions have not been reported in man. This anthracycline antibiotic with antineoplastic properties does not cross the blood–brain and blood–nerve barriers, but affects the neurones of peripheral ganglia. Changes are most pronounced in dorsal root ganglia of the lumbo-sacral region. Histological and ultrastructural studies indicate that the initial changes are in the nuclei which show clearing and reduction of stainable chromatin and finally karyolysis. Advanced nuclear changes are accompanied by perikaryal reactions such as loss of Nissl substance, increased neurofilaments and vacuolation. Wallerian degeneration secondary to loss of sensory neurones is found in spinal dorsal roots, posterior columns and peripheral nerves. Actinomycin D is reported to cause similar nuclear changes in experimental animals following intrathecal administration[18].

Excitatory neurotoxins also cause neuronal damage and death. These can be endogenous neurotransmitters which are released at excitatory synapses and in fact become excitotoxic by excessive stimulation of excitatory receptors on dendrosomal surfaces. Alternatively, administration of exogenous excitatory amino acids can have a similar toxic effect. Initially interest concentrated on the endogenous neurotransmitter glutamate as a potential excitotoxin[19]. Glutamate given parenterally or orally to immature and adult laboratory animals causes acute necrosis of neurones in selected areas of the brain. Such changes are reported in rats, mice, guinea pigs and monkeys. Ultrastructurally, the changes are characterized by swelling of dendrosomal components with degenerative changes in intracellular organelles and clumping of nuclear chromatin. The process rapidly leads to a nuclear pyknosis, cell death and phagocytosis. Pathological changes are not generally detected in the adjacent glia.

Numerous analogues of glutamate have a similar excitotoxic potential and many, particularly kainic acid, are exceedingly potent[20]. Many of these exogenous amino acids may be important in the human clinical situation, e.g. glutamate (as monosodium glutamate, MSG), aspartamine, alanosine and more recently β-N-oxalylamino-L-alanine (BOAA) and β-N-methylamino-L-alanine (L-BMAA). The importance of MSG in human safety assessment is controversial, particularly as brain lesions are not found in laboratory animals (immature or adult) when MSG is administered in water or diet[21]. Non-human primate studies with BOAA, in excitatory amino-acid present in the chickling pea (*Lathyrus sativus*), and with BMAA, found in seeds of *Cycas circinalis*, both show degenerative changes in neurones[22,23]. These studies suggest that repeated oral exposure to BMAA induces a disorder in primates similar to amyotrophic lateral sclerosis, and BOAA may be a cause of lathyrism.

Methylphenyltetrahydropyridine (MPTP) can enter the CNS and cause neuronal damage (Figure 9.5) in the zona compacta of the substantia nigra of monkey and man[24]. The many similarities between this intoxication and Parkinson's disease have led to the use of MPTP in the study of the pathophysiology of the disease and also to the development of MPTP animal models to study the efficacy of potential anti-parkinsonian drugs.

Axonopathies

Axons can extend considerable distances from their cell bodies and this may make them particularly sensitive to toxic damage. In fact, in routine toxicity testing in our laboratories damage to axons is encountered more frequently than neuronal damage. Axonal degeneration is followed by a secondary demyelination (myelinated axons) and chromatolysis of parent neurones. The cardinal signs of demyelination – myelin spheroids and myelinophages – are often indicators of axonal damage and are relatively easy to detect in routine H&E stained preparations. By convention, axonopathies are classified according to location of the lesion in the nervous system (central, peripheral) and to location in the axon (proximal, distal).

Proximal axonopathies are rare. Administration of β,β′-iminodiproprionitrile (IDPN) to rodents causes neurological disorders, impairment of slow axonal transport and proximal axonal swellings of anterior horn and brain stem neurones. These axonal swellings are composed of accumulations of 10 nm neurofilaments. Sequelae include atrophy of the distal axon, secondary demyelination, remyelination of proximal portions and extensive gliosis[25]. Similarities between the axonal changes in rodents with IDPN and the changes in various forms of human motor neurone disease may help elucidate the human disease. Proximal axonopathies are also recorded in experimental allergic neuritis (EAN) and occasionally in experimental allergic encephalomyelitis (EAE)[26]. In these examples, axonal damage is probably secondary to demyelination but there is a possibility that primary axonal damage may occur[27].

Distal axonopathies, mostly central-peripheral, are not uncommon in toxicology. The list of compounds which cause distal axonopathies in man and laboratory animals is now extensive[28] and includes pharmaceutical compounds (such as chloramphenicol, diphenylhydantoin, disulphiram, isoniazid, nitrofurantoin, vincristine) and chemicals (such as acrylide monomer, carbon disulphide, n-hexane, methyl-n-butyl ketone, organophosphates (Figure 9.6), arsenic, zinc pyridinethione, polychlorinated biphenyls and thallium salts). With these compounds, axonal lesions tend to occur multifocally in the distal portions of long and large diameter axons both in the PNS and the CNS.

Morphological lesions can usually be detected prior to the onset of neurological manifestations of intoxication. This relatively late development of clinical signs justifies the use of the term 'delayed neurotoxicity'. Cessation of treatment allows a certain amount of recovery both neurologically and histopathologically. During the course of treatment with these compounds, the histological picture in the CNS and PNS is similar. Silver impregnation stains show disruption, fragmentation and distortion of axons, some of which may be more argyrophilic than normal. Variation in thickness of axons may be noted together with the presence of large axon balls. Ultrastructurally, the picture is variable and depends on the neurotoxic compound, i.e. neurofilamentous accumulation with carbon disulphide, hexacarbon and acrylamide poisoning, disruption of neurotubules by vincristine, mitochondrial swelling by thallium and accumulation of tubulovesicular arrays derived from smooth endoplasmic reticulum by organophosphates and zinc pyridinethione[29].

In toxicology, delayed neurotoxicity is encountered in the routine assays of organophosphorous compounds in the hen[30]. The hen has been used for many years in these assays as a suitable and sensitive animal model for the detection of acute delayed neurotoxicity (Figures 9.7, 9.8 and 9.9). Teased nerve preparations can be a valuable technique for the demonstration of axonal degeneration (Figure 9.10). In order to assess the risks associated with all human 'in-life' situations, particularly repeated ingestion of small amounts of organo-

phosphorous insecticides, chronic hen studies with small daily doses are now required[31]. A useful adjunct to these standard tests is the neurotoxic esterase assay[32]. Axonopathic organophosphates react with neurotoxic esterase early in the intoxication process and cause an inhibition of the esterase which can be measured in brain, spinal cord and peripheral nerve.

A distal, but solely central, axonopathy is seen in beagle dogs following the administration of high doses of clioquinol (5-chloro-7-iodo-8-hydroxyquinoline)[33]. Axonal and secondary myelin changes are detected mainly in the cervical region of the spinal cord in the dorsal, ventro-medial and lateral columns (Figure 9.11). Optic tract degenerative changes are also detected.

Myelinopathies

Primary myelinopathies are encountered in routine toxicology but are, in our experience, less frequent than axonopathies. Compound-induced myelin damage is usually easily identifiable in standard H&E sections due to myelin vacuolation and the classical signs of myelin degradation. Long myelinated axons appear more susceptible to damage than shorter ones.

The pathogenesis of myelin change is usually described as direct action on myelin (hexachlorophene, isoniazid, triethyl tin, AETT) or secondary to interference of Schwann cell or oligodendrocyte metabolism (buckthorn toxin, tellurium). The former group of compounds produces a spongiform myelinopathy characterized by the splitting of lamellae at the intraperiod line and vacuolation and oedema of the myelin sheaths[34]. Histologically, myelin oedema can be quite marked and widespread (Figure 9.12). With this type of myelinopathy, peripheral nerves are generally less susceptible to damage. If the insult is not severe, clinical and morphological recovery without segmental demyelination may ensue. Other compounds are also known to produce spongiform myelinopathies but are associated with oligodendroglial degeneration, i.e. Cuprizone (*bis*-cyclohexane oxalyldihydrazone), ethidium bromide, actinomycin D, diphtheria toxin, inorganic lead and perhexiline maleate[34,35].

Compounds which interfere with the metabolism of the myelin producing cells, such as tellurium and buckthorn toxin, show myelin vacuolation followed by widespread segmental demyelination with some secondary axonal degeneration. Changes may be more pronounced in peripheral nerves than in the CNS, and ultrastructurally in the PNS cytoplasmic changes in Schwann cells appear before myelin sheath changes[35].

Experimental allergic encephalomyelitis (EAE) is an autoimmune inflammatory disease of the nervous system which can be induced by injection of whole CNS or myelin basic protein in complete Freund's adjuvant[26]. The histological changes consist of perivascular inflammation, mainly in the brain stem and spinal cord (Figure 9.13). In the acute form, demyelination is not prominent. However, a chronic relapsing–remitting form of EAE may be induced in guinea pigs and rats, which shows extensive demyelination. This form has some features in common with multiple sclerosis (MS) in man and is therefore used as a model to study MS pathogenesis and in screening immunosuppressive drugs for efficacy in such autoimmune conditions. We have observed inflammatory lesions in the peripheral nerves of rats treated with a novel immunostimulant (Figures 9.14 and 9.15).

Vacuolar encephalopathy (Figure 9.16) is a spontaneous age-related change in the white matter of rat

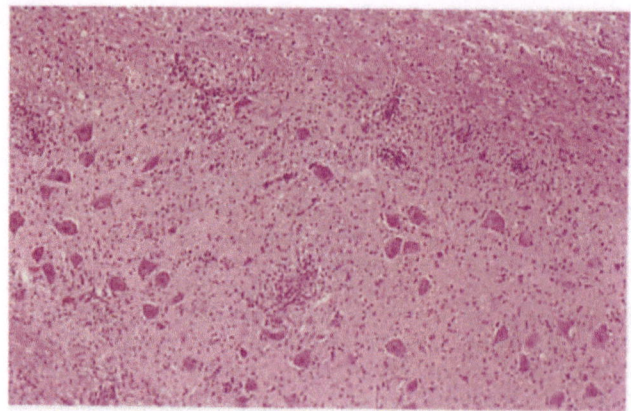

Figure 9.13 Experimental allergic encephalomyelitis (EAE) in a Lewis rat. Photomicrograph of a longitudinal section of the spinal cord showing widespread but focally intense infiltrations of mononuclear cells in both white and grey matter.   H & E

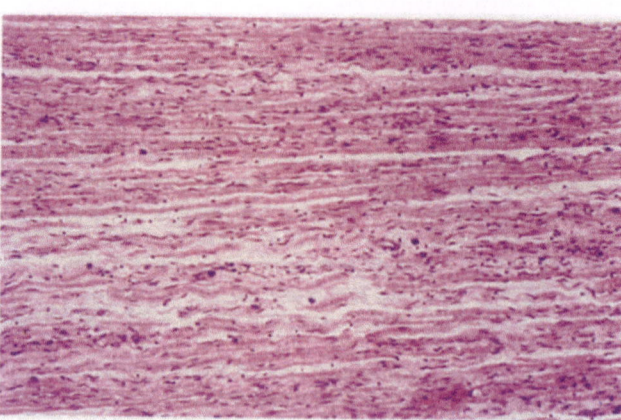

Figure 9.14 Peripheral neuritis in a rat treated with a novel immunostimulant. This longitudinal preparation of the sciatic nerve shows a diffuse increase in interfibre cellularity.   H & E

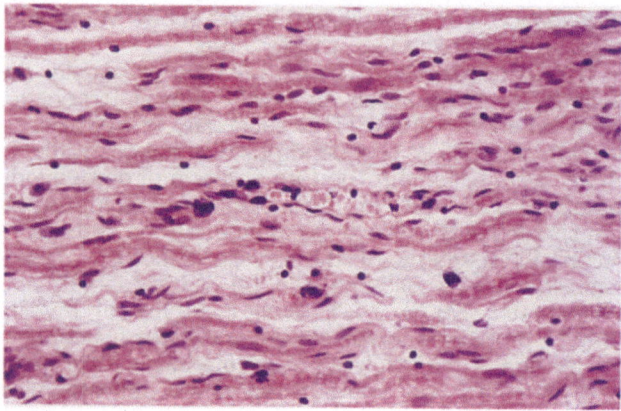

Figure 9.15 Peripheral neuritis in a rat. A higher magnification of Figure 9.14 showing evidence of myelin breakdown in addition to the cellular infiltrate.   H & E

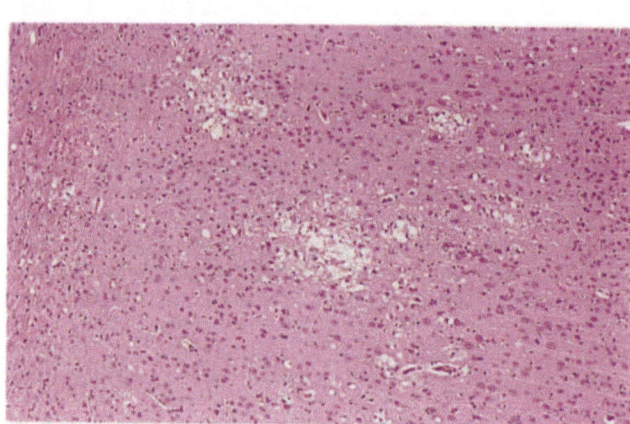

Figure 9.16 Vacuolar encephalopathy in midbrain in an aged rat. Focal vacuolation and oedema without inflammatory reaction occurs spontaneously in the white matter of various areas, particularly midbrain and cerebellum[36]. The significance of the lesion remains unknown but we have encountered an increase in both incidence and severity following long-term treatment with differing types of compounds.   H & E

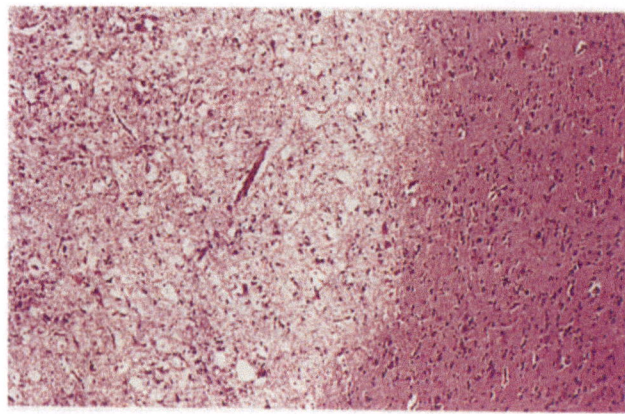

Figure 9.17 A large circumscribed area of vacuolation around a brain-stem nucleus in a rhesus monkey treated with a potential male antifertility compound[40]. The vacuoles are confined to the astrocyte population, and on cessation of treatment recovery appears to be complete both morphologically and clinically. Degenerative changes are not detected in this photomicrograph.   H & E

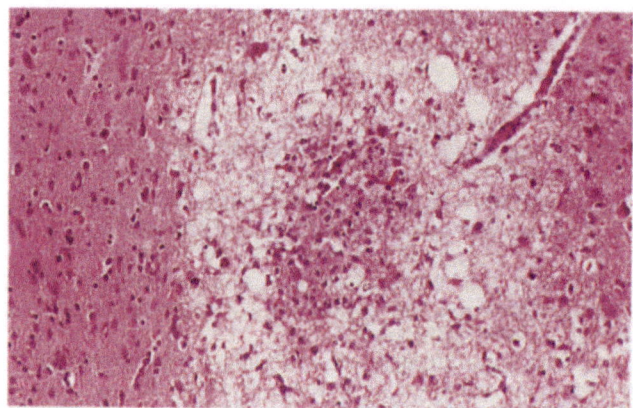

Figure 9.18 Circumscribed area of vacuolation and gliosis in a rhesus monkey treated with a potential male antifertility compound. This section is from a similar location to Figure 9.17 but here this monkey was treated for a longer period. Astrocytic changes are prominent but mild secondary neuronal and myelin degeneration are now present.   H & E

brains[36]. The aetiology and significance of the change remains unknown. Histologically, the vacuoles do not incite any reaction. However, chronic treatment with a variety of compounds has, in our laboratories, increased the incidence and severity of such changes.

Routinely prepared paraffin sections of brain may show numerous round spaces in white matter filled with an amorphous eosinophilic or basophilic material. These mucocytes (mucocoeles) are found in most laboratory animal species and are particularly prominent in the optic tract[37]. Their origin is obscure (perhaps artefactual) and they may mimic pathological change but from the toxicological pathology standpoint they are unimportant.

Gliopathies

Glial cell changes are uncommon in toxicology. Astrocytic changes and oligodendroglial changes are described in association with segmental demyelination. Toxic damage to astrocytes rarely occurs alone and is often accompanied by changes in other glial and nervous system elements. Methionine sulphoximine (MSO), an experimental epileptic agent, induces in rats and mice massive accumulations of glycogen granules in astrocytic bodies and processes[38]. As methionine can prevent the convulsions, and the ultrastructural changes are similar to those seen when ammonia plasma levels are raised, it is probable that MSO exerts its effect by inhibiting the enzyme glutamine synthetase.

Several compounds cause glial changes, particularly astrocytic swelling in laboratory rodents and primates. Histologically, the lesions appear as circumscribed regions of vacuolation in routine paraffin sections, usually within specific nuclei of the brain stem and spinal cord. Ultrastructurally, astrocytes contain extremely large vacuoles and possibly also enlarged mitochondria. The most severely affected astrocytes are found in perivascular locations. With prolonged treatment, secondary (or late primary) glial and neuronal changes become evident. Such compounds include potential male antifertility drugs, 6-chloro-6-deoxyglucose and 1-amino-3-chloro-2-propanol hydrochloride[39,40] (Figures 9.17 and 9.18), antiprotozoal nitroimidazoles[13,41] thiamine deficiency[42], monoamine oxidase inhibitors[43] and nicotinamide deficiency induced by 6-aminonicotinamide[44,45].

Vasculopathies

Toxic vasculopathies of the nervous system are rarely encountered in routine toxicity testing. However, minor or subtle alterations of the blood–brain and blood–nerve barriers may not be detectable by routine investigative methods and in this 'leaky' situation toxins may enter the nervous system. The stroke-prone hypertensive rat[46], which is used in pharmaceutical research as a model for human 'stroke', provides the toxicological pathologist with an opportunity to study CNS changes following thrombosis and haemorrhage.

Cadmium and inorganic lead cause vascular endothelial damage in the nervous system of adult rodents. The neonatal rat appears particularly susceptible to toxic vascular damage. Haemolytic encephalopathies of the neonate are recorded following administration of salts of indium, terbium, thallium and mercury and also of triethyl tin[47].

Choroid plexus vacuolation

Extensive vacuolation of the choroid plexus is reported in rats and monkeys, but not dogs, treated with the piperidine-ring drug disobutamide[48]. A high drug concentration is found in the choroid plexus of rats and monkeys but not in dogs. The demonstration of increased acid phosphatase activity suggests a lysosomal origin. Similar changes are reported with chloroquine, triparanol and chlorcyclizine[48].

References

1. Hirano, A., Iwata, M., Lhena, J. F. and Matsui, T. (1980). *Color Atlas of Pathology of the Nervous System.* (New York, Tokyo: Igaku-Shoin)
2. Spencer, P. S. and Schaumburg, H. H. (1980). Classification of neurotoxic disease: a morphological approach. In Spencer, P. S. and Schaumburg, H. H. (eds.) *Experimental and Clinical Neurotoxicology.* pp. 92–99. (Baltimore and London: Williams and Wilkins)
3. Tsubaki, T. (1975). Studies on the health effects of alkyl mercury in Japan. (Japan: Environmental Agency)
4. Bakir, F., Damluji, S. F., Amin-Zaki, L., Murtadha, M., Khalidi, A., Al-Rawi, N. Y., Tikriti, S., Dhahir, H. I., Clarkson, T. W., Smith, J. C. and Doherty, R. A. (1973). Methyl mercury poisoning in Iraq. *Science,* **181**, 230–241
5. Chang, L. W. (1980). Mercury. In Spencer, P. S. and Schaumburg, H. H. (eds.) *Experimental and Clinical Neurotoxicology.* pp. 508–526. (Baltimore and London: Williams and Wilkins)
6. Chang, L. W. (1977). Pathological effects of mercury – a review. *Environ. Res.,* **14**, 329–393
7. Chang, L. W. and Hartman, M. A. (1972). Blood–brain barrier dysfunction in experimental mercury intoxication. *Acta Neuropathol.,* **21**, 179–184
8. Crapper, D. R., Krishnan, S. S. and Quittkat, S. (1976). Aluminium, neurofibrillary degeneration and Alzheimer's disease. *Brain,* **99**, 67–79
9. Aldridge, W. N., Brown, A. W., Brierley, J. B., Verschoyle, R. D. and Street, B. W. (1981). Brain damage due to trimethyl tin compounds. *Lancet,* **2**, 692–693
10. Watanabe, I. (1980). Organo-tins (triethyl tin). In Spencer, P. S. and Schaumburg, H. H. (eds.) *Experimental and Clinical Neurotoxicology.* pp. 545–557. (Baltimore and London: Williams and Wilkins)
11. Krigman, M. R., Bouldin, T. W. and Mushak, P. (1980). Lead. In Spencer, P. S. and Schaumburg, H. H. (eds.) *Experimental and Clinical Neurotoxicology.* pp. 490–507. (Baltimore and London: Williams and Wilkins)
12. Seawright, A. A., Brown, A. W., Aldridge, W. N., Verschoyle, R. D. and Street, B. W. (1980). Neuropathological changes caused by trialkyl lead compounds in the rat. In Holmstedt, B., Lauwerys, R., Mercier, M. and Roberfroid, M. (eds.) *Mechanisms of Toxicity and Hazard Evaluation.* pp. 71–74. (Amsterdam: Elsevier, North Holland Biomedical Press)
13. Heywood, R., James, R. W. and Prentice, D. E. (1980). Chemical toxicity in the central nervous system of laboratory animals. In Clifford Rose, F. and Behan, P. O. (eds.) *Animal Models of Neurological Disease* pp. 317–321. (Bath: Pitman Medical Ltd)
14. Krinke, G., Schaumburg, H. H., Spencer, P. S., Suter, J., Thomann, P. and Hess, R. (1980). Pyridoxine megavitaminosis produces degeneration of peripheral sensory neurones (sensory neuronopathy) in the dog. *Neurotoxicology,* **2**, 13–24
15. Krinke, G., Heid, J., Bittiger, H. and Hess, R. (1978). Sensory denervation of the plantar lumbrical muscle spindles in pyridoxine neuropathy. *Acta Neuropathol. (Berl.),* **43**, 213–216
16. Spencer, P. S., Sterman, A. B., Horoupain, D., Bischoff, M. and Foster, G. (1979). Neurotoxic changes in rats exposed to the fragrance compound acetylethyltetramethyl tetralin. *Neurotoxicology,* **1**, 221–237
17. Cho, E. S. (1977). Toxic effects of adriamycin on the ganglia of the peripheral nervous system – a neuropathological study. *J. Neuropathol. Exp. Neurol.,* **36**, 907
18. Schwartz, H. S., Sternberg, S. S. and Phillips, F. S. (1968). Selective cytotoxicity of actinomycin in mammals. In Walksman, S. A. (ed.) *Actinomycin.* (New York: Wiley-Interscience Publishers)
19. Olney, J. W. (1980). Excitotoxic mechanisms of neurotoxicity. In Spencer, P. S. and Schaumberg, H. H. (eds.) *Experimental and Clinical Neurotoxicology.* pp. 272–294. (Baltimore and London: Williams and Wilkins)
20. Olney, J. W. and Price, M. T. (1978). Excitotoxic amino acids as neuroendocrine probes. In McGeer, E. G., Olney, J. W. and

McGeer, P. L. (eds.) *Kainic Acid as a Tool in Neurobiology*. pp. 239–264. (New York: Raven Press)

21. Heywood, R. and Worden, A. N. (1979). In Filer, L. J., Garaltini, S., Kare, M. R., Reynolds, W. A. and Wurtman, R. S. (eds.) *Glutamic Acid*. p. 203. (New York: Raven Press)

22. Spencer, P. S., Roy, D. N., Ludolph, A., Hugon, J., Dwivedi, M. P. and Schaumburg, H. H. (1986). Lathyrism – evidence for role of the neuroexcitatory amino-acid, BOAA. *Lancet*, **2**, 1066–1067

23. Spencer, P. S., Nunn, P., Hugon, J., Ludolph, A., Ross, S., Roy, D., Schaumburg, H. H. and Soiefer, A. (1986). Primate motor neurone disorders induced by chemically related excitatory neurotoxins isolated from Guamanian cycad and Indian chickling pea. *Muscle Nerve*, **9**, 108

24. Burns, R. S., Markey, S. P., Phillips, J. M. and Chiueh, C. C. (1984). The neurotoxicity of 1-methyl-4-phenyl-1,2,3,6-tetrahydropyridine in the monkey and man. *Can. J. Neurol. Sci.*, **11**, 166–168

25. Griffin, J. W. and Price, D. L. (1980). Proximal axonopathies induced by toxic chemicals. In Spencer, P. S. and Schaumburg, H. H. (eds.) *Experimental and Clinical Toxicology*. pp. 161–178. (Baltimore and London: Williams and Wilkins)

26. Raine, C. S. (1984). Biology of disease. Analysis of autoimmune demyelination: its impact upon multiple sclerosis. *Lab. Invest.*, **50**, 608–635

27. Brown, A., McFarlin, D. E. and Raine, C. S. (1982). Chronologic neuropathology of relapsing experimental allergic encephalomyelitis in the mouse. *Lab. Invest.*, **46**, 171–185

28. Schaumburg, H. H. and Spencer, P. S. (1979). Toxic models of certain disorders of the nervous system – a teaching monograph. *Neurotoxicology*, **1**, 209–220

29. Asbury, A. K. and Brown, M. J. (1980). The evolution of structural changes in distal axonopathies. In Spencer, P. S. and Schaumburg, M. D. (eds.) *Experimental and Clinical Neuropathology*. pp. 179–192. (Baltimore and London: Williams and Wilkins)

30. Crammer, J. M. and Hixson, E. J. (eds.) (1984). *Delayed Neurotoxicity*. Proceedings of the workshop presented June 27–30, 1982, at the University of Illinois at Urbana-Champagne. (Little Rock, Arkansas: Intox Press)

31. Prentice, D. E. and Majeed, S. K. (1983). A subchronic study (90 day) using multiple dose levels of tri-*ortho*-cresyl-phosphate (TOCP): Some neuropathological observations in the domestic hen. *Neurotoxicology*, **4**, 277–282

32. Johnson, M. K. and Richardson, R. J. (1983). Biochemical endpoints: Neurotoxic esterase assay. *Neurotoxicology*, **4**, 311–320

33. Worden, A. N., Heywood, R., Prentice, D. E., Chesterman, H., Skerrett, K. and Thomann, P. E. (1978). Clioquinol toxicity in the dog. *Toxicology*, **9**, 227–238

34. Powell, H. C., Myers, R. R. and Lampert, P. W. (1980). Edema in neurotoxic injury. In Spencer, P. S. and Schaumburg, H. H. (eds.) *Experimental and Clinical Neurotoxicology*. pp. 118–138. (Baltimore and London: Williams and Wilkins)

35. Cammer, W. (1980). Toxic demyelination: biochemical studies and hypothetical mechanisms. In Spencer, P. S. and Schaumburg, H. H. (eds.) *Experimental and Clinical Neurotoxicology*. pp. 239–256. (Baltimore and London: Williams and Wilkins)

36. Burek, J. D. (1978). *Pathology of the Aging Rat*. pp. 139–141. (Florida: CRC Press Inc.)

37. Sanders, L. Z. and Rubin, L. F. (1975). *Ophthalmic Pathology of Animals*. p. 156 (Basel: Karger)

38. Guttierrez, J. A. and Norenberg, M. D. (1977). Ultrastructural study of methionine sulfoximine-induced Alzheimer type II astrocytes. *Am. J. Pathol.*, **86**, 285

39. Jacobs, J. M. and Ford, W. C. L. (1981). The neurotoxicity and antifertility properties of 6-chloro-6-deoxyglucose in the mouse. *Neurotoxicology*, **2**, 405–417

40. Heywood, R., Sortwell, R. J. and Prentice, D. E. (1978). The toxicity of 1-amino-3-chloro-2-propanol hydrochloride (CL88,236) in the rhesus monkey. *Toxicology*, **9**, 219–225

41. Rogulja, P. V., Kovac, W. and Schmid, H. (1973). Metranidazol-Encephalopathie der Ratte. *Acta Neuropathol.*, **25**, 36–45

42. Robertson, D. M., Wasan, S. M. and Skinner, D. B. (1968). Ultrastructural features of early brain stem lesions of thiamine deficient rats. *Am. J. Pathol.*, **52**, 1081–1098

43. Palmer, A. L. and Noel, P. R. (1963). Neuropathological effects of prolonged administration of some hydrazine monoaminooxidase inhibitors in dogs. *J. Pathol. Bacteriol.*, **86**, 463–476

44. Schneider, H. and Cervos-Navarro, J. (1974). Acute gliopathy in spinal cord and brain stem induced by 6-aminonicotinamide. *Acta Neuropathol.*, **27**, 11–23

45. O'Sullivan, B. M. and Blakemore, W. F. (1980). Acute nicotinamide deficiency in the pig induced by 6-aminonicotinamide. *Vet. Pathol.*, **17**, 748–758

46. Rascher, W., Clough, D. and Garten, D. (eds.) (1981). *Hypertensive Mechanisms. The spontaneously hypertensive rat as a model to study human hypertension*. Proceedings of 4th International Symposium on Rats with Spontaneous Hypertension and Related Studies. Heidelberg, 1981. (Stuttgart and New York: Schattauer Verlag)

47. Jacobs, J. M. (1980). Vascular permeability and neural injury. In Spencer, P. S. and Schaumburg, H. H. (eds.) *Experimental and Clinical Neurotoxicity*. pp. 102–117. (Baltimore and London: Williams and Wilkins)

48. Koizumi, H., Watanabe, M., Numata, H., Sakai, T. and Morishita, H. (1986). Species differences in vacuolation of the choroid plexus induced by the piperidine-ring drug disobutamide in the rat, dog and monkey. *Toxicol. Appl. Pharmacol.*, **84**, 125–148

Eye

Adverse ocular side-effects in man, due to therapeutic agents, have received considerable attention and are widely reported[1-4]. The profusion of reports may give a disproportionate view of selective organ toxicity. In practice histopathologically detectable changes in the eyes are relatively rare in animal safety evaluation studies, although there is evidence of species variation and susceptibility, probably resulting from differences in metabolism[4].

Toxic changes may be induced in ocular tissues following both direct exposure and systemic administration. Agents involved include airborne pollutants, industrial (occupational) chemicals and pharmaceuticals[3-5]. It should also be noted that in addition to obvious toxic effects other reactions may be encountered which are undesirable manifestations of the pharmacological action of the compound[1,6].

Ocular tissues illustrate several unusual or unique histological and physiological features. These include: a large avascular lens composed of a high concentration of specific protein; a complex, metabolically active neural structure, the retina, which contains photosensitive pigments; the aqueous humour, an isolated CSF-like system containing choroid plexus analogues, the ciliary bodies; a blood–aqueous barrier similar to the blood–brain barrier; a high concentration of melanin – a potent electron acceptor with strong binding properties; and a transparent avascular window, the cornea which is maintained in a state of hydration. Consequently, a wide range of toxic changes may be encountered in ocular tissues which reflect these diverse specialized features (Table 10.1).

For simplicity, the lesions encountered in the eye and accessory tissues will be described with reference to their anatomical location. In addition to the eye itself, induced lesions of the ocular adnexa, including the lachrymal, harderian and meibomian glands are also included in this chapter.

Cornea

Induced changes in the cornea generally result from topical damage and are often associated with conjuctival lesions. The changes predominantly affect the epithelia and are characterized by degrees of inflammatory cell infiltration, oedema, epithelial hyperplasia, keratinization, epithelial erosion, ulceration and even perforation.

Systemic administration rarely induces selective changes in the cornea[5]. In order for lesions to be produced in this avascular tissue, entry of a toxic compound into the aqueous humour or its excretion in the tears is necessary[4]. However, in a few cases corneal lesions are

Table 10.1 Induced ocular lesions

Cornea
  Keratitis/conjuctivitis
  Epithelial ulceration
  Neovascularization
  Epithelial vacuolation

Lachrymal glands
  Keratoconjunctivitis sicca

Harderian glands
  Atrophy

Uveal tract
  Uveitis
  Vacuolation of ciliary body

Lens
  Cataract

Retina
  Atrophy
  Vascular changes
  Degeneration of tapetum lucidum

Optic disc and nerve
  Papilloedema
  Optic disc swelling

induced by the systemic route (Figures 10.1–10.3). The corneal epithelium has a high concentration of acetylcholine. Dietary administration of an anticholinesterase pesticide causes keratitis and purulent conjunctivitis with corneal ulceration[7]. In addition, denervation produces corneal lesions in rats [8] and stimulation of the sensory innervation has a trophic effect on the cornea. Administration of narcotic analgesics, which prevents closing of the eyelids, induces corneal opacities[4]. The administration of 1-α-acetylmethadol to rats causes epithelial thickening with hyalinization of the basement membrane and vascularization[8]. Excessive evaporation of corneal surface moisture during sedation is probably responsible for the development of the lesion; moistening of the cornea with saline reduces the severity.

The cornea is avascular, but following damage and in certain nutritional deficiencies, neovascularization takes place (Figure 10.4). Vascularization in the cornea indicates a long standing keratitis[9]. It is believed that leukocytes are an important mediating factor in the development of neovascularization[10].

Anterior synechias may develop in association with corneal inflammatory lesions, e.g. chronic administration of sulphonylurea derivatives to rats[11].

Pigmentation of the cornea results from both topical and systemic administration of silver[12]. Treatment of rats with silver lactate in the drinking water results in deposition of silver grains in the lysosomes and base-

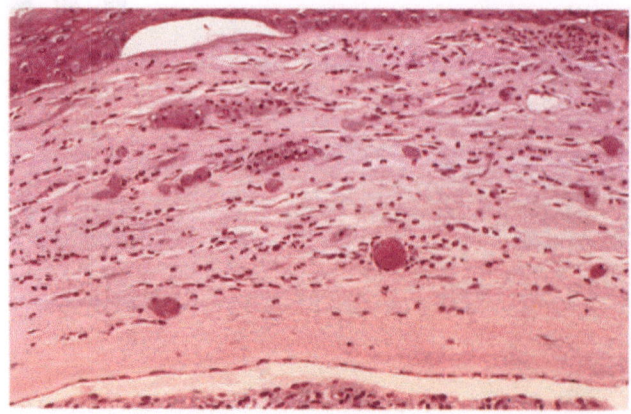

Figure 10.1 Keratitis in a rat eye following systemic administration of a novel pharmaceutical. The epithelium and underlying stroma are infiltrated by neutrophils. H & E

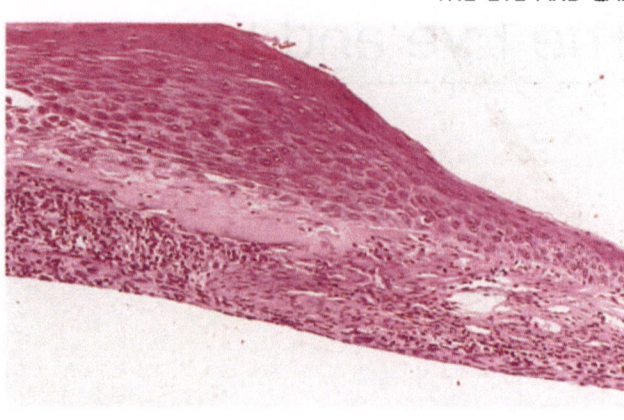

Figure 10.2 Keratitis in a rat induced by systemic administration of a novel pharmaceutical. The epithelium is hyperplasic. Note the subepithelial inflammatory cell infiltration. H & E

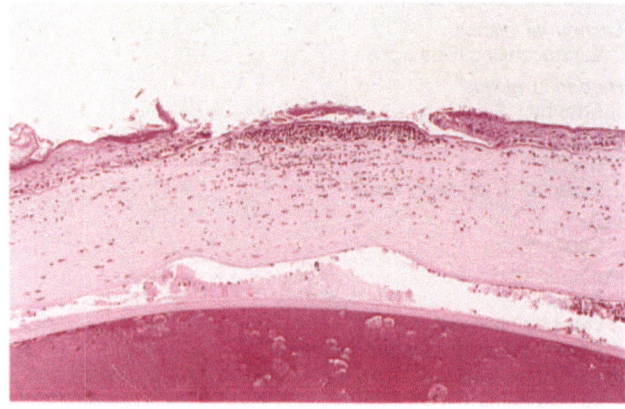

Figure 10.3 Focal corneal epithelial ulceration in a rat treated systemically with a novel agrochemical. The underlying stroma shows inflammatory infiltration. Note the early fibre swelling in the anterior portion of the lens. H & E

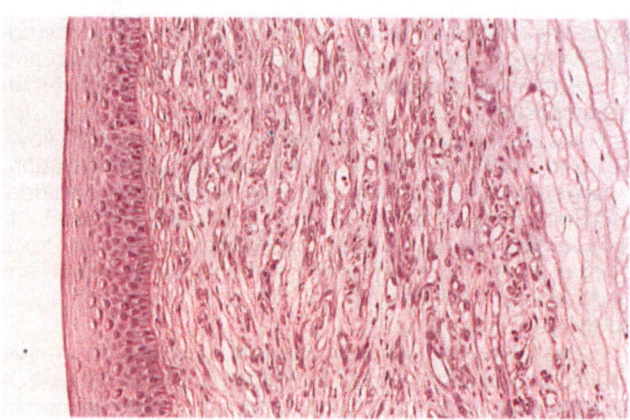

Figure 10.4 Vascularization of the cornea of a dog treated with a novel antispasmodic compound. The lesion developed following keratoconjunctivitis sicca and is characterized by neovascularization and fibroblasts in the stroma. Little inflammatory cell involvement is present and the overlying epithelium appears normal. H & E

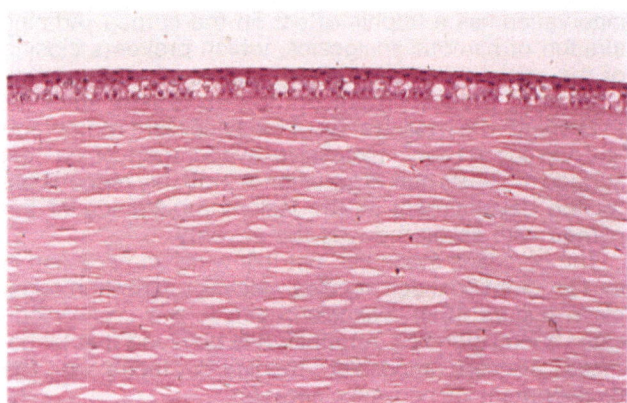

Figure 10.5 Vacuolation in the corneal epithelium of a monkey treated with an antineoplastic agent. The vacuoles are confined to the basal cells. H & E

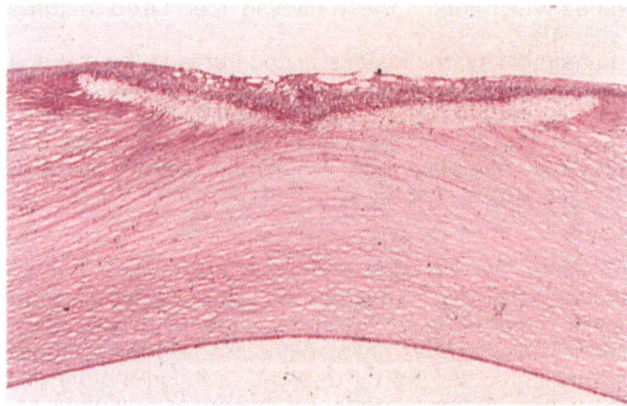

Figure 10.6 Cornea of a dog with keratoconjuntivitis sicca induced by a novel antispasmodic compound. The central depressed area probably represents the site of previous ulceration in which the epithelium has repaired. Note the pale area of degeneration beneath the epithelium. H & E

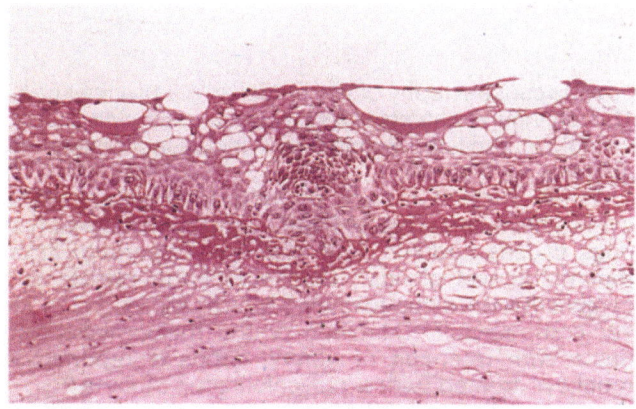

Figure 10.7 Higher magnification of Figure 10.6 to show vesiculation of the superficial epithelial cells and subepithelial swelling and necrosis. H & E

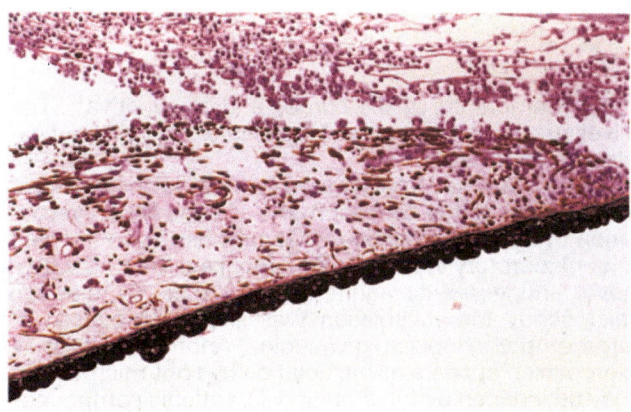

Figure 10.8 Uveitis which developed in the eye of a baboon following the systemic administration of an antiviral agent. Polymorphs and histiocytes are present in the anterior chamber and iris. H & E

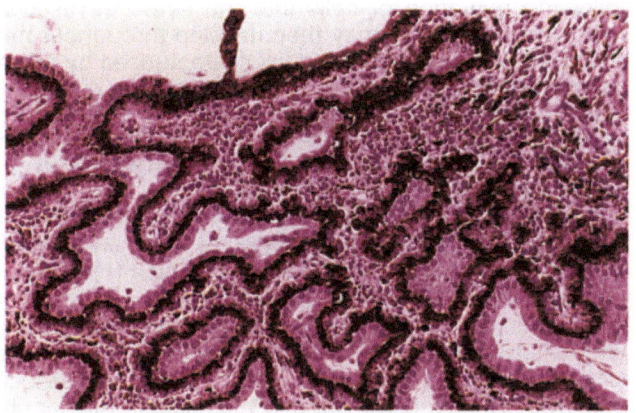

Figure 10.9 Uveitis in the eye of a baboon from same study as Figure 10.8. Inflammatory cell infiltration of the ciliary body. H & E

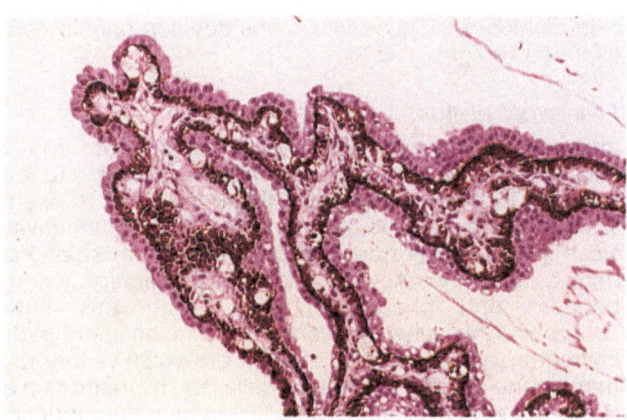

Figure 10.10 Minimal vacuolation of the ciliary body from a monkey treated with a novel anticancer agent. The vacuolation is largely confined to the pigmented cells. H & E

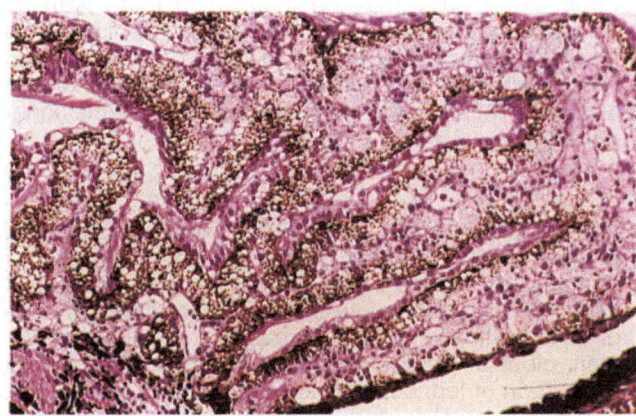

Figure 10.11 Pronounced vacuolation and swelling of the ciliary body of a monkey. The animal is from the same study as Figure 10.10 but received a higher dose of the test compound. H & E

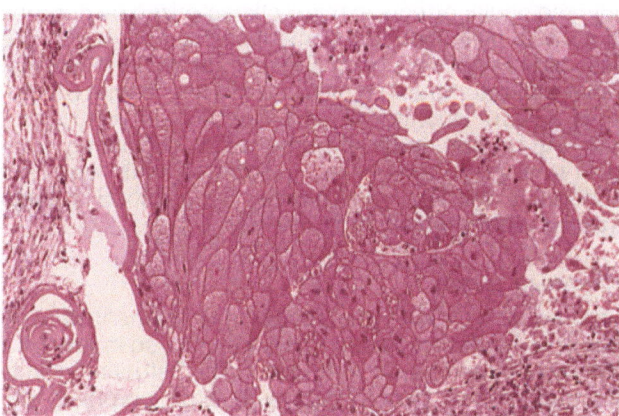

Figure 10.12 Severe swelling, rupture and degeneration of the lenticular fibres from the eye of a rat treated systemically with a novel herbicide. H & E

ment membranes of the cornea and conjunctiva[12]. The silver grains remain, even 15 months after discontinuation of treatment.

Other, less severe, induced corneal lesions involve vacuolation or the development of inclusions. Vacuolation of basal corneal epithelial cells has been induced in our laboratory in cynomolgus monkeys treated with a novel antineoplastic agent (Figure 10.5). By electron microscopy the vacuolation was shown to consist of large empty cytoplasmic vacuoles. Another form of lesion, which appears as vacuolation by light microscopy, may be induced by the amphiphilic, cationic compounds such as chlorphentermine and iprindole[13]. Ultrastructurally, these vacuoles are in fact multilamellar bodies typical of systemic phospholipidosis. The bodies are found in keratocytes, basal epithelial cells and endothelial cells. In comparison with chlorphentermine, multilamellar bodies are infrequently found with chloroquine, except when applied topically to the cornea[13].

Cytoplasmic inclusions, in the form of small yellow globules, develop in dogs treated orally with the fungicide dichloran[14]. These inclusions develop only in dogs exposed to light.

Lachrymal glands

Inflammatory and degenerative changes in the cornea and conjunctiva may also develop secondary to decreased lachrymal secretion (Figures 10.4, 10.6 and 10.7). This syndrome, known as keratoconjunctivitis sicca (KCS), is reported in dogs treated with sulphonamides, 5-aminosalicylic acid, antichlolinergic compounds[4] and phenazopyridine[15]. With this latter compound the lachrymal glands illustrate an adenopathy characterized by the presence of brownish-yellow pigment in the glandular epithelial cells, and by infiltration of inflammatory cells and some cell degeneration. Induced KCS is rarely encountered in rats but treatment with clonidine reduces lachrymal secretion and is associated with intracellular oedema and disorganization of the basal cell layer[16]. The lesions are diminished by pretreatment with phentolamine. KCS is also reported in dogs treated with an antispasmodic compound[17].

Administration of β-adrenergic receptor blocking agents induces a condition commonly referred to as 'dry eye', in dogs[4]. One such compound, practolol, induces adverse ocular effects in man[5] characterized by degrees of corneal ulceration and corneal perforation, which are associated with atrophic changes in the lachrymal gland. However, attempts to reproduce this lesion with proctolol in several laboratory animal species are unsuccessful[4]. An autoimmune disease with circulating anti-lachrymal gland antibodies, associated with lymphoid nodules in the lachrymal glands, is described in dogs treated with a β-blocker[18].

Harderian glands

Chromodacryorrhea – the secretion of pigmented tears from the harderian glands – may be induced in rats by a variety of experimental methods[19]. The harderian glands illustrate sexual dimorphism with large porphyrin deposits in female rats, mice and hamsters but not in males. Castration and the administration of oestrogens increases the porphyrin content of these glands in males[20]. Chromodacryorrhea may also be seen in inhalation studies with irritant compounds. The intravascular injection of acetylcholine or cholinergic drugs rapidly induces this condition[19] which can be prevented by atropine. In our experience some anticholinesterase com-

pounds cause atrophy of the harderian gland acinar cells. This change is characterized by decreased cytoplasmic vacuolation, dilated lumina and increased single cell necrosis.

A few isolated reports of induced changes in the eyelids have been traced. Paracetamol administration to dogs causes oedema, with decreased secretion from the meibomian glands[4]. Oedema of the eyelids and conjunctiva develops following topical application of silver compounds[12]. Dilatation of the meibomian gland ducts with retention of keratin debris is reported in monkeys treated with a polychlorinated biphenyl[21].

Uveal tract

The iris may be sensitive to chemical insult because of its high degree of vascularization[5]. However, in our experience and that of others[4], morphological changes are rarely detected in laboratory animals. Uveitis may be caused by chemicals or by immunological mechanisms[5]. The eye is unusual in normally having no resident lymphoid population and an immune response may only occur following migration of cells into the eye. Perivascular lymphoid aggregates may then develop throughout the choroid and ciliary body. Uveitis, characterized by acute inflammatory cell infiltrations in the anterior chamber, with neutrophil and lymphocytic infiltrations of the iris and the ciliary body (Figures 10.8 and 10.9), has been found in our laboratories in baboons treated with an antiviral agent[4].

Extensive cytoplasmic vacuolation of both the pigmented and non-pigmented cells of the cynomolgus monkey ciliary body (Figures 10.10 and 10.11) has been recorded in our laboratory following administration of a novel anticancer agent. In severe cases the vacuolation was associated with decreased pigmentation and the ciliary body appeared swollen. The condition was associated with widespread systemic vacuolation. Similar changes are described in rabbits following intraperitoneal administration of 6-aminonicotinamide[22].

Proliferation of melanin-containing cells in the iris may be induced in a strain of hooded rat treated neonatally with urethane [23] but similar lesions are not detected in Wistar rats. The change is due to the presence of melanin-containing cells between the two epithelia of the iris.

Thickening of the basement membrane between cells of the ciliary body may be induced in dogs with an anticholinesterase pesticide[7]. Systemic administration of silver lactate to rats results in silver grain deposition in the ciliary body and iris[12]. The silver is located on the basement membranes and intracellularly in the inner 'pigmented' epithelial cells.

Lens

The lens is essentially of simple uniform structure and because of this displays only a restricted number of reactions to induced injury. In practice most lenticular changes are degenerative (cataract formation). This involves opacification of the lens due to swelling, vacuolation, globular fragmentation, degeneration, rupture or liquefaction of lenticular fibres (Figures 10.3 and 10.12). In severe lenticular degeneration, distortion, collapse and calcification may take place (Figure 10.13). As the lens is avascular and the capsule is impermeable to inflammatory cells, inflammation does not usually play a role in lenticular degeneration. However, if the capsule becomes ruptured, neutrophils may become involved (Figure 10.14) and subsequently fibrosis may also develop. In some cases the histopathological interpretation of lenticular degeneration requires a note of caution since autolytic changes are virtually indistinguishable from genuine cataract.

Many types and classes of compound induce cataracts in laboratory animals and there is some evidence of species differences. Only a few examples are given in this chapter as cataract induction is comprehensively reviewed elsewhere[24]. Administration of high levels of galactose, xylose and glucose readily induce cataracts in rats[24]. The mechanism responsible for the cataractogenic action of these sugars is believed to involve formation of sugar alcohols and osmotic stress on the lens fibres. The influx of water necessary to maintain osmotic equilibrium causes swelling and rupture of the lenticular fibres. An association between cataract development and diabetes can be shown experimentally in alloxan-treated rats[25] and rhesus monkeys[24].

Lenticular changes develop secondary to induced keratitis and iridocyclitis in rats treated with 4-diethylaminoethoxy-α-ethyl-benzhydrol[26]. The first detectable change involves epithelial proliferation along the anterior lens capsule. Nuclear pyknosis and fibre degeneration subsequently occur. The pesticide mirex induces cataracts in suckling rats when administered postpartum[27]. This study describes and illustrates the sequential changes which occur during the development of lenticular degeneration. Cataracts are described in dogs treated with a styryl hexahydroindolinol, a hypolipidaemic agent[28]. Other hypolipidaemic agents, triparanol and AY-9944, also induce lenticular changes[24,28]. It is suggested that sudanophilic material, detected in the lens fibres, may represent a manifestation of phospholipidosis[4], and lamellar inclusion bodies are present in lenticular fibres of rats treated with AY-9944[29]. Other compounds which induce cataracts are diquat, dimethylsulphoxide and parachlorophenylalanine[4,24].

Retina

Atrophy or degeneration (Figure 10.15) is the most common of the induced retinopathies and is reported, usually in rats, following administration of a wide range of pharmaceuticals and industrial chemicals.

Albino rats' eyes are particulary sensitive to light and progressive retinal degeneration is repeatedly described in these nocturnal animals when exposed to fluorescent light at high and continuous intensities[4,9,30]. Pigmented rats are less susceptible to the development of light-induced retinopathy. In albino rats and mice the lesion involves thinning of the outer nuclear and plexiform layers with their subsequent loss. Severe retinal lesions may be induced within 40 hours in rats exposed to typical fluorescent illumination[6]. Light intensity is so critical in the development of this retinopathy that the position of the cage within a battery (and therefore the light intensity to which the animals are exposed) plays an important role[31]. Mice caged at the top of a battery develop a high incidence of retinal atrophy, whereas at the lower positions the lesion is rarely encountered.

Light may also have a potentiating effect on some compound-induced retinopathies[6]. In our experience potentiation of induced retinal lesions is difficult to achieve in the non-albino rat. Light-induced damage is also recorded in rhesus and cynomolgus monkeys[32]. A detailed standardized method of histological grading is described in this report and it is suggested that the system could be applied to toxic retinopathies in order to establish dose-response relationships[32].

The effects of experimental photocoagulation on the retina is demonstrable in dogs[33]. Lesions range from necrosis of all retinal layers with degeneration of the pigment epithelium to those which also involve the choroidal vessels, melanophores and the inner sclera.

An example of differential species susceptibility is provided by 1,5-di(p-aminophenoxy)pentane dihydrochloride. This compound produces retinopathies in cats, monkey and dog but not in mouse, rat, rabbit or guinea pig[34]. The sequence of retinal changes involves degeneration of the pigment epithelium, retinal arcade formation, loss of photoreceptors, intraretinal pigment deposition and loss of the outer nuclear layer. Retinal lesions are reported in dogs and albino rats treated with a 4-aminoquinoline compound – amopyroquin[35]. In rats the outer nuclear layer is lost with distortion of the rods and cones. The lesion in dogs consists of focal accumulation of pigment at the choroid–retinal junction with atrophy of the overlying rods and cones.

The sequence of morphological changes which occurs during photoreceptor damage, and which leads to retinal atrophy, is described following administration of propionic acid derivatives to rats[36]. Initially, nuclei from the outer nuclear layer appear to migrate focally into the photoreceptor layer; these migratory nuclei form crescent shaped domes, or arcades around remaining photoreceptors; the arcades then develop into rosettes. With the electron microscope, these remnants are found to be composed of fragmented photoreceptors with disrupted lamellar discs.

The retina is a highly complex structure in terms of its physiology, histology and metabolism; it is therefore not surprising that some compounds induce changes in specific retinal cells or layers. A few compounds induce changes in the ganglion cells. The phenothiazines, which cause a systemic lipofuscinosis, also result in pigmentation of the ganglion cells in the dog[6]. This pigmentation is not associated with degenerative changes in the ganglion cells and is unrelated to the development of a toxic retinopathy described elsewhere[6]. Hexachlorophene treatment causes a slightly decreased number of ganglion cells in rats. As this compound also induces severe degenerative changes in the optic nerve it is likely that the retinal changes are a secondary event[37]. Multilamellar inclusion bodies are recorded in the ganglion cells of rats treated with chloroquine[4,5]. Degeneration and necrosis of ganglion cells is reported following intraperitoneal injection of β-N-oxalyl-L-α,β-diaminopropionic acid to immature mice or sodium 1-glutamate to newborn rats[5].

Treatment with 6-aminonicotinamide produces vacuolation of the outer plexiform layer in rabbits[22]. We have observed vacuolation of the inner nuclear layer in monkeys treated with a novel antineoplastic agent (Figure 10.16). The lesion was associated with a widespread vacuolation of many tissues and organs.

Changes in the retinal pigment epithelium are detected with several compounds and many are believed to be related to the phagocytic function of these cells. With induced disintegration of the outer segment of the photoreceptors, the pigment epithelial cells phagocytose the debris. Examples include: chloroquine, phenothiazines, hexachlorophene and lead[6,36]. In dogs and cats treated with phenothiazines and in vitamin E deficient dogs, this phagocytic activity leads to pigmentation of the epithelial cells[6]. Following chloroquine administration markedly increased amounts of PAS positive substance and of free sulphydryl groups are detected in swollen pigment epithelial cells[5,6]. Some compounds which induce systemic phospholipidosis, such as triparanol, cause the development of multilamellar inclusion bodies in the pigment epithelial cells[4].

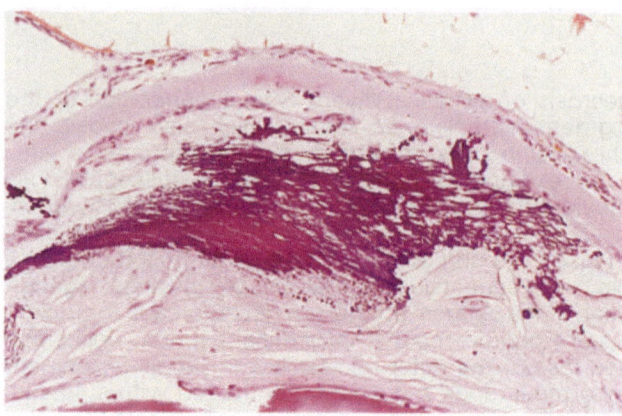

Figure 10.13 Severe lenticular disruption with calcification in the eye of a rat treated systemically with a herbicide.   H & E

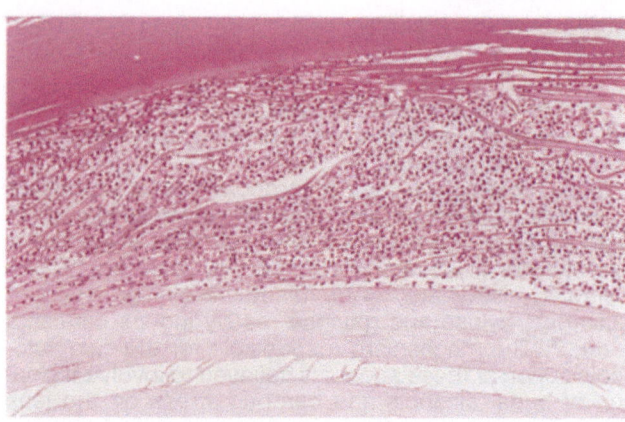

Figure 10.14 Pronounced inflammatory cell infiltration in the lens of a rat following systemic treatment with a novel agrochemical. Rupture of the lens capsule has allowed entrance of inflammatory cells.   H & E

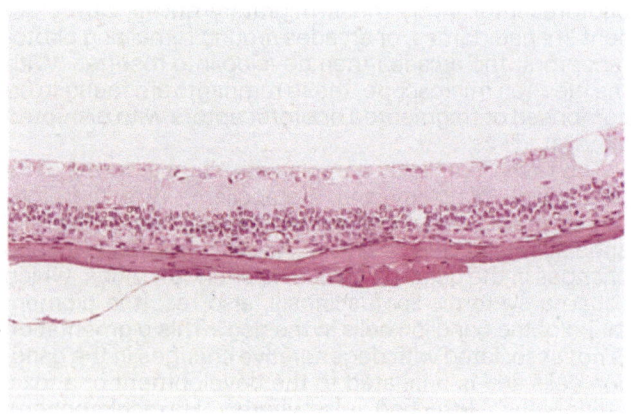

Figure 10.15 Retinal atrophy in a rat treated with an industrial chemical. The outer nuclear and photoreceptor layers have been lost.   H & E

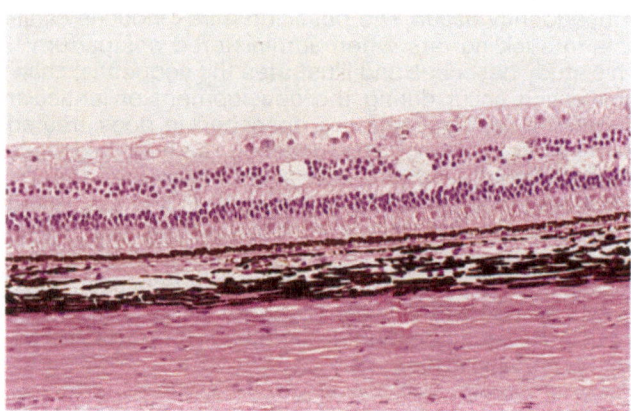

Figure 10.16 Vacuolar degeneration in the retina, primarily affecting the inner nuclear layer, from a monkey treated with an antineoplastic compound.   H & E

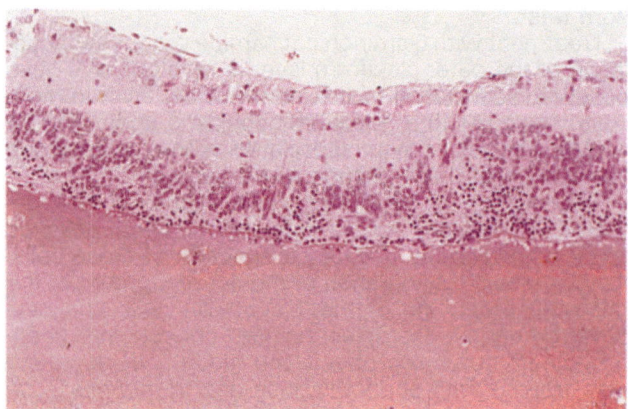

Figure 10.17 Subretinal haemorrhage in a rat given a vitamin K deficient diet. The retina is detached with atrophy of the outer nuclear and photoreceptor layers.   H & E

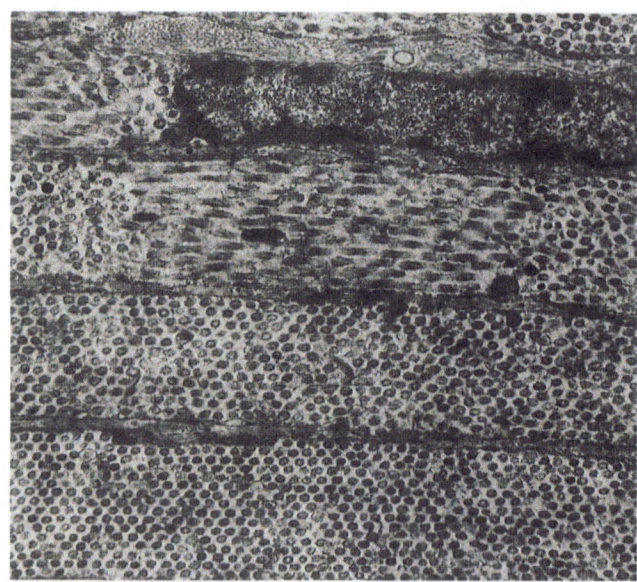

Figure 10.18 Tapetum lucidum from the eye of a normal dog. The tapetal cells are packed with electron-dense rods. Electron micrograph

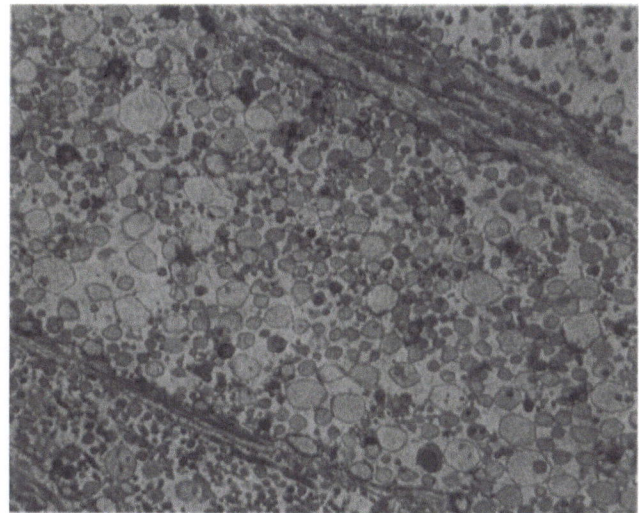

Figure 10.19 Degeneration of the tapetum lucidum from the eye of a dog treated with a compound with chelating properties. The cells are swollen and the orderly arrangement has been lost. Rods are decreased in number and swollen. Compare with Figure 10.18. Electron micrograph

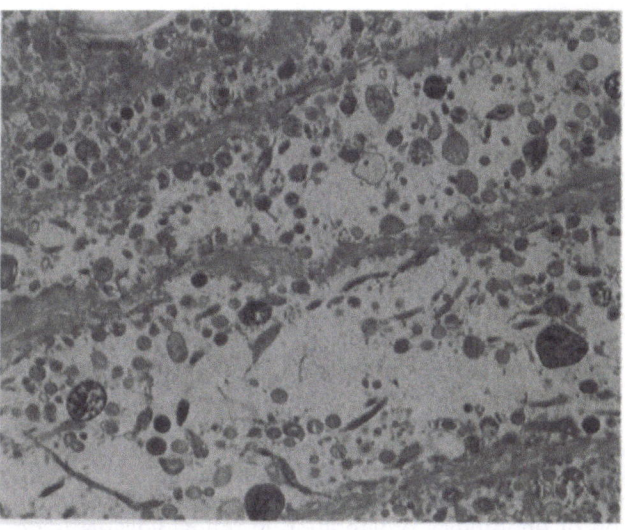

Figure 10.20 Severe degeneration of the tapetum lucidum of the eye of a dog treated with a chelating compound. Marked loss of rods. Compare with Figure 10.18. Electron micrograph

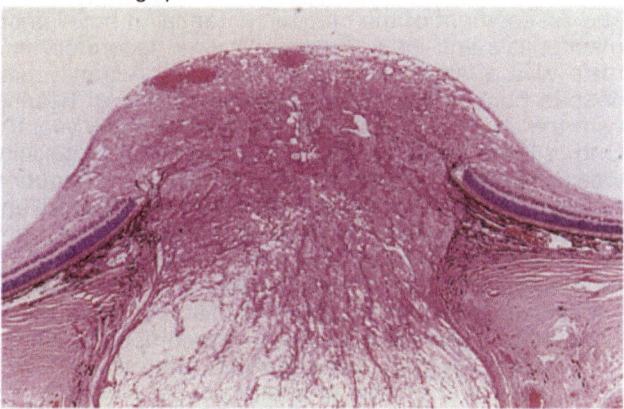

Figure 10.21 Papilloedema which developed in the eye of a dog following systemic administration of a novel agrochemical. The swollen optic disc projects into the posterior chamber

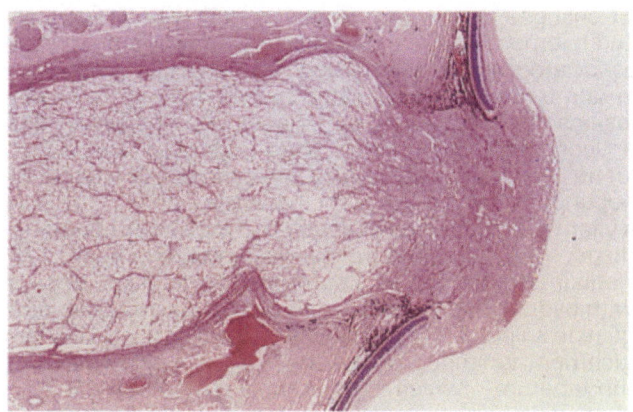

Figure 10.22 Papilloedema in the eye of a dog from the same study as Figure 10.21. The protrusion of the optic disc into the posterior chamber is associated with severe swelling, oedema and vacuolation of the optic nerve.   H & E

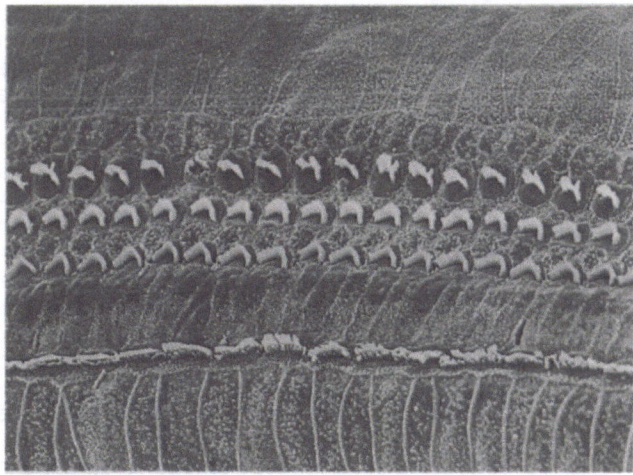

Figure 10.23 Cochlea from an untreated guinea pig showing the three rows of outer hair cells and one row of inner hair cells. A single hair cell has been lost in the outer hair cells. The high degree of organization and regimentation of the hair cells shown in this photomicrograph is a consistent finding in untreated animals. Scanning electron micrograph

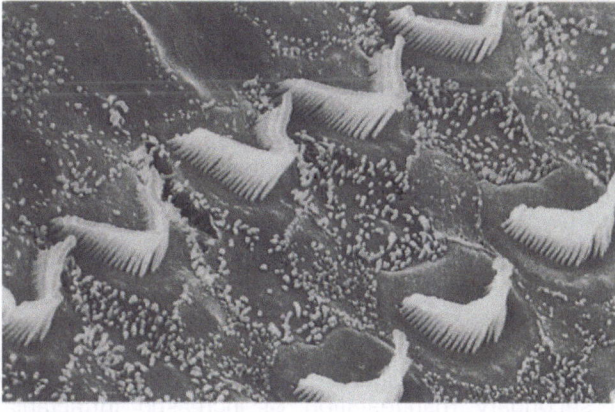

Figure 10.24 High power magnification of the outer hair cells from the cochlea of an untreated guinea pig. Note the consistent, highly organized arrangement of the stereocilia of individual hair cells. Scanning electron micrograph

Necrosis of retinal pigment epithelial cells is described in rabbits treated with sodium fluoride[38].

Chorioretinal vascular disease with subsequent retinal degeneration is known to occur in man, secondary to diabetes mellitus. The condition involves microvascular changes with loss of retinal pericytes, thickening of capillary basal lamina, capillary aneurysms and retinal haemorrhages. A retinal angiopathy is described in rats following a single oral dose of β,β'-iminodipropionitrile[39]. The condition is characterized by deposition of PAS positive material and endothelial proliferation in the arteries. Retinal micro-aneurysms are not found frequently in laboratory animals with induced diabetes[39]. However, a form of retinopathy is described in dogs with alloxan or somatotrophin-induced diabetes[39] and in alloxan-induced diabetes in rhesus monkeys[25]. A method for the induction of endothelial proliferation in retinal vessels is described[39], which involves administration of β-aminopropionitrile to alloxan-diabetic rats. The substitution of β,β'-iminodipropionitrile in this model results in the development of capillary micro-aneurysms[39].

Spontaneously hypertensive rats show retinal vascular changes which may be associated with aneurysms and haemorrhage[30,40]. Ocular haemorrhage is described associated with a generalized haemorrhagic syndrome, in rats treated with butylated hydroxytoluene[41]. Similar lesions are induced by other compounds such as the anticoagulant dicoumarol. Both butylated hydroxytoluene and dicoumarol reduce the activities of vitamin K-dependent clotting factors[42]. In our laboratory, rats given a vitamin K-deficient diet developed intra-ocular haemorrhage, with secondary retinal disruption (Figure 10.17). Retinal detachment is also described in dogs treated with hydroxypyridinethione, an imidazo-quinazoline, and quinine sulphate[43,44]. With hydroxypyridinethione the detachment is limited to the area of the retina overlying the tapetum – which is necrotic and associated with a choroiditis. With the imidazo-quinazoline the detachment is due to haemorrhage between the rods and cones and the pigment epithelium. Little work to determine the degree of reversibility of retinal detachments has been reported but it is suggested that, in some cases, such retinas may re-attach[44].

Changes are reported in the dog tapetum lucidum with several compounds including: ethambutol, dithizone, hydroxypyridinethione and diethyldithiocarbamate[5,43]. The tapetal cells contain a high concentration of zinc, probably as a zinc–cysteine complex or as zinc cysteinate[45]. All these administered compounds are believed to have chelating properties and it is probable that they chelate the zinc with consequent disruption of the rods within the tapetal cells (Figures 10.18–10.20). In some cases, e.g. with dithizone, severe tapetal damage leads to an associated secondary retinopathy[5,43]. With an imidazo-quinaline, retinal lesions can be induced in normal but not in red-eyed beagles which lack a tapetum lucidum[43].

Optic disc and nerve

Papilloedema, in which the optic disc projects into the posterior chamber (Figures 10.21 and 10.22), is generally a secondary manifestation of increased intracranial pressure[46]. This condition is reported in man with ethylene glycol, vitamin A, lead and nalidixic acid[2,3]. In primates, but not lower mammals, papilloedema can be induced with methanol. This differential species susceptibility is due to differences in metabolism. Papilloedema is described in monkeys with trimethyl tin acetate and in dogs with a salicylanilide[4]. With the latter, there is increased CSF pressure and secondary retinal detachment develops[9].

A lesion similar to papilloedema, in that it also involves protrusion of the head of the optic nerve into the vitreous humour, is generally referred to as optic disc swelling[47]. Administration of β,β'-iminodipropionitrile systemically to guinea pigs, dogs and primates produces swelling of the optic disc which regresses after cessation of treatment. Ultrastructural investigation shows that the swelling is due to massive accumulation of neurofilaments[47].

In man, optic nerve damage has been reported with more than 40 compounds[3]. Optic nerve axonopathies, with secondary demyelination, develop in dogs treated with ethylthioemeton, or cloquinol and in monkeys with ethambutol[4]. The optic nerves of dogs treated with organophosphate pesticides show reduced numbers of axons, thin myelin sheaths and in some cases glial cell proliferation[48].

Ear

The assessment of the ototoxic potential of novel pharmaceuticals and industrial chemicals in laboratory animals was a largely neglected field until recent years, despite human clinical observations of loss of hearing with the aminoglycosides and quinine for many years[49]. One of the reasons for the lack of interest in ototoxicity was undoubtedly the technical difficulties of routine examination of the inner ear. However, with the advent of the scanning electron microscope and plastic 1 μm sectioning techniques, it is now possible to perform morphological examinations in routine toxicity studies. Consequently, a considerable expansion of the number of reported investigations has been recorded recently[50–52]. However, despite this enhanced interest, relatively few chemical or groups of chemicals have been identified as having ototoxic potential. The best known of these are the aminoglycoside antibiotics. Other ototoxic compounds include quinine, the salicylates and furosemide[49,50]. The morphological examination of the inner ear is relatively unusual in that it is the only tissue in routine toxicity studies for which the scanning electron microscope has become the method of choice. With this technique the whole organ of Corti may be examined, enabling both qualitative (Figures 10.23–10.30) and quantitative assessment of hair cell damage[52,53].

Although several laboratory animal species are used as models for ototoxicity the guinea pig is the most common because of the relative ease with which the cochlea may be dissected and removed. Three possible sites of morphologically detectable damage have been identified: the hair cells; the cochlear ganglion with nerve fibres; and the stria vascularis[50].

As a class, aminoglycoside antibiotics show differences in terms of their ototoxic potential[50]. A comparison of the ototoxic effects of amikacin, gentamicin, tobramycin and netilmicin in guinea pigs shows the latter induce less severe lesions[52]. There is also evidence of differential susceptibility amongst the hair cells. With netilmicin, for example, the outer hair cells in the basal turns are more severely and consistently damaged but this differential susceptibility decreased towards the apex. The inner hair cells show greatest damage in the apical turns[52]. In rats, kanamycin induces extensive damage to the organ of Corti with the outer hair cells more severely affected than the inner ones[54]. The initial changes include distortion of the cuticular plates and irregular and fused stereocilia. The hair cells appear to be lost in a sequential manner, commencing at the base of the cochlea with

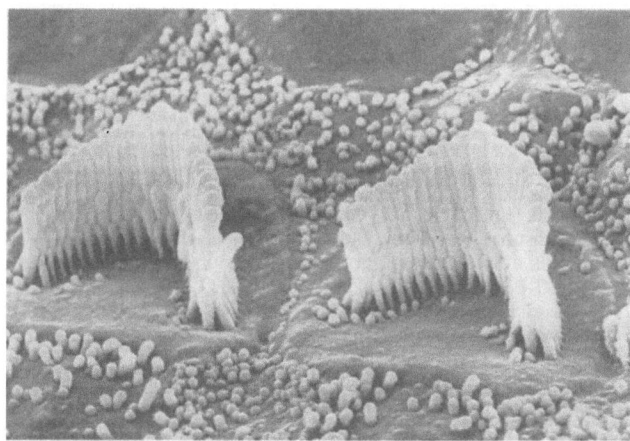

Figure 10.25 Higher power photomicrograph showing the characteristic normal arrangement of the different length stereocilia of outer hair cells of the guinea pig cochlea. Scanning electron micrograph

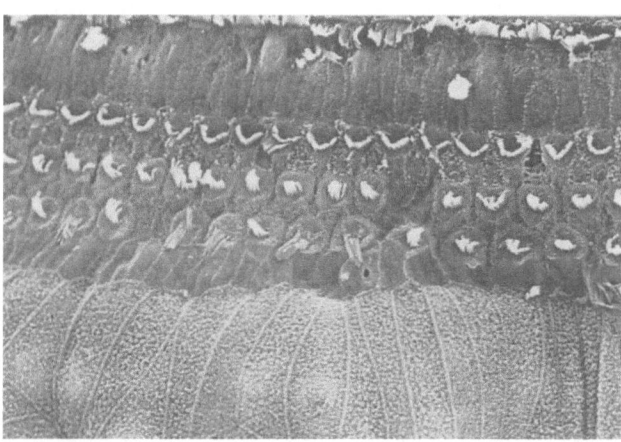

Figure 10.26 Low power photomicrograph showing damage to the outer hair cells of a cochlea from a guinea pig treated with gentamicin. Scanning electron micrograph

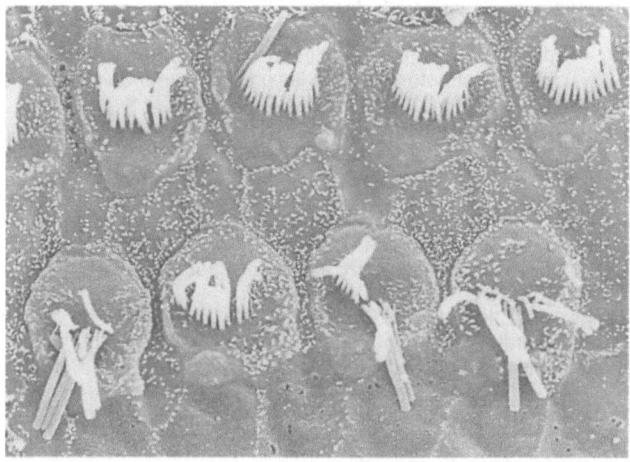

Figure 10.27 Early damage to the outer hair cells of the cochlea of a guinea pig treated with a novel pharmaceutical. There is disruption of the usual organization and orientation of the stereocilia. Scanning electron micrograph

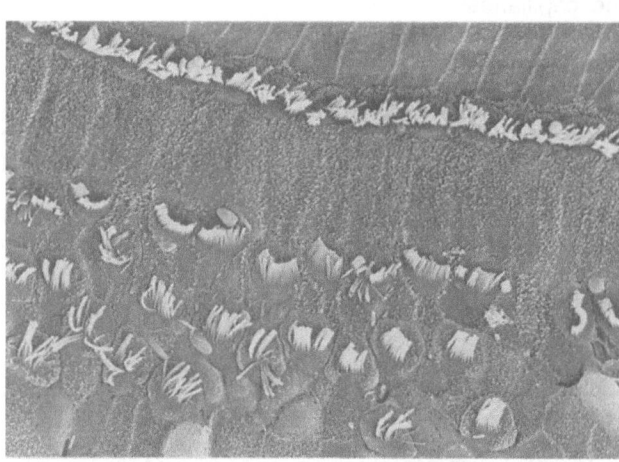

Figure 10.28 Focal loss of stereocilia from the outer hair cells of the cochlea from a gentamicin-treated guinea pig. Remaining hair cells show disruption, collapse and clumping of stereocilia. Scanning electron micrograph

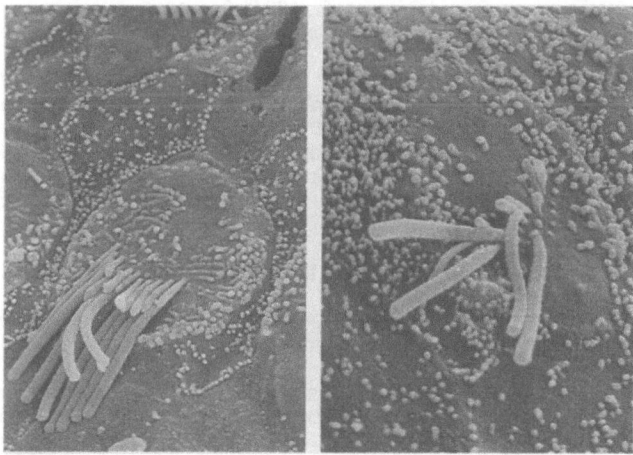

Figure 10.29 Higher power photomicrograph showing normal, collapsed and damaged stereocilia from the outer hair cells of a gentamicin-treated guinea pig. Scanning electron micrograph

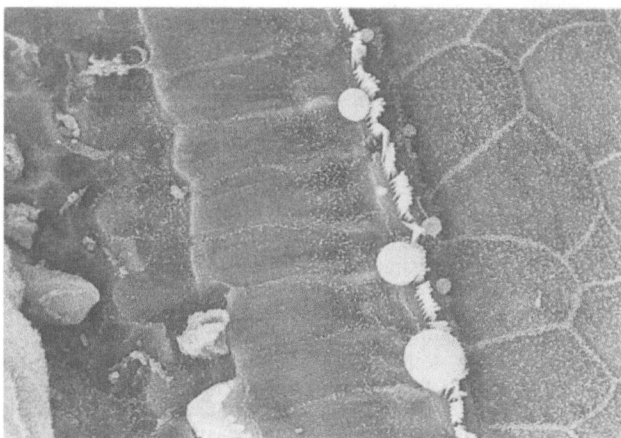

Figure 10.30 Complete loss of stereocilia of the outer hair cells from the cochlea of a gentamicin-treated guinea pig. The inner hair cells are unaffected. Scanning electron micrograph

progression towards the apex. Inner hair cells are then lost. The cell degeneration continues after cessation of drug administration. Streptomycin can be ototoxic in rats[55], cats, squirrel monkeys and mice[49]. Damage to cochlea hair cells is also reported with sodium arsanilicum, cyclophosphamide, cisplatin, vinblastine, vincristine, methyl mercury, nitrogen mustard, chloramphenicol, quinine and in hypothyroidism[49-51, 56, 57].

A few ototoxic compounds exert their primary effect on the stria vascularis. This structure is responsible for maintaining the high potassium content of the endolymph[58] and the loop diuretics ethacrynic acid, furosemide and bumetanide cause both inter- and intra-cellular oedema[49,50,56,58]. The oedema is detected within minutes of an intravenous dose[51]. The salicylates produce reversible loss of hearing in squirrel monkeys[49] but there is no morphological evidence of damage. However, labelled salicylate is rapidly detectable in the blood vessels of the stria vascularis[56]. The physiological changes are considered consistent with ischaemia[51] and it is suggested that swollen endothelial cells cause partial occlusion of the capillaries[58].

In man, chloroquine administration is known to induce inner ear damage[59]. Melanin binding may be responsible for the ototoxic changes. Melanin is present in the stria vascularis of the cochlea and the planum semilunatum of the ampullae, and a high concentration of labelled chloroquine is recorded in these structures of hooded rats, but not of albino rats[59].

Ototoxicity due to damage to the neural structures of the cochlea is rarely reported. However, mercury induces primary changes in the nerve terminals of the spiral ganglion[50].

References

1. Henkes, H. E. (1972). Drug-induced opthalmological changes. In Meyler, L. and Peck, H. M. (eds.) *Drug-Induced Diseases*. Vol. 4, pp. 524–533. (Amsterdam: Excerpta Medica)
2. Henkes, H. E. and Canta, L. R. (1973). Drug-induced disorders of the eye. *Proc. Eur. Soc. Study Drug Toxic.*, **14**, 146–153
3. McCaa, C. S. (1985). Anatomy, physiology and toxicology of the eye. In Hayes, A. C. (ed.) *Toxicology of the Eye, Ear and Other Special Sense Organs*. pp. 1–15. (New York: Raven)
4. Heywood, R. (1985). Clinical and laboratory assessment of visual dysfunction. In Hayes, A. C. (ed.) *Toxicology of the Eye, Ear and Other Special Sense Organs*. pp. 61–77. (New York: Raven)
5. Potts, A. M. and Gonasun, L. M. (1980). Toxic responses of the eye. In Klaassen, C. D., Amdur, M. O. and Doull, J. (eds.) *Toxicology*. (New York: MacMillan)
6. Meier-Ruge, W. (1973). Eye toxicity. *Proc. Eur. Soc. Study Drug Toxic.*, **14**, 133–145
7. Plestina, R. and Puikovic-Plestina, M. (1978). Effect of anticholinesterase pesticides on the eye and on vision. *CRC Crit. Rev. Toxicol.*, **6**, 1–24
8. Roerig, D. L., Hasegawa, A. T., Harris, G. J., Lynch, K. L. and Wang, R. I. H. (1980). Occurrence of corneal opacities in rats after acute administration of 1-α-acetylmethadol. *Toxicol. Appl. Pharmacol.*, **56**, 155–163
9. Saunders, L. Z. and Rubin, L. F. (1975). *Opthalmic Pathology of Animals*. (New York: Karger)
10. Leure-Dupree, A. E. (1986). Vascularization of the rat cornea after prolonged zinc deficiency. *Anat. Rec.*, **216**, 27–32
11. Wright, H. N. (1963). Corneal and lenticular opacities in the eyes of rats following long-term administration of sulfonylurea derivatives. *Diabetes*, **12**, 550–554
12. Rungby, J. (1986). Experimental argyrosis: ultrastructural localisation of silver in rat eye. *Exp. Mol. Pathol.*, **45**, 22–30
13. Drenckhahn, D., Jacobi, B. and Lüllman-Rauch, R. (1983). Corneal lipidosis in rats treated with amphiphilic cationic drugs. *Arzneim.-Forsch. (Drug. Res.)*, **33**, 827–831
14. Earl, F. L., Curtis, J. M., Bernstein, H. W. and Smalley, H. E. (1971). Ocular effects in dogs and pigs treated with dichloran (2,6-dichloro-4-nitroaniline). *Food Cosmet. Toxicol.*, **9**, 819–828
15. Slatter, D. H. (1973). Keratoconjunctivitis sicca in the dog produced by oral phenazopyridine hydrochloride. *J. Small. Anim. Pract.*, **14**, 749–771
16. Weisse, I., Hoefke, W., Greenberg, S., Gaidal, W., Stötzer, H. and Kreuzer, H. (1978). Ophthalmological and pharmacological studies after administration of clonidine in rats. *Arch. Toxicol.*, **41**, 89–98
17. Majeed, S. K., Prentice, D. E. and Heywood, R. (1983). A form of kerato-conjuctivitis sicca in dogs treated with an antispasmodic compound. *J. Pathol.*, **140**, 133
18. Wachsmuth, E. D. (1983). Evaluating immuno-pathological effects of new drugs. In Gibson, G. G., Hubbard, R. and Parke, D. V. (eds.) *Immunotoxicology*. pp. 237–250. (London: Academic Press)
19. Harkness, J. E. and Ridgway, M. D. (1980). Chromodacryorrhea in laboratory rats: etiologic considerations. *Lab. Anim. Sci.*, **30**, 841–844
20. Shirama, K., Furuya, T., Takeo, Y., Shimiza, K. and Maekawa, K. (1981). Sex and strain differences in porphyrin content of Harderian glands in mice. *Zool. Mag.*, **90**, 247–250
21. Tryphonas, L., Arnold, D. L., Zawidzka, Z., Mes, J., Charbonneau, S. and Wong, J. (1986). A pilot study in adult rhesus monkeys treated with Aroclor 1254 for two years. *Toxicol. Pathol.*, **14**, 1–10
22. Render, J. A., Turek, J. J., Hinsman, E. J. and Carlton W. W. (1985). Ultrastructural ocular lesions of 6-aminonicotinamide toxicosis in rabbits. *Vet. Pathol.*, **22**, 475–482
23. Roe, F. J. C., Millican, D. and Mallet, J. M. (1963). Induction of melanotic lesions of the iris in rats by urethane given during the neonatal period. *Nature*, No. 4899, 1201–1202
24. Gehring, P. J. (1971). The cataractogenic activity of chemical agents. *CRC Crit. Rev. Toxicol.*, **1**, 93–118
25. Gibbs, G. E., Wilson, R. B. and Gifford, H. (1966). Glomerulosclerosis in the long-term alloxan diabetic monkey. *Diabetes*, **15**, 258–261
26. Bencz, Z., Iván, É. and Cholnoky, E. (1985). Analysis of cataract and keratotic damage induced by 4-diethylaminoethoxy-α-ethyl-benzhydrol (RGH-6201) in rats. *Arch. Toxicol.*, Suppl. 8, 476–479
27. Scotti, T. M., Chernoff, N., Linder, R. and McElroy, W. K. (1981). Histopathologic lens changes in mirex-exposed rats. *Toxicol. Lett.*, **9**, 289–294
28. Bagdon, R. E., Engstrom, R. G., Kelly, L. A., Hartman, H. A., Robison, R. L. and Visscher, G. E. (1983). Hypolipidaemic activity and toxicity studies of a styryl-hexahydroindoliol, 34-250. *Toxicol. Appl. Pharmacol.*, **69**, 12–28
29. Sakuragawa, N., Sakuragawa, M., Kuwabara, T., Pentcher, P. G., Barranger, J. A. and Brady, R. O. (1977) Niemann–Pick disease experimental model: sphingomyelin reduction induced by AY-9944. *Science*, **196**, 317–319
30. Taradach, C. and Greaves, P. (1984). Spontaneous eye lesions in laboratory animals: incidence in relation to age. *CRC Crit. Rev. Toxicol.*, **12**, 121–147
31. Greenman, D. L., Bryant, P., Kodell, R. L. and Sheldon, W. (1982). Influence of cage shelf level on retinal atrophy in mice. *Lab. Anim. Sci.*, **32**, 353–356
32. Currier, G., Crockett, R. S. and Lawwill, T. (1983). A standardized method for the description and grading of histologic changes in the monkey retina: specific case of light-induced damage. *Invest. Ophthalmol. Vis. Sci.*, **24**, 270–276
33. Okum, E. and Collins, E. M. (1962). Histopathology of experimental photocoagulation in the dog eye. *Am. J. Ophthalmol.*, **54**, 3–18
34. Ashton, N. (1957). Degeneration of the retina due to 1:5-di(p-aminophenoxy)pentane dihydrochloride. *J. Pathol. Bacteriol.*, **74**, 103–114
35. Kurtz, S. M., Kaump, D. H., Schardein, J. L., Roll, D. E., Reutzer, T. F. and Fisken, R. A. (1967). The effect of long-term administration of amopyroquin, a 4-aminoquinoline compound, on the retina of pigmented and non-pigmented laboratory animals. *Invest. Ophthalmol.*, **6**, 420–425
36. Lee, K. P., Gibson, J. R. and Sherman, H. (1979). Retinopathic effects of 2-aminooxy propionic acid derivatives in the rat. *Toxicol. Appl. Pharmacol.*, **51**, 219–232
37. Towfighi, J., Gonatas, N. K. and McCree, L. (1975). Hexachlorophene retinopathy in rats. *Lab. Invest.*, **32**, 330–338

38. Orzalesi, N., Grignolo, A. and Calabria, S. A. (1967). Experimental degeneration of the rabbit retina induced by sodium fluoride. *Exp. Eye Res.*, **6**, 165–170

39. Heath, H. and Rutter, A. C. (1966). Retinal angiopathy in the imino-dipropionitrile-treated alloxan-diabetic rat. *Br. J. Exp. Pathol.*, **47**, 116–120

40. Parr, J. C. (1978). Retinal arterioles in the New Zealand strain of genetically hypertensive rat. *Aust. J. Ophthalmol.*, **4**, 58–65

41. Takahashi, O. and Hiraga, K. (1978). Dose-response study of haemorrhagic death by dietary butylated hydroxytoluene (BHT) in male rats. *Toxicol. Appl. Pharmacol.*, **43**, 399–406

42. Suzuki, H., Nakao, T. and Hirago, K. (1979). Vitamin K deficiency in male rats fed diets containing butylated hydroxytoluene (BHT). *Toxicol. Appl. Pharmacol.*, **50**, 261–266

43. Schiavo, D. M. (1972). Retinopathy from administration of an imidazo-quinozoline to beagles. *Toxicol. Appl. Pharmacol.*, **23**, 782–783

44. Heywood, R. (1974). Drug-induced retinopathies in the beagle dog. *Br. Vet. J.*, **130**, 564–568

45. Wen, G. Y., Sturman, J. A., Wisniewski, H. M., MacDonald, A. and Niemann, W. H. (1982). Chemical and ultrastructural changes in tapetum of beagles with a hereditary abnormality. *Invest. Ophthalmol. Vis. Sci.*, **23**, 733–742

46. Brown, W. R., Rubin, L., Hite, M. and Zwickery, R. E. (1972). Experimental papilledema in the dog induced by a salicylanilide. *Toxicol. Appl. Pharmacol.*, **21**, 532–541

47. Parhad, I. M., Griffin, J. W. and Miller, N. R. (1986). Optic disc swelling. *Comp. Pathol. Bull. AFIP*, **18**, 2–3

48. Uga, S., Iskikawa, S. and Mukuno, K. (1977). Histopathological study of canine optic nerve and retina treated by organophosphate pesticide. *Invest. Ophthalmol.*, **16**, 877–881

49. Schukneckt, H. F. (1974). *Pathology of the Ear.* (Cambridge, Mass.: Harvard University Press)

50. Anniko, M. (1985). Principles in cochlea toxicity. *Arch. Toxicol.*, Suppl. 8, 221–239

51. Brown, R. D., Henley, C. M., Penny, J. E. and Kupetz, S. (1985). Link between functional and morphological changes in the inner ear – functional changes produced by ototoxic agents and their interactions. *Arch. Toxicol.*, Suppl. 8, 240–250

52. Parravicini, L., Arpine, A., Bamonte, F., Marzanatti, M. and Ongini, E. (1982). Comparative ototoxicity of amikacin, gentamicin, netilmicin and tobramycin in guinea pigs. *Toxicol. Appl. Pharmacol.*, **65**, 222–230

53. Voelker, F. A., Henderson, C. M., Macklin, A. W. and Tucker, W. E. (1980). Evaluating the rat inner ear. *Arch. Otolaryngol.*, **106**, 613–617

54. Astbury, P. J. and Read, N. G. (1982). Kanamycin induced ototoxicity in the laboratory rat. *Arch. Toxicol.*, **50**, 267–278

55. Myhre, J. L., De Paoli, A. and Keim, G. R. (1985). Ototoxicity of subcutaneously administered aztreonam in neonatal rats. *Toxicol. Appl. Pharmacol.*, **77**, 108–115

56. Rybak, L. P. (1986). Drug ototoxicity. *Annu. Rev. Pharmacol. Toxicol.*, **26**, 79–99

57. Falk, S. A., Klein, R., Haseman, J. K., Sanders, G. M. and Talley, F. A. (1974). Acute methyl mercury intoxication and ototoxicity in guinea pigs. *Arch. Pathol.*, **97**, 297–305

58. Lawrence, M. (1985). Structure and function of the ear and auditory nervous system. In Hayes, A. W. (ed.) *Toxicology of the Eye, Ear and Other Special Senses.* pp. 17–23. (New York: Raven Press)

59. Dencker, L., Lindquist, N. G. and Ullberg, S. (1976). Chloroquine ototoxicity. *Proc. Eur. Soc. Toxicol.*, **17**, 356-367 (Amsterdam: Excerpta Medica)

The Musculoskeletal System and Skin 11

Skeletal System

Lesions of the skeletal system, as compared with many other organ systems, are only rarely encountered during routine toxicity screening studies. Most published reports of induced lesions of these tissues originate from studies in which dietary manipulation is used to develop animal models of human conditions. However, several compound-induced lesions and examples of exacerbation of spontaneous lesions are documented (Table 11.1). A factor which may have some influence on the frequency of detected induced lesions is the relatively sparse histological investigations carried out in some studies. For example, induced arthropathies do not always manifest in every joint and therefore may be missed if only one joint is examined.

Table 11.1 Induced lesions of the skeletal system

Arthropathy
Synovitis and synovial reduplication
Arthritis and polyarthritis
Osteoarthrosis
Haemarthrosis
Osteodystrophia fibrosa
Osteomalacia
Osteosclerosis
Osteoporosis
Osteolathyrism

Although often regarded as an inert tissue in the adult animal, bone is continuously being remodelled with an equilibrium maintained between osteogenesis and osteolysis. Interference with this equilibrium leads to the development of proliferation or resorption and accounts for many of the induced lesions.

Despite the infrequent occurrence of toxic changes in the skeletal system, bone may sometimes play a role in the development or exacerbation of toxic changes in other organs since it acts as a reservoir for some xenobiotic compounds, such as fluoride, and lead[1]. Although stored in bone, some xenobiotics are not irreversibly held there and may be released into the plasma by ion exchange or dissolution of bone by osteoclasis.

Within the skeletal system, induced lesions may be simply and conveniently divided into those which affect the joints and those which act on the bones.

Lesions which affect the joints

A form of arthropathy in young beagles is induced by alkyl pyridone carboxylic acid analogues, such as nalidixic, oxolinic and pipemidic acids or cinoxacin[2]. The pathogenesis of the lesion is unknown. Grossly, the lesions are detected on the articular cartilage surfaces and are characterized by single or multiple vesiculations,

bullae, erosion or detachment. Many joints are involved but the head of the humerus, distal femur and patella are consistently affected[2]. The lesions may be graded in a semi-quantitative manner and involve degrees of cartilaginous matrix loss and rarefaction, abnormal clustering of chondrocytes, cavitation, cartilage fibrillation, vesicle or bullae formation with inflammation, tissue degeneration and erosion. In our experience these lesions are also induced in dogs treated with some novel immunostimulants (Figures 11.1 and 11.2). Similar changes are reported following injection of filipin, an antibiotic which is a potent releaser of β-glucuronidase[3].

Synovitis, with synovial hyperplasia and villus formation and reduplication were observed in our laboratories, in dogs, following administration of novel immunostimulants (Figures 11.3 and 11.4). The reduplication of the villi became extensive in some cases and the inflammation was characterized by diffuse infiltration of plasma cells and lymphocytes, with the development of follicles. Apparently similar reactions, described as activation of mesothelial cells in the knee joints of dogs, are found following subcutaneous or intravascular administration of a muramyl peptide – an immunostimulant[4]. A haemorrhagic synovitis, characterized by synovial cell proliferation with focal erosions, proteinaceous exudation and also fibrinoid vascular necrosis, associated with a form of arthropathy, is reported in dogs treated with pipemidic acid[2]. Grossly, the synovial membranes are thickened and discoloured with petechia and the synovial fluid is blood-tinged.

Some drugs such as trimethoprim and sulfadiazine are implicated in the development of immune-mediated non-erosive polyarthritis[5]. Circulating immune complexes are believed to be involved in the development of the synovitis and synovial hyperplasia.

The intra-articular injection of polysaccharides also induces synovitis and synovial proliferation[6]. The ability of these polysaccharides to induce changes is related to their molecular weight and viscosity, with the degree of sulphation also playing a part. Direct intra-articular injections of rabbits with Congo Red also produces synovial hyperplasia with reduplication and lymphoid cell aggregations[6].

Arthritis in laboratory animals is usually induced in animal models of the human condition to assess the efficacy of therapeutic compounds[7]. Many of these models involve direct intra-articular injections of agents such as formaldehyde and histamine.

Arthritis is also induced by systemic administration of some compounds, for example oral treatment of rats with 6-sulphanil-aminoindazole[8]. Polyarthritis may be induced experimentally by endocrine manipulation. In adrenalectomized or hypophysectomized rats treated with both prolactin and growth hormone acute inflammatory

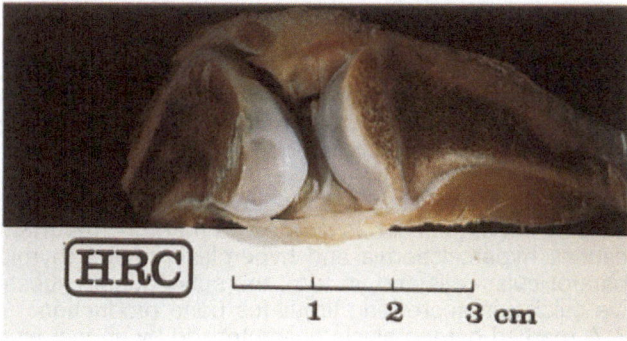

Figure 11.1 Vesicle formation of the articular surface of a joint from a dog treated with a novel immunostimulant drug. H & E

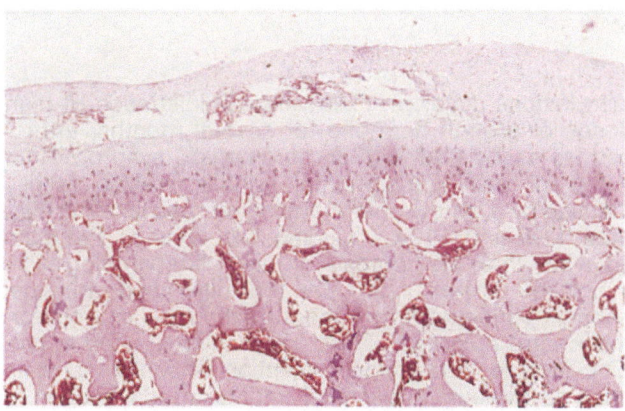

Figure 11.2 Photomicrograph of vesicle from the same study as Figure 11.1. H & E

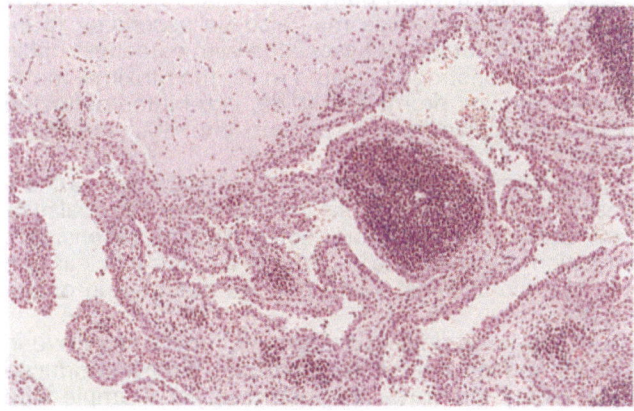

Figure 11.3 Synovial hyperplasia, villus formation and reduplication in the joint of a dog treated with a novel immunostimulant drug. Infiltration by lymphoid cells with follicle formation is also shown. H & E

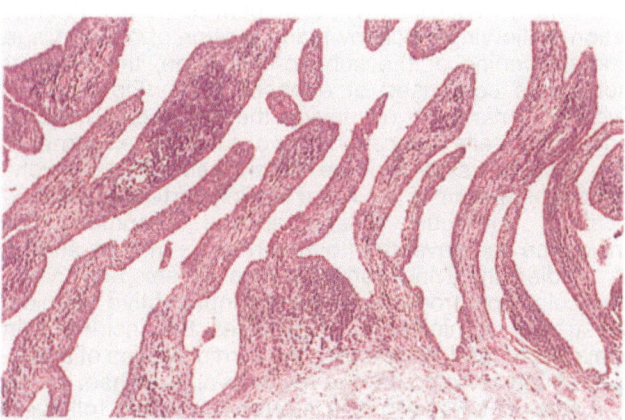

Figure 11.4 From the same study as Figure 11.3. Synovial hyperplasia with extensive villus formation and reduplication. An associated lymphocytic infiltrate is also present. H & E

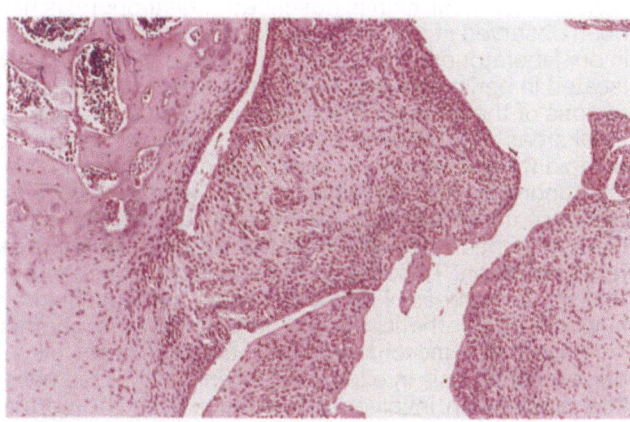

Figure 11.5 Arthritis in a rat induced by Freund's adjuvant. Synovial hyperplasia and inflammatory cell infiltration. H & E

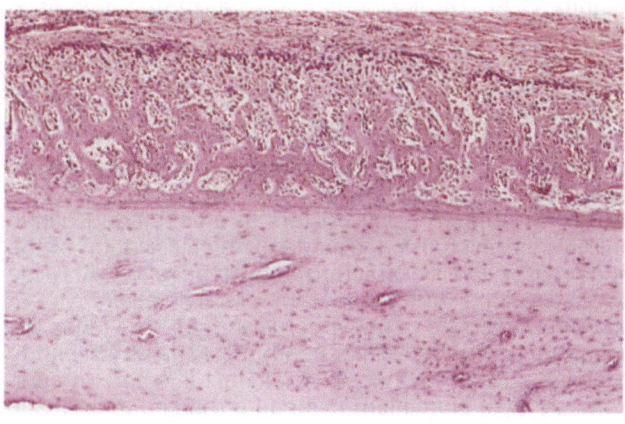

Figure 11.6 From the same study as Figure 11.5. Periosteal new bone formation from an animal with severe arthritis. H & E

joint lesions develop[8]. Following administration of high doses of growth hormone for several months, arthropathies associated with an acromegalic syndrome develop in rats[8]. Experimental arthritis is also readily induced by a variety of immunological mechanisms (Figures 11.5 and 11.6), including injections of Freund's adjuvant into the footpad or tail. Histopathologically, synovitis, peri-arthritis, peri-tendinitis and bursitis, pannus, periosteal new bone formation and osteoid formation are recorded[8]. Other mechanisms, used in rabbits, include intra-articular injection of foreign protein such as ovalbumin, bacterial endotoxin and antigen in immunised animals[7]. The synthetic adjuvant, N-acetyl-muramyl-L-alanyl-D-isoglutamine induces a severe polyarthritis[9]. Congenitally athymic nude rats do not develop polyarthritis with this synthetic adjuvant, which indicates a possible immunological mechanism.

Osteoarthrosis, a degenerative joint disease, is described in mice[10]. The condition occurs spontaneously and is more prevalent in males. The initial change involves alteration of the staining characteristics of the cartilage with acellularity, development of clefts and fibrillation. Following breakdown and erosion of the cartilage and thickening of the subchondral bone, the articular surface is composed of exposed bone (Figure 11.7) with sclerotic bone occupying the entire epiphysis. In addition, patella dislocation may occur and the ligaments and synovial tissue undergo metaplastic changes involving development of fibro- and hyaline-cartilage and ossification. Although a spontaneous condition, the incidence and severity of osteoarthrosis may be altered in studies involving administration of sex hormones, particularly oestrogen-containing contraceptive steroids. Oestradiol administration decreases the incidence in male mice[11] and, conversely, the administration of androgens such as testosterone leads to an increase.

A form of haemarthrosis is produced in rats following intraperitoneal injection of high molecular weight dextran[12]. Dextran also causes thrombocytopenia, hypofibrinogenaemia and hypoprothrombinaemia.

Lesions which affect the bones

In our experience, osteodystrophia fibrosa may be seen in rats as a treatment-related lesion, secondary to induced chronic renal changes and hyperparathyroidism (Figure 11.8). The lesion is characterized by increased bone resorption by active osteoclasis. The most common site for this increased osteoclasis is the endosteum of the long bones, where the osteoclasts often appear in a single row along the osseous margin (Figure 11.9). Subsequently, behind this osteoclastic front, fibroblasts and variable degrees of collagenization occur. In severe cases the bones become thin and brittle.

The term osteomalacia refers to a condition in adult animals in which there is inadequate calcification of the bone matrix and is characterized by trabeculae with wide osteoid seams. It is induced by dietary deficiencies of vitamin D, calcium or phosphorus and often involves the accumulation of osteoid beneath the periosteum and to a lesser extent the endosteum. In rats injected intraperitoneally with aluminium chloride a marked increase in bone aluminium content is detected together with a defect in bone mineralization. An increased amount of osteoid, typical of osteomalacia, with abnormally wide seams and no calcification front is present on the cancellous trabeculae[13]. Osteomalacic changes are also reported in rats following long term cadmium administration[14].

Reports of induced, unequivocal osteopetrosis in tox-icity studies have not been traced. This condition, in which large unresorbed bones develop, may be the result of either increased osteoblastic or decreased osteoclastic activity[15]. However, an osteopetrosis-like condition can be induced in mice treated from birth with parathyroid extract[15]. It is suggested that this treatment causes hypercalcaemia and hyperplasia of the thyroid parafollicular cells and, in turn, the subsequent excessive calcitonin secretion stimulates bone production.

A marked osteomalacia characterized by an increase in the trabecular surface covered by active and inactive osteoid seams is reported in uraemic rats[16]. Ethane-1-hydroxy-1,1-diphosphonate (EHDP), a synthetic analogue of pyrophosphate, reduces bone resorption and increases osteoid in metaphyseal and diaphyseal bone in rats and dogs[17]. In our laboratories, several compounds known to decrease bone resorption have been found to result in increased trabecular bone in the marrow cavity of rats and mice. In severe cases the bone formed a complex meshwork which occupied most of the marrow cavity and replaced the haemopoietic elements (Figure 11.10). Proliferation of bony trabeculae into the marrow cavity or osteosclerosis may also be secondary to induced myelofibrosis or associated with osteodystrophia fibrosa[18]. In oestrogen-treated mice, the proximal metaphysis contains prominent, wide, large interconnected bone trabeculae which project into the medullary cavity[19].

Lead administration to dogs and primates causes changes in the distal metaphysis in which thick trabeculae of new bone on cartilaginous cores become extensive[15]. Inhibition of osteocytic osteolysis and intranuclear and cytoplasmic acid-fast inclusions are detected in osteoclasts.

Osteoporosis develops when an imbalance between bone formation and resorption occurs. It may be induced by a variety of hormonal imbalances, for example with increased levels of oestrogens. Most of the hormones are believed to affect osteoblast activity. Protein deficiency, calcium deficiency and hypervitaminosis A are thought to induce osteoporosis by promotion of osteolysis by osteoclasts. The osteolysis may occur in periosteal, endosteal and intracortical locations. Intracortical resorption in the long bones usually occurs along vascular channels. With high oral doses of retinoic acid, dissolution of bone matrix by osteolysis and increased osteoclastic resorption is described[20]. Osteoporosis has been observed in rats treated with a novel agrochemical in our laboratories. The lesion, which was predominantly located in peri-osteal and to a lesser extent in endosteal regions of the femur, was characterized histologically by focal areas of prominent osteoclasts along the irregular osteoid margin and by periosteal fibrosis (Figure 11.11). Osteoporosis may develop in dogs treated with high doses of corticosteroids. Glucocorticoids decrease calcium absorption from the intestine and also increase its renal excretion. This results in secondary hyperparathyroidism and increases bone resorption. Heparin, dextran sulphate (a synthetic heparin substitute) and another sulphated polysaccharide, laminarin sulphate, all induce osteoporosis in experimental animals[21]. One possible mechanism involves interference with the normal ossification by competition between the exogenous sulphated polysaccharide and endogenous ones. The bones are brittle and fracture readily and the cortical bone is thinned at the metaphysis and in the mid-diaphysis. Histologically, the rats show evidence of osteoclastic resorption. Guinea pigs and rabbits develop a more severe and widespread osteoporosis than rats, which is attributed to inanition and anorexia. No evidence of parathyroid hyperplasia is present and parathyroidectomy has no effect on the development of the lesion.

Occasionally unusual toxic manifestations, apparently due to skeletal changes, may be detected in toxicological studies. In rats given oral prizidilol, thoracic spinal deformation causes lordosis of the spine into the thoracic cavity with consequent dyspnoea[22]. Abnormal vertebrae are detected on X-ray investigation, but the results of histopathological investigations are not included in the report. Similar spinal lesions are described in rats treated with benserazide[23].

Osteolathyrism is one of the more spectacular of the induced lesions of the skeletal system. The condition is induced in most laboratory animal species by feeding with *Lathyrus odoratus* seeds or by enteric or systemic administration of lathyrogens, such as aminopropionitrile aminoacetonitrile or methyleneaminoacetonitrile[24]. In its more acute form the condition in rats is characterized by peri-osteal proliferation with bone and cartilaginous metaplasia of peri-osteal connective tissue. The chronic lesions involve gross deformation of tubular bone with exostoses, callus formation, widening of the marrow cavity due to peri-osteal bone production and endosteal absorption, enlargement of the epiphyseal cartilages and retarded long bone growth[24].

Skin

The skin is obviously one of the most extensive tissues in the body and is exposed to a wide variety of environmental agents. Most cutaneous lesions which are encountered in toxicity studies involve topical application of the test substance. However, in a few instances, systemic administration of compounds may also result in skin lesions. There are only a limited number of reactions or combinations of reactions which may be

Table 11.2 Induced skin lesions

Epidermal hyperplasia
Epidermal ulceration
Chloracne
Otitis externa
Toxic epidermal necrolysis
Xanthoma

induced in the skin (Table 11.2).These reactions involve three basic processes: inflammation, degeneration and proliferation. With topical administration of compounds, the epidermis may show single or combinations of lesions such as: inflammation, acanthosis, hyperkeratosis, parakeratosis, erosion, ulceration or necrosis. The lesion observed is often dependent on the time scale after the initial insult, the dose employed, the species used and of course the potency of the agent under test. These lesions are the subject of two detailed reviews[25,26]. Much of the work to assess primary irritation is limited to macroscopic observation, with scoring of reactions such as erythema and oedema[27].

Inflammation is induced in mice by a wide range of topically applied chemicals including: phenol, croton oil, benzalkonium chloride, ethylphenylpropionate and methylsalicylate[26]. Histologically, all these compounds produce oedema, cellular inflammatory infiltrates and vascular dilatation, but the developmental time-scale differs.

The epidermis has a remarkable capacity for proliferation and regeneration and numerous chemicals induce epidermal hyperplasia[25]. Hyperplasia may be subdivided into two mechanistic forms: one, which follows ulceration or necrosis, is considered a regenerative hyper-

plasia; the second develops without appreciable degenerative epidermal change and therefore is considered likely to represent a primary reactive form[25]. However, this is only an arbitrary classification as the development of lesions is dependent on the dose administered[25]. 12-O-tetradecanoyl-phorbol-13-acetate (TPA) is generally believed to cause epidermal hyperplasia without degenerative changes. After application the epidermal cells become hypertrophic, with decreased basophilia, widened intercellular spaces and a prominent stratum granulosum. In comparison, treatment of mouse skin with 3-methylcholanthrene or benzo[a]pyrene causes an initial epidermal degeneration followed by a regenerative hyperplasia. A single topical application of the divalent cation ionophore A23187 to mouse skin induces epidermal hyperplasia[28]. A rapid rise in prostaglandin E_2 levels is detectable 10 minutes after application of A23187[29] and the development of the hyperplastic epidermis can be completely inhibited by the prior application of prostaglandin synthetase inhibitors, such as indomethacin[28]. This shows that an early increase in PGE_2 levels is necessary and probably triggers the epidermal hyperplasia. A wide range of cosmetic preparations including sodium lauryl sulphate, sun-tan lotions and antiperspirants induced epidermal hyperplasia in rabbit skin[30].

Administration of 6-aminonicotinamide to newborn mice is used as an animal model for pellagra. These mice, in addition to showing intestinal and nervous changes, also develop skin acanthosis and hyperkeratosis[31].

One of the most unusual induced changes in cutaneous tissues is produced in laboratory animals treated with chloracnegens[32]. A widely known chloracnegen is 2,3,7,8-tetrachlorodibenzo-p-dioxin (TCDD), but other polyhalogenated aromatic hydrocarbons induce chloracne or chloracne-like conditions in animal models. In addition, the non-halogenated hydrocarbons 3-methylchloanthrene and benzo[a]pyrene produce chloracne-like lesions in rabbit pinnae[32], but are less potent than TCDD. Most of the work on the development of chloracne is performed on models of the human condition and for screening possible chloracnegens. Three models used are: the inner surface of the rabbit pinnae; the facial skin of the rhesus monkey; and the skin of the hairless mouse[32,33]. The rabbit ear is generally considered the most sensitive and reliable model[32–34] and even after systemic exposure chloracne develops on the inner surfaces. Interestingly, it is not possible to produce chloracne on any other part of the rabbit's skin; predilection sites are also found in human cases[34]. During the development of chloracne the epithelium of the hair sheath and sebaceous gland ducts become hyperkeratotic, the pilosebaceous follicles dilate and keratin-filled cysts develop (Figures 11.12 and 11.13). The sebaceous cells undergo squamous metaplasia and the glands involute and atrophy. With the accumulation of keratinaceous debris, impaction occurs and the occluded cyst, or comedone, enlarges[33]. The transformation of the pilosebaceous tissue into keratin cysts is considered pathognomonic for chloracnegens[34].

An otitis externa-like condition is described in beagle dogs treated orally with an aromatic retinoid[35]. The lesions involve epidermal acanthosis in the external auditory meatus and hyperplasia, hypertrophy and hypersecretion of the ceruminous glands. These are followed by an inflammatory reaction. The external ear canal appears a distinct predilection site for the compound, as changes are not detected elsewhere on the body.

Toxic epidermal necrolysis is a severe, widespread

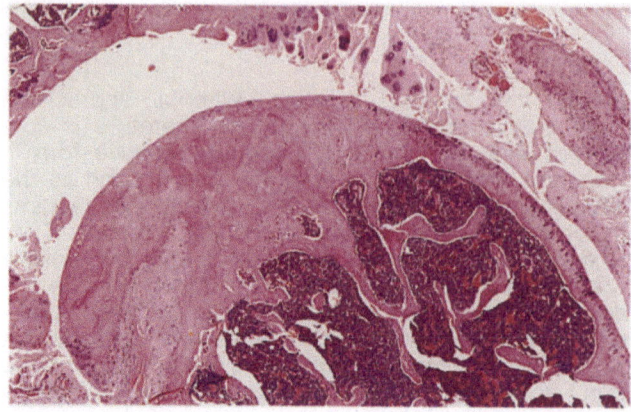

Figure 11.7 Osteoarthrosis in the knee joint of a mouse exposed to an androgenic compound. Superficial cartilage has been eroded from the articular surface which is composed of exposed bone. H & E

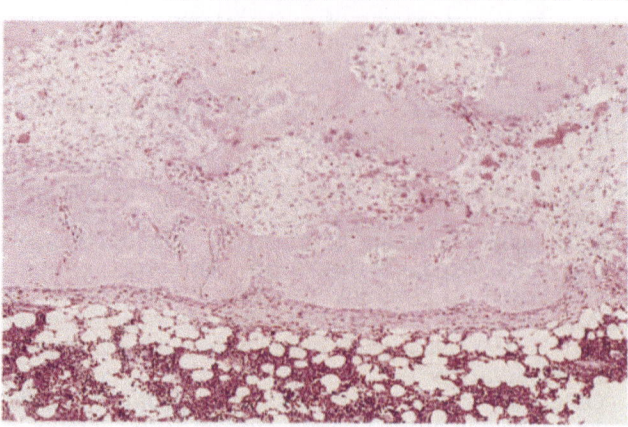

Figure 11.8 Osteodystrophia fibrosa in a rat with induced chronic renal damage and parathyroid hyperplasia. Resorption of bone, with fibrosis, along the endosteum and focally in cortical areas. H & E

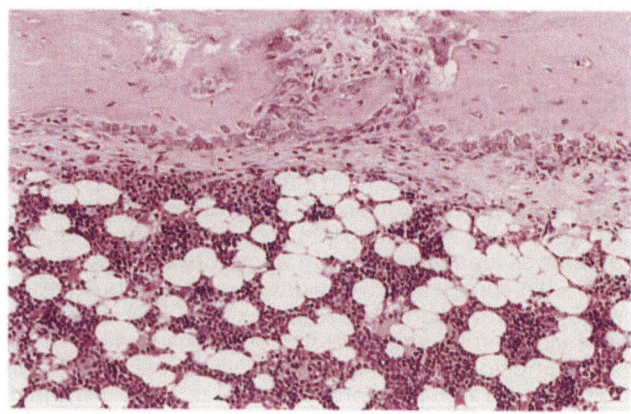

Figure 11.9 From the same study as Figure 11.8. Higher magnification shows a distinct orientation of osteoclasts along the endosteum. H & E

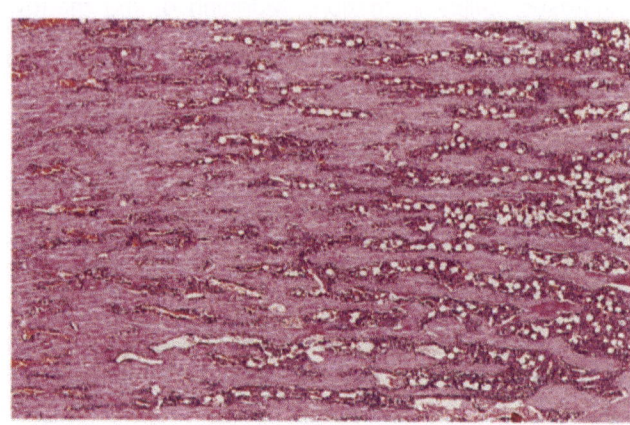

Figure 11.10 Pronounced bone trabeculae in the marrow cavity of a rat treated with a compound known to decrease bone resorption. H & E

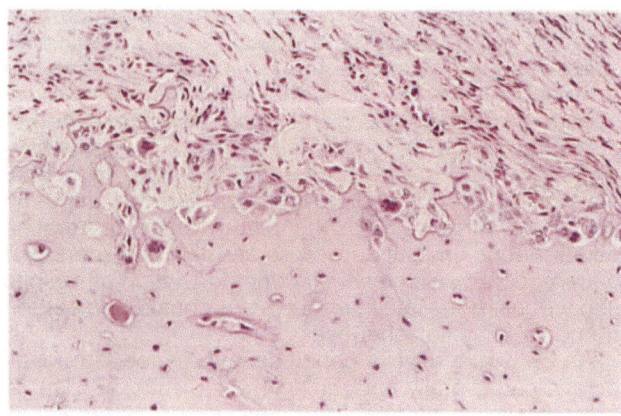

Figure 11.11 Osteoporosis in a rat treated with a novel agrochemical. Active osteoclasis along the periosteum with periosteal fibrosis. H & E

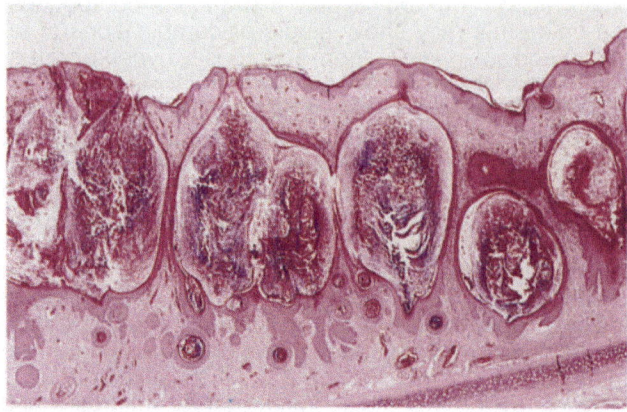

Figure 11.12 Chloracne in a rabbit pinna induced by a potent chloracnegen. The pilosebaceous follicles are grossly distended with keratin debris. The lining epithelium shows acanthosis and hyperkeratosis. Note the absence of sebaceous glands. H & E

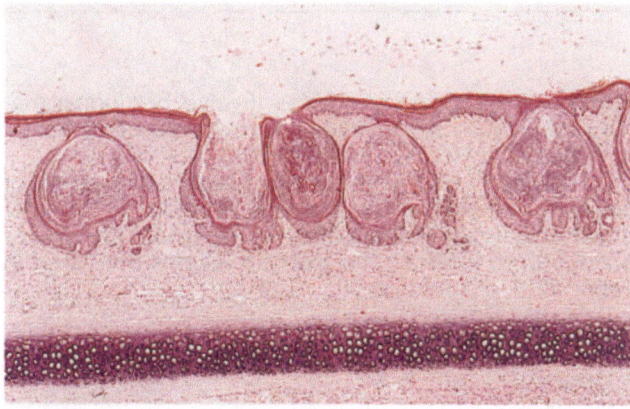

Figure 11.13 The same condition as in Figure 11.12 but with a lower dose of the chloracnegen. The follicles are slightly dilated with acanthosis and hyperkeratosis of the lining epithelium. H & E

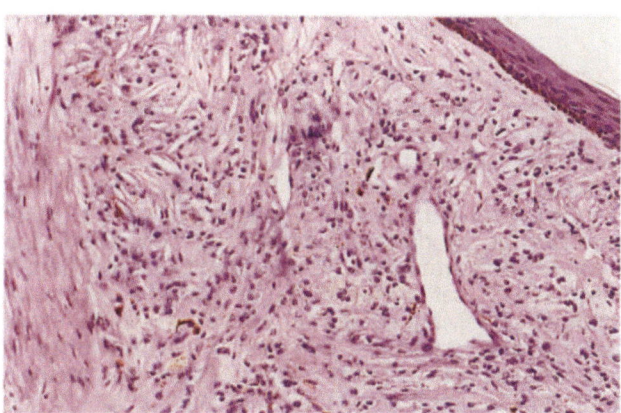

Figure 11.14 Xanthomatous change in the dermis of a rhesus monkey with diet-induced atherosclerosis. The reaction is characterized by histiocyte infiltration and cholesterol clefts. H & E

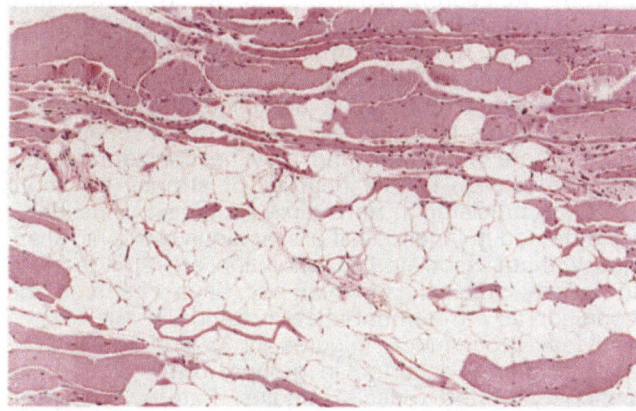

Figure 11.15 Atrophic fibres in the skeletal muscle of a rat treated with a novel agrochemical. The atrophic fibres appear narrow and more intensely eosinophilic than adjacent normal fibres. Note the extensive replacement of muscle by adipose tissue. H & E

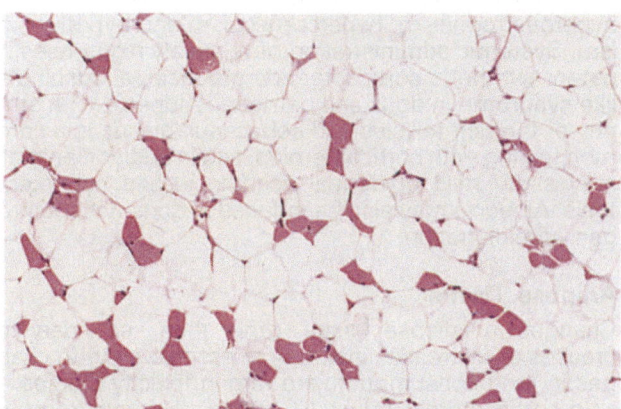

Figure 11.16 From the same study as Figure 11.15. In transverse section the atrophic muscle fibres appear small and slightly distorted. Note the extensive adipose replacement. H & E

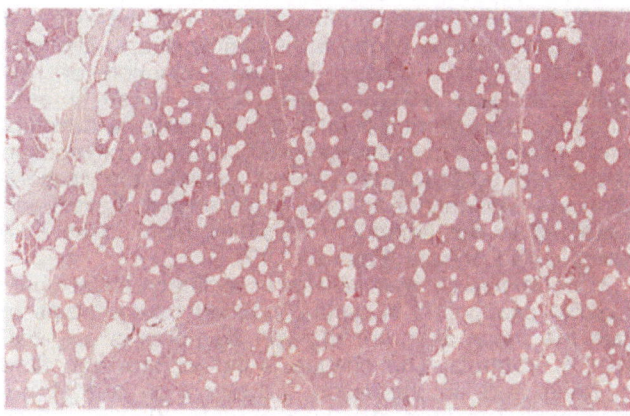

Figure 11.17 Skeletal muscle from a cynomolgus monkey treated with high doses of a potent novel corticosteroid. Adipose tissue replacement of muscle fibres. H & E

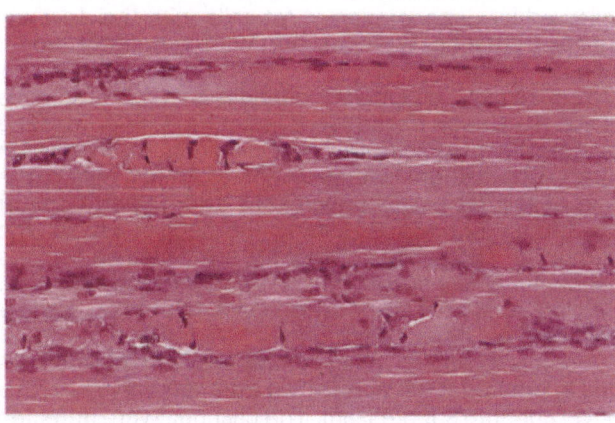

Figure 11.18 Induced segmental necrosis in skeletal muscle. The necrotic fibres are strongly eosinophilic and homogeneous with loss of striations. H & E

bullous condition of the skin. In man many drugs are implicated in its occurrence, including antibiotics such as penicillin and tetracycline, anti-epileptic drugs such as phenytoin, and indomethacin[36]. The condition involves coagulative epidermal necrosis, with clefts and blister formation at the dermo-epidermal junction. The lesion is rarely encountered in routine toxicity studies but is described in a cat treated with cephaloridine[37]. A similar condition involving epidermal necrosis, subepidermal blisters, and liquefactive degeneration is described in dogs treated with sulphonamides[37]. Epidermal necrosis is induced in rabbit skin by sodium lauryl sulphate and hexachlorophene[30].

Xanthomas consisting of foamy macrophages with cholesterol clefts (Figure 11.14), with an associated slight lymphocytic infiltrate, were detected in the dermis of rhesus monkeys given an atherogenic diet in our laboratories. Similar xanthomatous changes are reported in hypercholesterolaemic rabbits[38]. The xanthomas begin in the dermis as small collections of foam cells.

Dermatoses may be detected as secondary events following the induction of endocrinopathies, including hyperoestrogenism, hypercortisonism and hypothyroidism. Systemic administration of relatively high doses of potent synthetic corticosteroids produces a Cushing's-like syndrome in dogs and primates. Alopecia with atrophy of the hair follicles and sebaceous glands is a common finding with corticosteroids, and in addition animals may show mild epidermal acanthosis and hyperkeratosis. Alopecia may also be induced in dogs with oestrogen administration.

Adipose Tissue

Changes in adipose tissue, other than secondary increases or decreases in amounts associated with changes in food consumption, are rare in toxicity studies.

In corticosteroid-induced Cushing's-like syndrome in cynomolgus monkeys, we observed increased deposits of subcutaneous and abdominal adipose tissue with extensive fat necrosis. The cause of the fat necrosis is uncertain but trauma is a possible explanation.

'Yellow fat disease' is a condition induced in rats given a vitamin E-deficient diet, supplemented with fish oil[39]. The lesion is found predominantly in subcutaneous fat depots. Initially, lipofuscin-containing macrophages infiltrate the interstitium of the adipose tissue and this is followed by degeneration of fat cells with the development of steatitis. The condition does not affect brown adipose tissue[39].

Few reports of induced changes in brown adipose tissue have been traced in the literature. One compound to affect this tissue is dioxin, which induces changes in rats[40]. This change develops in three phases. Initially the size of the fat droplets increases with hypertrophy of the brown adipocytes. During the second phase, the number of fat droplets decreases and some adipocytes become spindle-shaped, with glycogen accumulation. Subsequently, the adipocytes appear shrunken and devoid of both fat and glycogen.

In our laboratories, macroscopic and histological changes in brown fat were detected from rats treated with a novel appetite suppressant. The changes were detected microscopically as a consistent, generalized decrease in the size of the fat droplets within the adipocytes.

Skeletal Muscle

In spite of its volume (approximately 40% of total body mass)[41], skeletal muscle is relatively rarely involved in toxic injury in routine safety evaluation studies. Most reports of induced myopathies involve nutritional manipulation. Such myopathies are reviewed elsewhere[42] and are not described in this text.

In common with some other tissues, the range of possible pathological reactions is limited. Briefly, atrophy, necrosis and hypertrophy are the most commonly encountered lesions. The induced lesions are listed in Table 11.3.

Table 11.3 Induced lesions of skeletal muscle

Atrophy
Hypertrophy
Increased capillarization
Degeneration/necrosis
Phospholipidosis
Muscular dystrophy-like conditions
Regeneration
Fatty degeneration

Changes may be induced by four general mechanisms: by a direct effect on muscle fibres; by interference with the function of peripheral nerves; by disturbance of neuromuscular transmission; or by ischaemia[41].

Atrophy of muscle fibres may be induced by five main mechanisms: malnutrition, denervation, vascular insufficiency, direct action and disuse. Histologically atrophic fibres become angular in cross-section, their nuclei more prominent and may be considerably decreased in size. Lesser degrees of atrophy are more readily appreciated in transverse sections but may also be detected in longitudinal preparations. Atrophic changes, without associated degeneration, are rarely induced in toxicity studies. However, we have observed the condition as a treatment-related change in rats treated with an agrochemical (Figures 11.15 and 11.16). The atrophic fibres occurred in groups, often around the periphery of the muscle bundles. Extensive adipose tissue replaced the atrophic fibres. No evidence of a neurogenic origin was detected.

Muscle atrophy is also induced in rats following administration of emetine[41,43]. Decreased numbers of Type II fibres in the soleus muscle are associated with loss of myofibrillar ATPase and activity. The atrophy is considered to be due to a direct effect on the muscle fibres; innervation appears normal.

In man, the most commonly encountered drug-induced myopathy is due to corticosteroid administration[41]. Dexamethasone-induced atrophy of the extensor digitorum muscles of the rat is mainly due to changes in fast glycolytic fibres. Marked reduction of myophosphorylase activity is detected in these fibres[44]. Anabolic steroids and B vitamins prevent the development of steroid myopathy in rats[41]. Atrophic changes in muscles of cynomolgus monkeys, subsequently associated with extensive adipose replacement, have been detected in our laboratory following high doses of a novel corticosteroid (Figure 11.17).

Osteomalacia in man is often associated with atrophic muscle changes[45]. In dietary-induced osteomalacia in rats the mean diameter of Type 2B fibres is only half that of controls. The change is associated with fibre splitting and an increased incidence of central nucleation[45]. The fibre atrophy resembles that of disuse atrophy.

Atrophy secondary to interruption of the normal innervation may arise from damage to any part of the lower motor neurone. The histological features of denervation-induced atrophy are considered pathognomonic[46]. Affected fibres are thinner and shorter and the nuclei become more crowded. The striations are usually retained. Myopathies, due to induced peripheral neuropathies, include perhexiline which causes granular inclusions and tubular aggregates in myofibrils[41]. In chickens treated with tri-*ortho*-cresyl phosphate, diffuse atrophy is induced in the limb muscles.

Thyrotoxicosis induces atrophy of skeletal muscle in several species. Experimentally, administration of L- or D-thyroxine produces similar changes in rabbits[47]. It is suggested that these changes may be due to the actions of thyroid hormones on some lysosomal enzymes and pronounced increases in cathepsins B and D are found[47].

Hypertrophy of muscle occurs in cases of increased workload. The increase in size of individual fibres appears to be due to increased amounts of inter-myofibrillar material and numbers of myofibrils[42]. Anabolic steroids readily induce hypertrophy in laboratory animals. The change is best appreciated macroscopically but may be easily assessed microscopically with a comparison–head microscope or by using morphometric techniques. Pronounced hypertrophy, particularly of the hind limbs, has been found in our laboratories in rats treated with a novel pharmaceutical. Microscopically, a generalized hypertrophy of all muscle fibres is present. Apart from their increased size, the hypertrophied fibres are indistinguishable from normal fibres. Individual groups of hypertrophic fibres may also be found as a compensatory mechanism in some cases of atrophy[46].

Hypertrophy induced in rats by growth hormone is due to increased protein synthesis, increased numbers of myonuclei and increased length and diameter of muscle fibres[48,49]. The increased number of myonuclei is thought to follow proliferation of satellite cells and their subsequent fusion with myofibres. This process is considered to be the mechanism by which the fibres elongate[50]. The growth hormone effect may be mediated by somatomedins which act as satellite cell mitogens[49]. Administration of T_4 to rats causes an increased number of satellite cell nuclei and also of the number of satellite cells per muscle fibre[50].

Increased capillarization of skeletal muscle develops in rats treated with dipyridamole[51]. This is due to proliferation of capillary wall cells. The aetiology of the lesion is uncertain but would appear most likely to be related to the potent vasodilatation caused by dipyridamole.

Muscle necrosis is rarely encountered in toxicity studies, except in those involving intramuscular injections where a spectrum of pathological changes are observed, the extent and severity of which may range from a slight focal reaction, due to the mechanical trauma of the injection procedure, to severe cases of widespread necrosis. Inflammatory cell infiltration, fibre degeneration, mineralization and phagocytosis may all occur. With resolution, granulation tissue and fibrosis may develop.

Degenerative changes following systemic administration of compounds may be divided into two types dependent upon the extent and severity of the damage. In both types, infiltration of inflammatory cells may be associated with the degenerative changes. The first type of degenerative change is dependent on the unusual features of myocytes. Individual muscle cells are multinucleate, extremely long[52], and sometimes only show focal injury. This leads to a phenomenon of partial or segmental necrosis in which the remaining portion of the cell 'seals-off' the damage and remains unaffected. In segmental degeneration parts of individual fibres undergo hyaline or coagulative necrosis and appear homogeneous and strongly eosinophilic (Figures 11.18 and 11.19). The sarcolemma remains intact and the degenerate sarcoplasm is removed by infiltration of mac-

rophages (myophagia), leaving 'myocyte ghosts' (Figures 11.20 and 11.21). Sarcolemmal nuclei of adjacent fibres often become central and oriented in characteristic rows (Figure 11.22). This is a common finding in myopathies in man[52] and is the main feature of a congenital centronuclear myopathy[46]. The second type of degeneration is characterized by a distinctly granular appearance of the affected fibres. This type is generally more severe and granulomatous inflammation and calcification may develop. This form of skeletal muscle degeneration is well illustrated in mice treated with an antimalarial drug[42]. A form of myopathy, associated with generalized phospholipidosis and characterized by multilamellar bodies and autophagic vacuoles with associated fibre necrosis, is reported in rats treated with choroquine and chlorphentermine[41,53].

The antibiotic monensin, which is used as a coccidiostat, produces myotoxicity in poultry, pigs and dogs[54]. The coincident administration of another antibiotic tiamulin enhances the myopathy. In chickens type I fibres are believed to be predominantly affected, but in pigs both I and II are involved. The degeneration is characterized by hyalinization of the sarcoplasm with proliferation of nuclei, phagocytosis of debris and empty sarcolemmal sheaths ('ghosts').

Compounds such as pyridostigmine, soman, paraoxan and phospholine induce necrosis of muscle fibres[55] in the region of endplates. Distinct differences exist in the incidence and severity of the lesions between different muscles; the diaphragm being identified as the most vulnerable[56]. These compounds act by inhibiting acetylcholinesterase at the neuromuscular junction and it is suggested that the consequent hyperactivity causes a loss of muscle fibre integrity which may be mediated by Ca^{2+} influx[41,57]. Staining of the motor endplates shows that the ramifications are rarified, shortened and plump[56]. Ultrastructural changes are present at the neuromuscular junction prior to the development of the necrosis[57]. An intact nerve supply is necessary for the development of the necrosis and nerve stimulation enhances the effect[55].

In man, the most common cause of induced muscle necrosis is ε-aminocaproic acid; however this lesion is not apparently reproducible in rats or guinea pigs[41].

Skeletal muscle has an extensive blood supply with good collateral circulation[46]. However, infarction may occur and vasoactive amines, such as serotonin, induce a form of myopathy in which ischaemia is believed to be involved[41,58]. Focal fibre necrosis is induced by amines alone, amines in conjunction with aortic ligation, amines with imipramine, or the monoamine oxidase inhibitor, pargyline[58].

A muscular dystrophy-like syndrome is described in rats injected subcutaneously with 6-mercaptopurine[59]. The muscles are atrophic with proliferation of sarcolemmal nuclei, focal necrosis and inflammatory cell infiltration and adipose replacement. Another muscular dystrophy-like syndrome is produced in most species of laboratory animals by vitamin E deficiency[60]. The rabbit is especially susceptible and the hyaline degeneration is associated with myositis. The degeneration regresses upon dietary vitamin E supplementation.

Muscle has a considerable capacity to regenerate[46,52] following injury, but the success of this repair is dependent on the severity of the initial lesion. Regeneration may occur quickly in cases of hyaline degeneration and evidence of both degenerative and regenerative processes may be seen simultaneously. Regeneration is believed to involve a similar myoblast fusion to that seen during embryogenesis[52]. Regeneration is possible when

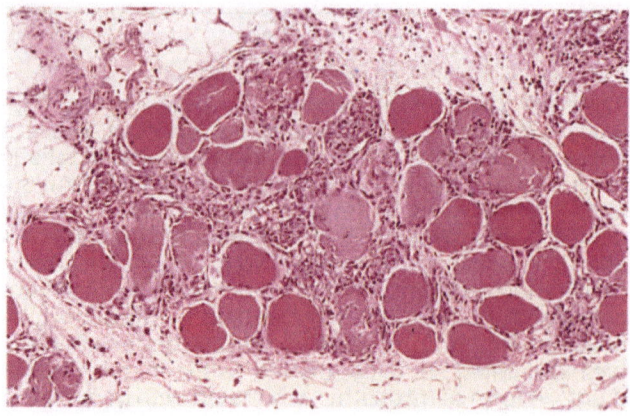

Figure 11.19 Segmental necrosis of muscle fibres from a chicken treated with an antibiotic. The necrosis is associated with an inflammatory infiltrate. H & E

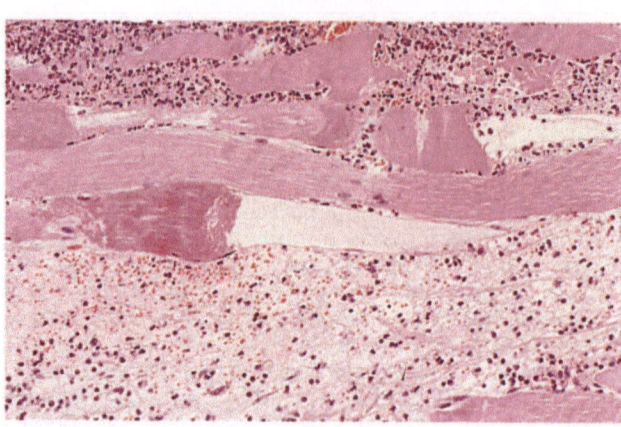

Figure 11.20 Skeletal muscle necrosis in a rabbit, with pronounced inflammation and oedema. In the centre, the sarcolemma of one affected fibre clearly remains intact, despite loss of sarcoplasm, appearing as a myocyte 'ghost'. H & E

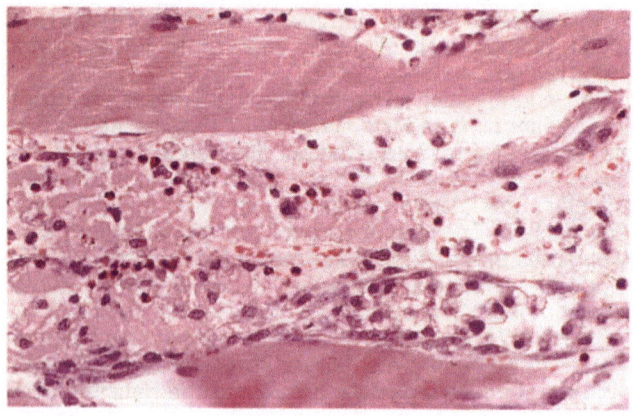

Figure 11.21 From the same study as Figure 11.20. Segmental necrosis with infiltration of macrophages into muscle cells (myophagia). The phagocytic cells digest and remove the damaged sarcoplasm, leaving the sarcolemma intact which results in the myocyte 'ghost' appearance shown in Figure 11.20. H & E

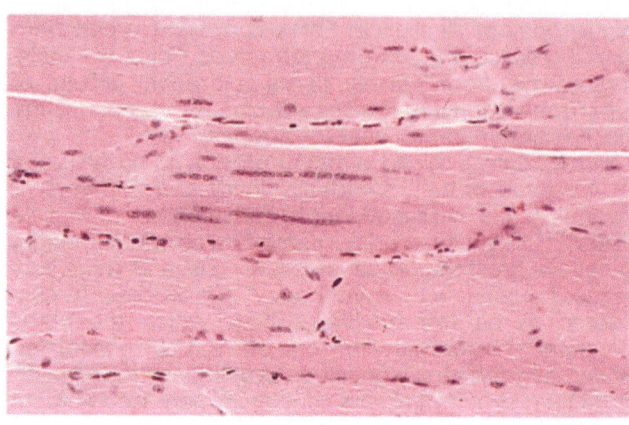

Figure 11.22 Skeletal muscle from a mouse, adjacent to an area of induced segmental necrosis. The sarcolemmal nuclei have proliferated, become central and are arranged in distinct rows. H & E

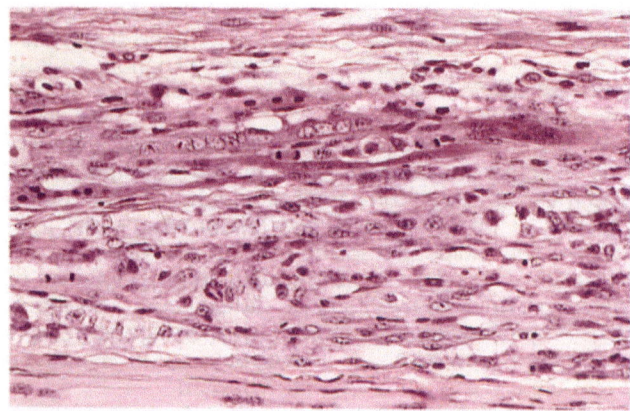

Figure 11.23 Early regeneration of skeletal muscle following induced segmental necrosis in a mouse. Prominent numbers of mitotic cells. Note the overall basophilia. H & E

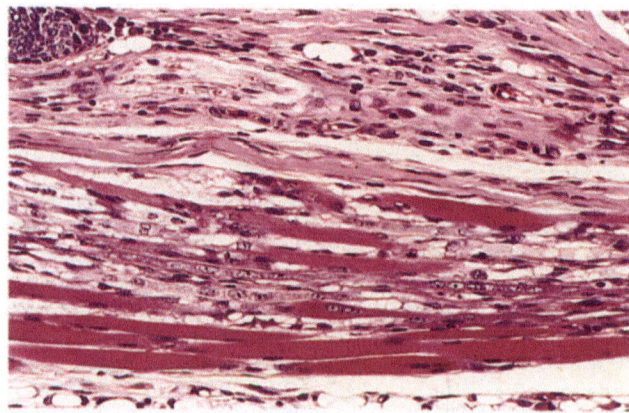

Figure 11.24 Basophilic myotubes in the skeletal muscle of a mouse following segmental necrosis. During regeneration the myotubes are believed to arise from satellite cells and fuse with damaged myocytes. H & E

viable satellite cells and the reticulin framework of the affected muscle fibre are preserved. The satellite cells, which lie between the basement membrane and the sarcolemma, proliferate (Figure 11.23), migrate along the necrotic fibre, and fuse to form characteristic thin, basophilic myotubes (Figure 11.24), which in turn fuse with the ends (Figure 11.24) of the damaged muscle fibre[52]. In cases of severe necrosis, regeneration may be impaired and fibrosis and scar tissue develop.

Fatty degeneration may be induced in muscle fibres either as a primary lesion or secondary to granular degeneration. The antineoplastic antibiotic, adriamycin, induces a myopathy in mice[61] which is characterized by increased numbers and size of lipid droplets in the red fibres of the gastrocnemius muscle but without evidence of other damage.

References

1. Klaassen, C. D. (1986). Distribution, excretion and absorption of toxicants. In Klaassen, C. D., Amdur, M. O. and Doull, J. (eds.) *Toxicology*. pp. 33–63. (New York: Macmillan)
2. Gough, A., Barsoum, N. J., Mitchell, L., McGuire, E. J. and de la Iglesia, F. A. (1979). Juvenile canine drug-induced arthropathy: clinicopathological studies on articular lesions caused by oxolinic and pipemidic acids. *Toxicol. Appl. Pharmacol.*, **51**, 177–187
3. Lack, C. H. (1969). Lysosomes in relation to arthritis. In Dingle, J. T. and Fell, H. B. (eds.) *Lysosomes in Biology and Pathology*. Vol. 1, pp. 493–508. (London: North Holland)
4. Wachsmuth, E. D. (1983). Evaluating immuno-pathological effects of new drugs. In Gibson, G. G., Hubbard, R. and Parke, D. V. (eds.) *Immunotoxicology*. pp. 237–250. (London: Academic Press)
5. Gorman, N. T. and Werner, L. L. (1986). Immune-mediated diseases of the dog and cat. II. Immune-mediated diseases of the haemolymphatic and musculoskeletal system. *Br. Vet. J.*, **142**, 403–410
6. Page-Thomas, D. P. (1969). Lysosomal enzymes in experimental and rheumatoid arthritis. In Dingle, J. T. and Fell, H. B. (eds.) *Lysosomes in Biology and Pathology*. Vol. 2, pp. 87–110. (London: North Holland)
7. Wepsic, H. T. and Hollingsworth, J. W. (1968). Effects of drugs on different types of synovial inflammation in the rabbit. *Yale J. Biol. Med.*, **41**, 273–281
8. Alspaugh, M. A. and van Hoosier, G. L. (1973). Naturally-occurring and experimentally-induced arthritides in rodents: a review of the literature. *Lab. Anim. Sci.*, **23**, 724–742
9. Kohaishi, O., Aihara, K., Ozowa, A., Kotani, S. and Azuma, I. (1982). New model of a synthetic adjuvant, N-acetylmuramyl-L-alanyl-D-isoglutamine-induced arthritis. *Lab. Invest.*, **47**, 27–36
10. Walton, M. (1977). Degenerative joint disease in the mouse knee: histological observations. *J. Pathol.*, **123**, 109–224
11. Silberberg, M. and Silberberg, R. (1970). Age-linked modification of the effect of estrogen on joints and cortical bone of female mice. *Geronotologia*, **16**, 201–211
12. Hall, C. E., Hall, O. and Ayachi, S. (1971). Experimental hemorrhagic disease and haemarthrosis produced in the rat by dextran injections. *Lab. Invest.*, **24**, 67–73
13. Ellis, H. A., McCarthy, J. H. and Herrington, J. (1979). Bone aluminium in haemodialysed patients and in rats injected with aluminium chloride: relationship to impaired bone mineralisation. *J. Clin. Pathol.*, **32**, 832–844
14. Takoshima, M., Moriwaki, S. and Itokawa, Y. (1980). Osteomalacic change induced by long-term administration of cadmium to rats. *Toxicol. Appl. Pharmacol.*, **54**, 223–228
15. Woodward, J. C. (1978). The musculoskeletal system. In Benirschke, K., Garner, F. M. and Jones, T. C. (eds.) *Pathology of Laboratory Animals*. pp. 663–820. (New York: Springer Verlag)
16. Weisbrode, S. E. (1981). Short term effects of vitamin D_3 and 1,25-dihydroxyvitamin D_3 on osteomalacia in uremic rats fed a low-calcium-low phosphorus diet. *Am. J. Pathol.*, **104**, 35–40
17. Yarrington, J. T., Capen, C. C., Black, H. E., Re, R., Potts, J. T. and Geho, W. B. (1977). Effect of ethane-1-hydroxy-1,1-diphosphonate (EHDP) on the ultrastructure of parathyroid glands and plasma immunoreactive parathyroid hormone in pregnant cows fed a low calcium diet. *Lab. Invest.*, **36**, 402–412
18. Itakura, C., Iida, M. and Goto, M. (1977). Renal secondary hyperparathyroidism in aged Sprague-Dawley rats. *Vet. Pathol.*, **14**, 463–469
19. Gaunt, S. D. and Pierce, K. R. (1985). Myelopoiesis and marrow adherent cells in estradiol-treated mice. *Vet. Pathol.*, **22**, 403–408
20. Dhem, A. and Goret-Nicaise, M. (1984). Effects of retinoic acid on rat bone. *Food Chem. Toxicol.*, **22**, 199–206
21. Ellis, H. A. and Peart, K. M. (1971). Dextran sulphate osteopathy in parathyroidectomised rats. *Br. J. Exp. Pathol.*, **52**, 684–695
22. Sutton, T. J., Darby, A. J., Johnson, P., Leslie, G. B. and Walker, T. F. (1986). Dyspnoea and thoracic spinal deformation in rats after oral prizidilol (SK&F 92657-A2). *Hum. Toxicol.*, **5**, 183–187
23. Schärerm, K. (1974). Special developmental derangements of the rat skeleton after administration of DL-serine-(2,3,4-trihydroxybenzyl)hydrazide. *Beitr. Pathol. Bd.*, **152**, 127–150
24. Selye, H. (1957). Lathyrism. *Rev. Can. Biol.*, **16**, 1–82
25. Argyris, T. S. (1981). The regulation of epidermal hyperplastic growth. *CRC Crit. Rev. Toxicol.*, **9**, 151–200
26. Patrick, E., Maibach, H. I. and Burkhalter, A. (1985). Mechanisms of chemically induced skin irritation. *Toxicol. Appl. Pharmacol.*, **81**, 476–490
27. Marzulli, F. N. and Maibach, H. I. (1975). The rabbit as a model for evaluating skin irritants: a comparison of results obtained on animals and man using repeated skin exposures. *Food Cosmet. Toxicol.*, **13**, 533–540
28. Marks, F., Fürstenberger, G. and Kownatzki, E. (1981). Prostaglandin E-mediated stimulation of mouse epidermis *in vivo* by divalent cation inophore A 23187 and by tumor promoter 12-o-tetradecanoylphorbol-13-acetate. *Cancer Res.*, **41**, 696–702
29. Marks, F., Fürstenberger, G., Ganss, M., Richter, H. and Seemann, D. (1983). Hyperplastic transformation: the response of mouse skin to irritation. *Br. J. Dermatol.*, **109**, Suppl. 25, 18–21
30. Stebbins, R. B. (1975). Data cited by Marzulli and Maibach (see footnote 27 above)
31. Aikawa, H. and Suzuki, K. (1986). Lesions in the skin, intestine and central nervous system induced by an antimetabolite of niacin. *Am. J. Pathol.*, **122**, 255–342
32. Vos, J. G., van Leeuwen, F. X. R. and De Jong, P. (1982). Acnegenic activity of 3-methylcholanthrene and benzo[a]pyrene, and a comparative study with 2,3,7,8-tetrachlorodibenzo-p-dioxin in the rabbit and hairless mouse. *Toxicology*, **23**, 187–196
33. Horton, V. L. and Yeary, R. A. (1985). Assessment of the chloracnegenic response induced by 3,4,3′,4′-tetrachloroazoxybenzene. *J. Toxicol. Environ. Health*, **15**, 215–227
34. Crow, K. D. (1982). Chloracne. *Sem. Dermatol.*, **1**, 305–314
35. Teelmann, K. (1986). Reversible, retinoid-induced secretion of canine ceruminous glands. *Toxicol. Lett.*, **34**, 33–39
36. Heng, M. C. Y. (1985). Drug-induced toxic epidermal necrolysis. *Br. J. Dermatol.*, **113**, 579–600
37. Scott, D. W., Wolfe, M. J., Smith, C. A. and Lewis, R. M. (1980). The comparative pathology of non-viral bullous skin diseases in domestic animals. *Vet. Pathol.*, **17**, 257–281
38. Armstrong, M. L., Mathur, S. N., Sando, G. N. and Megan, M. B. (1986). Lipid metabolism in xanthomatous skin of hypercholesterolemic rabbits. *Am. J. Pathol.*, **125**, 339–348
39. Danse, L. H. J. C. and Verschuren, P. M. (1978). Fish oil-induced yellow fat disease in rats. *Vet. Pathol.*, **15**, 114–124
40. Rozman, K., Pereira, D. and Iatropoulos, M. J. (1986). Histopathology of interscapular brown adipose tissue, thyroid and pancreas in 2,3,7,8-tetrachlorodibenzo-p-dioxin (TCDD)-treated rats. *Toxicol. Appl. Pharmacol.*, **82**, 551–559
41. Mastaglia, F. L. (1982). Adverse effects of drugs on muscle. *Drugs*, **24**, 304–321
42. Montgomery, C. A. (1978). Muscle diseases. In Benirschke, K., Garner, F. M. and Jones T. C. (eds.) *Pathology of Laboratory Animals*. pp. 821–887. (New York: Springer Verlag)
43. Bradley, W. G., Fewings, J. D., Harris, J. B. and Johnson, M. A. (1976). Emitine myopathy in the rat. *Br. J. Pharmacol.*, **57**, 29–41
44. Livingstone, I., Johnson, M. A. and Mastaglia, F. L. (1981). Effects of dexamethasone on fibre subtypes in rat muscle. *Neuropathol. Appl. Neurobiol.*, **7**, 381–398

45. Swash, M., Schwartz, M. S. and Sargeant, M. K. (1979). Oste-
    omalacic myopathy: an experimental approach. *Neuropathol.
    Appl. Neurobiol.*, **5**, 295–302
46. Anderson J. R. (1985). *Atlas of Skeletal Muscle Pathology.*
    (Lancaster: MTP)
47. Decker, R. S. and Wildenthal, K. (1981). Lysosomal alterations
    in heart, skeletal muscle and liver of hyperthyroid rabbits. *Lab.
    Invest.*, **44**, 455–465
48. Prysor-Jones, R. A. and Jenkins, J. S. (1980). Effect of excessive
    secretion of growth hormone in tissues of the rat, with particu-
    lar reference to the heart and skeletal muscle. *J. Endocrinol.*,
    85, 75–82
49. McCasker, R. H. and Campion, D. R. (1986). Effect of growth
    hormone-secreting tumours in skeletal muscle cellularity in
    the rat. *J. Endocrinol.*, **111**, 279–285
50. Beermann, D. H., Liboff, M., Wilson, D. B. and Hood, L. F.
    (1983). Effects of exogenous thyroxine and growth hormone
    on satellite cell and myonuclei populations in rapidly growing
    rat skeletal muscle. *Growth*, **47**, 426–436
51. Adolfsson, J. (1986). Time dependence of dipyridamole-in-
    duced increase in skeletal muscle capillarisation. *Arzneim.-
    Forsch.*, **36**, 1768–1769
52. Sloper, J. C. and Partridge, T. A. (1980). Skeletal muscle:
    regeneration and transplantation studies. *Br. Med. Bull.*, **36**,
    153–158
53. Schmalbruch, H. (1980). The early changes in experimental
    myopathy induced by chloroquine and chlorphentermine. *J.
    Neuropathol. Exp. Neurol.*, **39**, 65–81

54. Umemura, T., Kawaminami, A., Goryo, M. and Itakura, C.
    (1985). Enhanced myotoxicity and involvement of both type I
    and II fibres in momensin-tiamulin toxicosis in pigs. *Vet. Pathol.*,
    22, 409–414
55. Dettbarn, W.-D. (1984). Pesticide induced muscle necrosis:
    mechanisms and prevention. *Fundam. Appl. Toxicol.*, **4**, S18–
    S26
56. Gebbers, J-O., Lötscher, M., Kobel, W., Portmann, R. and
    Laissue, J.-A. (1986). Acute toxicity of pyridostigmine in rats:
    histological findings. *Arch. Toxicol.*, **58**, 271–275
57. Leonard, J. P. and Salpeter, M. M. (1979). Agonist-induced
    myopathy at the neuromuscular junction is mediated by cal-
    cium. *J. Cell Biol.*, **82**, 811–819
58. Laskowski, M. B. and Dettbarn, W-D. (1977). The pharmacology
    of experimental myopathies. *Annu. Rev. Pharmacol. Toxicol.*,
    17, 387–409
59. Slaughter, L. J., Alleva, F. R., Haberman, B. H. and Balazs,
    T. (1981). Muscular dystrophy-like syndrome in young adult
    Sprague-Dawley rats following neonatal treatment with 6-mer-
    captopurine. *Toxicol. Pathol.*, **9**, 38
60. Ringler, D. H. and Abrams, G. D. (1971). Laboratory diagnosis
    of vitamin E deficiency in rabbits fed a faulty commercial ration.
    Lab. Anim. Sci., **21**, 383–387
61. Doroshow, J. H., Tallent, C. and Schechter, J. E. (1985).
    Ultrastructural features of adriamycin-induced skeletal and car-
    diac muscle toxicity. *Am. J. Pathol.*, **118**, 288–297

Index

Italic references are to figures.